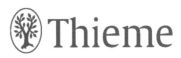

Management of Complications in Common Hand and Wrist Procedures

FESSH Instructional Course Book 2021

Brigitte van der Heijden, MSc, MD, PhD
Plastic Surgeon and Chairman
Department of Plastic Surgery
Jeroen Bosch Hospital
's-Hertogenbosch, the Netherlands;
Radboud University Medical Center
Nijmegen, the Netherlands

Jan-Ragnar Haugstvedt, MD, PhD
Division Chair of Hand Surgery and Consultant Hand Surgery
Department of Orthopaedics
Østfold Hospital Trust
Moss, Norway

Henk Coert, MD, PhD
Professor and Chairman
Department of Plastic Surgery
UMC Utrecht
Utrecht, the Netherlands

251 illustrations

Thieme
Stuttgart • New York • Delhi • Rio de Janeiro

Library of Congress Cataloging-in-Publication Data is available from the publisher.

© 2022 Thieme. All rights reserved.

Georg Thieme Verlag KG
Rüdigerstrasse 14, 70469 Stuttgart, Germany
+49 [0]711 8931 421, customerservice@thieme.de

Illustrator: Massimiliano Crespi
Cover design: © Thieme
Cover image source: Massimiliano Crespi
Typesetting by DiTech Process Solutions Pvt. Ltd., India

Printed in Germany by Beltz Grafische Betriebe   5 4 3 2 1

ISBN 978-3-13-243603-9

Also available as an e-book:
eISBN 978-3-13-243604-6

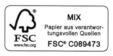

Contents

Section 1   Tendon Surgery

Contents

Contents

Preface

There would be none amongst us who hasn't witnessed complications in our profession. Even the greatest of us will have to face complications at some point in time. Colleagues who claim that they haven't faced complications most likely do not perform surgery, do not see their patients back, or are in denial.

Complications can have a major impact on both patient and surgeon. While nearly every textbook lists the complications that can occur after performing an operation, in general we prefer not to talk about them. This does not do appropriate justice to the complication, and moreover also not to the patient and the surgeon.

Complications are inherent to our profession and deserve the same attention as other aspects, specifically in order to learn from them and to improve the quality of future care.

With this book, we want to open up the discussion on complications!

We have focused on complications of common hand and wrist surgical procedures. Prevention as well as treatment of complications will be discussed. In addition, management of expectations, impact of complications on both the patient and surgeon will be presented.

We hope that this FESSH book will provide tools for handling complications to both senior and junior surgeons.

Being willing to acknowledge complications and subsequently discussing with patients and colleagues is essential for ultimately improving the quality of care.

Finally, we would like to thank all authors who have made an enormous effort to contribute to this book and share their expertise and knowledge, despite the hectic time of COVID.

Brigitte van der Heijden, MSc, MD, PhD
Jan-Ragnar Haugstvedt, MD, PhD
Henk Coert, MD, PhD

Contributors

Peter C. Amadio, MD
Lloyd A and Barbara A Amundson Professor of
  Orthopedic Surgery
Mayo Clinic
Rochester, Minnesota, USA

Andrea Atzei, MD
PRO-Mano
Treviso, Italy;
Hand Surgery Unit
Ospedale Koelliker
Torino, Italy

Peter Axelsson, MD, PhD
Senior Consultant
Department of Hand Surgery
Sahlgrens University Hospital
Sahlgrenska Academy
Institute of Clinical Sciences
University of Gothenburg
Gothenburg, Sweden

Greg I. Bain, MD
APWA President
Professor of Upper Limb and Research
Department of Orthopaedic Surgery
Flinders University
Adelaide, South Australia, Australia

Eva-Maria Baur, MD
Practice
Department for Plastic and Hand Surgery Murnau
Penzberg, Germany

Randy Bindra, FRACS
Professor of Orthopaedic Surgery
Griffith University School of Medicine and Dentistry
Southport, Australia

Michel E. H. Boeckstyns, MD, PhD
Consultant Hand Surgeon
Capio Private Hospital
Senior Researcher
Clinic for Hand Surgery
Herlev–Gentofte Hospital
University of Copenhagen
Hellerup, Denmark

Elske Bonhof-Jansen, MSc
European Certified Hand Therapist
Clinical Epidemiologist
Isala Zwolle
Zwolle, the Netherlands

Geert Alexander Buijze, MD, PhD
Hand & Upper Limb Surgery Unit
Department of Orthopaedic Surgery
Clinique Générale
Annecy, France;
Lapeyronie University Hospital
University of Montpellier
Montpellier, France;
Amsterdam University Medical Center
University of Amsterdam
Amsterdam, the Netherlands

Anne Eva J. Bulstra, MD, PhD
Department of Surgery
Red Cross Hospital
Beverwijk, the Netherlands

Marion Burnier, MD
Wrist Surgery Unit
Department of Orthopaedics
Claude-Bernard Lyon 1 University
Herriot Hospital
Lyon, France

Maurizio Calcagni, MD
Department of Plastic Surgery and Hand Surgery
University Hospital Zurich
Zurich, Switzerland

Alessandro Crosio, MD
Hand Surgery and Reconstructive Microsurgery
  Department
ASST-Orthopedic Institute, Gaetano Pini–CTO
Milan, Italy

Paul De Buck, MSc Manual Therapy
European Certified Hand Therapist
Department of Rehabilitation Sciences
Campus UZ Gent
Gent, Belgium

Ilse Degreef, MD, PhD
Professor of Orthopedic Surgery
University of Leuven
Leuven, Belgium

Godard C.W. de Ruiter, MD, PhD
Neurosurgeon
Department of Neurosurgery
Haaglanden Medical Center
The Hague, the Netherlands

Francisco del Piñal, MD, PhD
Hand and Microvascular Surgeon
Madrid and Santander, Spain

J.G.G. Dobbe, MD
Department of Biomedical Engineering and Physics
Amsterdam University Medical Center
Amsterdam, the Netherlands

David Elliot, MA, FRCS, BM, BCh
Consultant Hand and Plastic Surgeon (Retd.)
Essex, UK

Mireia Esplugas, MD
Consultant Hand Surgeon
Kaplan Hand Institute
Barcelona, Spain

Florian S. Frueh, MD, PhD
Department of Plastic Surgery and Hand Surgery
University Hospital Zurich
Zurich, Switzerland

Marc Garcia-Elias, MD, PhD
Consultant and Co-Founder
Kaplan Hand Institute;
Vall d'Hebron Institut de Recerca (VHIR)
Barcelona, Spain

Thomas Giesen, MD
Orthopaedic Surgeon
Clinica Ars Medica
Centro Manoegomito
Gravesano, Switzerland;
Clinic for Hand and Plastic Surgery
Luzerner Kantonsspital
Lucern, Switzerland

Max Haerle, MD
Professor
Director of Hand and Plastic Surgery Department
Orthopädische Klinik Markgröningen
Markgröningen, Germany

Daniel B. Herren, MD, MHA
Department of Hand Surgery
Schulthess Klinik
Zurich, Switzerland

Guillaume Herzberg, MD, PhD
Professor of Orthopaedic Surgery
Lyon Claude Bernard University
Herriot Hospital
Lyon, France

Pak Cheong Ho, MBBS, FRCS (Edinburgh), FHKAM (Orthopaedic Surgery), FHKCOS
Chief of Service
Department of Orthopaedic & Traumatology
Prince of Wales Hospital
Chinese University of Hong Kong
Hong Kong SAR

Ayla Hohenstein, MD
Hand and Plastic Surgery
Orthopädische Klinik Markgröningen
Markgröningen, Germany

Mick Kreulen, MD, PhD
Department of Hand Surgery
Rode Kruis Ziekenhuis
Beverwijk, the Netherlands

Gertjan Kroon, MD
European Certified Hand Therapist
Isala Zwolle
Zwolle, the Netherlands

Florian M.D. Lampert, PD, MD
Senior Consultant
Orthopädische Klinik Markgröningen
Markgröningen, Germany

Alex Lluch, MD
Kaplan Hand Institute;
Vall d'Hebron Institut de Recerca (VHIR);
Hand & Wrist Unit
Vall d'Hebron Hospitals
Barcelona, Spain

Riccardo Luchetti, MD
Rimini Hand Surgery and Rehabilitation Center
Rimini, Italy

Simon B.M. MacLean, MBChB, FRCS(Tr&Orth), PGDipCE
Consultant Orthopaedic and Upper Limb Surgeon
Tauranga Hospital, BOPDHB
Tauranga, New Zealand

Luke McCarron, BOcc. Thy., MSc. Hand
Assistant Professor, Orthopaedic Conjoint Position
Bond University Occupational Therapy Department
Gold Coast Hospital and Health Service Orthopaedic
  Department
Gold Coast, Queensland, Australia

Duncan Angus McGrouther, MD, PhD
Professor and Senior Consultant Hand Surgeon
Director Cell and Tissue Bioengineering Laboratory
Singapore General Hospital;
Adjunct Professor
Duke-NUS Medical School
Singapore

Daniel J. Nagle, MD, FAAOS, FACS
Professor Emeritus
Clinical Orthopedic Surgery
Northwestern Feinberg School of Medicine
Chicago, Illinois, USA

Ridzwan Namazie, FRACS
Gold Coast University Hospital
Southport, Australia

Simona Odella, MD
Hand Surgery and Reconstructive Microsurgery
  Department
ASST-Orthopedic Institute, Gaetano Pini–CTO
Milan, Italy

Dominic Power, MD
Peripheral Nerve Injury Service
Birmingham Hand Centre
Queen Elizabeth University Hospital
Birmingham, UK

Mike Ruettermann, MD
Consultant Plastic Surgeon—Hand Surgeon
University Medical Center Groningen—UMCG
Groningen, the Netherlands;
Institute for Hand and Plastic Surgery
Oldenburg, Germany

Niels W.L. Schep, MD, PhD, MSc
Trauma—Hand and Wrist Surgeon
Maasstad Hospital
Rotterdam, the Netherlands

Ton A. R. Schreuders, PT, PhD
Erasmus Medical Center
Department of Rehabilitation Medicine
Rotterdam, the Netherlands

S.D. Strackee, MD
Department of Plastic, Reconstructive and Hand
  surgery
Amsterdam University Medical Center
Amsterdam, the Netherlands

Filip Stockmans, MD, PhD
Campus Kulak Kortrijk
Kortrijk, Belgium

Jin Bo Tang, MD
Professor and Chair
Department of Hand Surgery
The Hand Surgery Research Center
Affiliated Hospital of Nantong University
Nantong, Jiangsu, China

Pierluigi Tos, MD, PhD
Director
Hand Surgery and Reconstructive Microsurgery
  Department
ASST-Orthopedic Institute, Gaetano Pini–CTO
Milan, Italy

Gwendolyn van Strien, PT, CHT-NL
Hand Therapist
The Hague, the Netherlands

Thomas Verschueren, MD
Department of Orthopedic Surgery
AZ Monica Hospital
Antwerp, Belgium

Frederik Verstreken, MD
Department of Orthopedic Suegery
Antwerp University Hospital
Edegem, Belgium

Erik Walbeehm, MD
Radboud Peripheral Nerve Centre
Department of Plastic, Reconstructive and Hand
  Surgery
Radboudumc
Nijmegen, the Netherlands

Marjolaine Walle, MD
Pediatric Surgery Department
University Hospital Estaing
Clermont-Ferrand, France

**David Warwick, MD, BM, DIMC, FRCS, FRSCS(Orth),
  Eur Dip Hand Surg**
Professor
Consultant Hand Surgeon
University Hospital Southampton
Southampton, Hampshire, UK

Paul M.N. Werker, MD, PhD, FEBOPRAS, FEBHS
Professor and Chief
Department of Plastic Surgery
University of Groningen and University Medical
  Center Groningen
Groningen, the Netherlands

Terry L. Whipple, MD
Chief of Orthopaedics
Hillelson-Whipple (H-W) Clinic;
Associate Professor of Orthopaedic Surgery
University of VA and VA Commonwealth University;
Director, Orthopaedic Research of Virginia
Richmond, Virginia, USA

Section 1

Tendon Surgery

1 Management of Complications of Flexor Tendon Surgery

Peter C. Amadio and Duncan Angus McGrouther

Abstract

Adhesions are the most common and troubling complication after flexor tendon repair in the hand. Aside from small children, essentially every tendon repair is complicated by adhesions that limit motion; the only real question is whether these will be severe enough to require surgical intervention in an attempt to improve function. Pulley loss can be the result either of direct injury or a decision by the surgeon to trim pulleys to improve motion. Usually, if the contiguous loss is less than 2 cm, reconstruction is not needed. Management of flexor tendon repair rupture will be focused by the history, exploration, and forensic examination of the wound to establish causation and identification of preventable factors. Key technique changes for primary or re-repair have been the move toward stronger repairs by multistranded core suture configurations, better anchorage points, and pulley release. Most therapy regimes aim at active mobilization and this is also indicated for a re-repair as the stuck tendon is vulnerable to rupture from later mobilization. The key to managing infection lies in understanding how the time-honored surgical principles of drainage, decompression, and dilution fit into modern understanding of inflammation and bacterial virulence factors. Infection in a tendon repair is uncommon and usually due to inadequate debridement or comorbidities. It is best managed by antibiotics, drainage, and catheter irrigation. If the tendon is necrotic, it should be excised and reconstruction considered.

Keywords: tendon, adhesion, bowstringing, pulley, rupture, infection

1.1 Management of Flexor Tendon Adhesions

1.1.1 Definition/Problem: Current Understanding of the Biology of Adhesion Formation

The observation "one wound, one scar" as it pertains to tendon repair is nearly as old as the specialty of hand surgery itself, and of course is a truism that reflects wound healing biology for nearly all tissues in nearly all mammalian species beyond the fetal stage. The functional implications and severity will vary depending on location, mechanism of injury, and the specific tissues that are injured. The flexor tendons in the hand are especially at risk for the negative consequences of this dictum—the gliding tendon fixed in place by scar to adjacent pulley and bone, limiting tendon excursion and impairing function.

The unique anatomy and nutritional arrangement of the flexor tendons in the hand particularly predispose them to adhesion formation because, even normally, the nutritional supply is precarious. The flexor profundus excursion is around 2.5 cm in the adult finger. This long excursion is made possible by a special nutritional arrangement. Instead of a circumferential paratenon to supply nutrients to the tendon, the blood supply of the finger flexors in the fingers is segmental, through the vincula, which arise from the digital arteries at the joint level, and enter the tendons through their dorsal surfaces (▸ Fig. 1.1). The feeding vessels enter just lateral and anterior to the bone, just proximal and distal to each joint. These feeding vessels must be carefully protected during dissection at the time of repair or tenolysis. If they are cut, even with a physically intact vinculum, the tendon will be effectively devascularized. To supplement this nutritional source, the tendons are surrounded by a synovial sheath also, so that synovial diffusion can provide nutrition as well. Both systems are commonly injured when the flexor tendon is lacerated, the synovial sheath by the same injury that injured the tendon, and the vincula either by that mechanism or by rupture with muscular contraction, pulling the proximal tendon stump out of the finger.

Unsurprisingly, this loss of nutrition has consequences, and one of the major drivers of adhesion severity is vascularity. Well-vascularized tendons have better motion than poorly vascularized ones, strongly suggesting that a good tendon blood supply is an important factor in reducing adhesion severity.[1] This is not only true for severely devascularized tendons, as occurs with amputation/replantation, but also with damage to the vincular system in an otherwise well-perfused finger. Avascular or hypovascular tendons, like any other vascularly impaired tissue, will release cytokines such as vascular endothelial growth factor (VEGF) that will stimulate neovascularization and new vascular ingrowth into the tendon. These new vascular connections, occurring in parts of the tendon normally nourished either by synovial fluid or the vincular system, do good in restoring nutrition to the tendons and aiding tendon healing, but at the same time do harm by binding the tendon to the surrounding tissues and limiting tendon motion. Usually, unfortunately, there is little that can be done to reverse this aspect of the initial injury—though as noted in the next section, there are some things that can be done to try to minimize the impact of tendon hypovascularity on tendon motion.

A second anatomical feature predisposing finger tendons to adhesions is the fibro-osseous sheath, which holds the tendons close to bone and allows the tendon excursion to drive a remarkable 270 degrees of combined active motion of the finger joints. These narrow confines

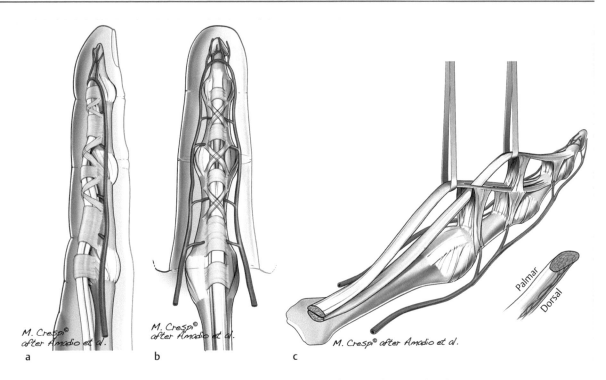

Fig. 1.1 (a–c) Blood supply of the flexor tendons. SV, short vinculum; LV, long vinculum; DA, digital artery.

can easily limit gliding of even the smoothest tendon repair, and provide an extremely short leash for any adhesions that do form. However, unlike vascularity, whose loss is currently irretrievable, there are some things that the surgeon can do to mitigate the impact of the sheath on adhesion formation, as discussed below.

Other anatomic factors predisposing to adhesions relate to associated injuries, which may affect tendon vascularity at a distance, require immobilization or otherwise compromise the physical aspects of tendon rehabilitation (fracture, nerve repair, proximal limb injury), or otherwise limit patient ability to participate in rehabilitation (polytrauma, head injury).

The second main group of factors affecting adhesion formation represents those under the control of the surgeon. These include tendon handling, the tidiness of the repair, decisions regarding pulley preservation, and the important question of postoperative rehabilitation. All these areas have seen notable advances in the past decade. The result has been an important reduction in the severity of postoperative adhesions after tendon injury, and the consequent need for tenolysis. These are discussed below.

1.1.2 Treatment

Surgical Techniques to Minimize Adhesions

It has been known for many years that rough handling of the lacerated tendon in Zone 2 can worsen adhesion for-

mation, by disrupting the smooth gliding surface of the tendon. For this reason it is important to *handle the tendon gently*, and grasp it only by the cut end. If the tendon has retracted into the palm, it should be retrieved with some sort of tendon carrier or passer, such as a narrow catheter. Any vincula that have survived the initial injury should be carefully preserved; indeed, if immediate repair is not possible then the finger should be splinted in wrist and finger flexion, to minimize the risk of rupturing any remaining vincula, until such time as surgical exploration can proceed. Active motion of the affected digit or digits should also be discouraged during this time.

A tidy repair, with the tendon ends coapted with slight bunching and normal rotational alignment, is critical to the smooth passage of the repaired tendon beneath any pulleys that are preserved. A tidy repair should also be a "low profile repair," with the least possible amount of suture material on the anterior surface of the tendon. Knots and even suture loops are sources of friction that will initially score the overlying pulley (▶ Fig. 1.2), and later this scoring will lead to inflammation and adhesions.

Initially, pulleys were sometimes resected to allow room for the tendon repair, only to result in bowstringing and flexion contracture. This clinical problem will be discussed in another section of this chapter. To avoid this problem, for many years there was a strong emphasis among hand surgeons to preserve the pulleys, and even to close the sheath completely. Unfortunately, this too led to adhesions and limited tendon gliding, even with well-performed, low-profile, tidy repairs. The problem was that even the

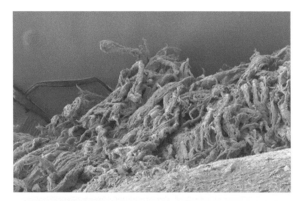

Fig. 1.2 Pulley scoring from a tendon suture knot in an animal model of tendon repair.

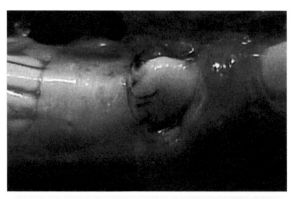

Fig. 1.3 Even the most tidy repair can catch on a pulley edge. The best solution is to make room for the repair, either by pulley excision or resection of one slip of the FDS.

best repair could not reproduce the dimensions of an intact tendon, and even a cursory examination of the tendons as they slide under the A2 pulley will confirm that there is no room for any additional bulk at all. Thus, more recently there has been a push again for judicious pulley resection, including, if need be, all the A4 pulley and even part of the A2 pulley.[2] Usually the amount of bowstringing after A4 excision is modest, because of the short segment affected (essentially, the length of P2), and the modest concave curvature of the palmar P2 surface. This is true even if, as is often the case with Zone 2 injury, the A3 pulley is not intact. In contrast, the P1 segment is longer, and its concavity deeper, resulting in more important bowing with A2 loss, especially if this is associated with A3 loss. Thus, it is important to preserve at least half of A2. An alternative strategy, which we prefer, is to resect (or excise rather than repair) one slip of the flexor digitorum superficialis (FDS), which creates adequate gliding space under the A2 pulley for even a somewhat bulky flexor digitorum profundus (FDP) repair.[3]

One may ask, how tidy is tidy enough, or how can one tell if enough pulley has been resected? Here the answer is clear. "Wide-awake" surgery, which allows the patient to actively move the tendon after it is repaired, but before the wound is closed, will reveal any deficiency in technique, including not only catching of a tendon repair on a pulley edge (▶ Fig. 1.3) but also a sloppy knot that unravels unexpectedly![4]

Adhesion Barriers

In addition to techniques of surgical approach and tendon repair, hand surgeons have often attempted to reduce the risk of adhesion formation through the use of various lubricant and adhesion barriers. In theory, these can make useful adjuncts, and, in practice, where there is room for them, protective sheets and films can block adhesions from, for example, an underlying fracture and a tendon repair. Unfortunately, there are two main problems that

have limited the usefulness of such barriers: first, their bulk often precludes using them just where they are needed most, between a tendon and its pulley; and second, because, as noted above, adhesions are a quite appropriate physiological response to bring blood supply to a damaged tendon. Thus, blocking adhesions often also means a persistently ischemic tendon, and one more likely to fail by rupture, as covered elsewhere in this chapter.

Liquid lubricants, such as hyaluronic acid, have also been used to block adhesions. These fluids, typically characterized as devices rather than drugs because their effect is mechanical and does not affect cellular processes, may at least allow the diffusion of nutrients, if not vascular ingrowth. In most cases though, these lubricants are either metabolized away or simply moved away by tendon motion, and therefore provide little benefit over the course of tendon healing. Lubricants that can be chemically bonded in molecularly thin layers to the tendon surface may one day overcome these problems, and have shown promise in animal models, but not yet in humans.

Drugs have also been used to block or mechanically weaken adhesions, most notably in the past, beta-aminopropionitrile, which interferes with collagen crosslinking. Unfortunately, it has not been possible to simply block crosslinking in the adhesions and not, for example, in the nearby tendon laceration or overlying skin. Thus these drugs end with unacceptable wound-healing complications; when used in experimental animals over longer terms, even the collagen in large vessels can be affected, leading to catastrophic hemorrhage.

Tenolysis

As noted above, advances in tendon surgery over the past two decades have reduced the need for tenolysis considerably, from over 20% in the 1970s and 1980s to under 10% today. Nonetheless, tenolysis is still needed for some patients, and the indications remain as they have always been: functionally disabling loss of active tendon motion in the presence of a supple finger (i.e., a mismatch between active and passive motion), an intact, healed tendon with a normal proximal muscle, and a cooperative patient. If the finger is not supple, there is no mismatch and thus no motion to be gained; if the tendon is not healed or the muscle is damaged then the solution is tendon reconstruction, not tenolysis; and of course without patient cooperation during postoperative rehabilitation the whole effort will be unrewarding.

A second factor in considering tenolysis is the risk/reward equation. What is the current functional limitation, and how bothersome is it? Is it worth jeopardizing current function for a chance at improvement? Neither full extension nor full flexion of a PIP joint is a realistic goal. Indeed, in general only about half of any intraoperative gain in active motion is maintained after tenolysis, so that, too, must be considered when determining if the procedure is worth considering.

In the preoperative assessment of a patient for tenolysis, it is important to determine if any joint contractures can be resolved with splinting, stretching, or serial casting preoperatively. It is also important for the surgeon to know that joint contractures can be the consequence of major pulley loss; in cases where pulley reconstruction and tenolysis are both under consideration, the surgeon should consider instead a staged reconstruction, since pulley reconstruction requires prolonged protection, while tenolysis demands early active mobilization postoperatively, to avoid the re-establishment of adhesions. This is especially true if a raw, tenolysed tendon surface is in contact with a reconstructed pulley. Recurrent adhesions are nearly inevitable. Finally, the surgeon should also verify that the tendon is healed—in addition to clinical assessment, ultrasound or magnetic resonance (MR) imaging is useful to confirm tendon integrity preoperatively, and they can also provide useful information on pulley loss.

Tenolysis is a procedure which carries substantial risks. The tendon and pulley may be deeply entwined in scar. Stray away from the tendon, and pulley loss may condemn the patient to a severe flexion contracture; get too close to the tendon and it may rupture. Because of this risk of intraoperative rupture, any patient consented for tenolysis should also be consented for a possible staged tendon reconstruction as well. At the very least, a plan for dealing with intraoperative rupture should be discussed in detail with the patient preoperatively. Tenolysis is an operation where there is a realistic probability that the result could be worse postoperatively.

The literature on the results of tenolysis is not particularly robust, likely reflecting the wide variety in the underlying cases, as well as the often mediocre results, which may make surgeons less enthusiastic about reporting their results.[5] All emphasize that one should expect the final result to be less good than whatever intraoperative gain is noted, and that tendon rupture may occur during or immediately following tenolysis.

1.1.3 Rehabilitation

After tenolysis, early active mobilization is important, but it is also wise not to be aggressive in the first few days, so as not to provoke any bleeding, and to minimize edema. In my experience, a close working relationship between the patient, the hand surgeon, and an experienced hand therapist is essential to a good clinical result after tenolysis. Each patient's care must be customized to the specifics of the underlying pathology and the details of the tenolysis that was performed. Edema control, passive joint mobilization, and graded active motion are all key elements of a successful rehabilitation program.

Early active flexion, usually through a "short arc" of partial motion that gradually increases over time postrepair, has generally replaced most passive flexion/active extension programs, which were popularized in the 1970s and 1980s. Passive motion and edema control measures still have an important role to play, to maintain a supple soft tissue sleeve and supple joints, but they, in and of themselves, do little to induce tendon gliding, even with various synergistic motion maneuvers. Protective splinting has also changed, as it has become clear that wrist immobilization does little to unload the flexor tendons in the fingers beyond what finger flexion can achieve. Thus, more and more, splinting after flexor tendon repair is hand based, at least after the initial surgical dressing is removed.

Together, the good fortune of a well-vascularized tendon injured by a sharp laceration, combined with modern methods of tendon repair, pulley release, and early active motion therapy, have gone a long way toward eliminating the need for tenolysis, which is often reserved now for complex combined injuries, such as replantation, where the anatomic ground and postoperative milieu are unfavorable.

1.1.4 Tips and Tricks

Each tenolysis case is in many ways unique, but there are still common features of tenolysis that allow the discussion of general principles. One of the most important and fundamental principles is that, since the goal is to restore active motion, it is important to assess active motion during the procedure. For this reason I prefer, and recommend to my patients, the "wide-awake" approach, without sedation, a tourniquet, or muscle-paralyzing agents to interfere with active contraction of the affected muscle tendon units. In many cases, an active contraction will rupture the final adhesions and allow the desired restoration of motion. In other cases, a traction check with the surgeon putting tension on the tendon will show full passive tendon motion through the zone of injury, but no active result when the patient attempts to flex the digit. This is a sign that adhesions may have formed outside the zone of injury. These can be distal, but proximal adhesions can also develop, even as far proximal as the distal forearm, between the profundus or superficialis muscle bellies.

Skin quality is important to surgical planning as well. A scarred digit with atrophic skin is unlikely to tolerate an extensive dissection, and thus represents a contraindication to tenolysis. Supple overlying skin is essential. Dissection must preserve whatever circulation remains, to both the digit and tendon. I prefer to use existing incisions, and to extend them proximally and distally as needed to get areas beyond the zone of injury, so that dissection can begin where anatomy is normal, and move from there into the zone of injury.

When exposing the tendon and sheath, it is important to avoid any further injury to the neurovascular bundles, or to their branches that feed the tendon and sheath, as noted in ▸ Fig. 1.1. The extent of remaining pulleys should be noted. To preserve these pulleys, dissection under them can be done through transverse windows, no closer than 1 cm apart. A variety of special narrow knives and elevators can be used for this purpose; however it is done, it is important to preserve tendon integrity. Just as with digging a tunnel under a mountain from both sides, coaxial alignment of the work is essential, so that when the proximal and distal dissections join they still define a robust tendon in continuity. In some cases with severe adhesions it may be necessary to sacrifice the superficialis tendon and preserve the profundus tendon, especially with severe adhesions under the A2 pulley.

For wound closure after tenolysis, hemostasis is another critical factor; another reason to favor the wide-awake approach, since the epinephrine that allows prolonged local anesthesia also provides excellent hemostasis. The skin must be closed carefully and without tension, so that early motion will not jeopardize wound healing.

1.1.5 Conclusions

In summary, tendon adhesions are an important but fortunately increasingly infrequent complication following flexor tendon injury. When tenolysis is required, care is necessary to be sure that the potential benefits of surgery outweigh the risks. Surgery using wide-awake anesthesia can facilitate complete release of the limiting adhesions. Postoperatively, a coordinated team of patient, therapist, and surgeon is required to optimize outcomes.

1.2 Bowstringing
1.2.1 Definition/Problem

Tendon bowstringing, strictly speaking, occurs any time a tendon loses its close contact with the underlying bone. This is a particular aspect of the anatomy of finger flexor tendons, because of the curved anterior surface of the phalanges. Without the bony A2 and A4 pulleys, the flexor tendons will naturally bow away from the curved phalanx, regardless of joint angle.[6] This is more so for the proximal phalanx, because it is both more bowed and longer than the middle phalanx. Bowstringing is exacerbated with joint flexion if the joint related A1, A3, or A5 pulleys are also affected. Basically, the longer the affected segment the greater the problem. Of note, the palmar condyles of the phalanges create a palmar bowing of the tendon at the joint so that the path of the tendon at the proximal interphalangeal (PIP) joint, as seen from a lateral view, does not actually become straight until the joint is flexed about 45 degrees; joint related bowstringing, even in the absence of pulleys, only occurs after this point. The more joint motion is restricted, then, by arthritis, intra-articular injury, or periarticular fibrosis, the less bowstringing is actually possible, and, by extension, the less critical it is to restore pulley function. The converse though is also true: the more a patient requires full flexion at the PIP joint to perform important functions, the more important it is to have an intact pulley system.

Why Do We Have Pulleys?

Pulleys are necessary to keep the tendon close to the bone, especially in places where large angular joint motion is needed. Tendon excursion is fixed, based on the ability of actin and myosin molecules in the muscle to contract. To get more angular motion with a fixed excursion, the tendon must be as close to the axis of motion of the joint as possible. Remember that the circumference of a circle is two times the radius, so if a rope (or tendon) is turning a circular joint with a radius of 5 mm, for every 5 mm of tendon excursion the joint angle will move 360/2 degrees, or about 60 degrees. If the tendon is bowing away from the joint by an additional 5 mm, then the same 5 mm excursion will only move the joint around 30 degrees. Because of the increased lever arm (10 mm vs. 5 mm) the tendon will exert twice as much force on the joint, but the joint will only move half as far. This is the tradeoff in pulley preservation or reconstruction, and, by the way, underlines one of the beauties of pulley anatomy—the A2 and A4 pulleys are fixed, but the A1, A3, and A5 pulleys connect to the volar plates, so they naturally allow some bowstringing with joint flexion, reducing potential joint angular motion a little but adding some strength. A very important point that we did not fully appreciate earlier in my career is that while normal pulley anatomy is necessary for perfect finger motion, in essentially all cases of pulley loss we are not realistically trying for normal. Usually a bit less motion and a bit more strength is a fair tradeoff for some residual bowing, and of course in the context of flexor tendon laceration normal motion is anyway almost never achieved in adults—the loss of a few degrees of active motion due to bowstringing caused by pulley trimming is well worth if the alternative is a stuck tendon, and no motion at all. This imbalance will nearly always result in a flexion contracture of some degree, but unless pulley loss is extensive, again, this may well be an acceptable tradeoff, compared to striving for perfect reconstruction, with its attendant risks of adhesions and stiffness.

Etiology of Pulley Loss

Pulley injury may be closed or open, and open injury may be due to direct trauma or be the result of a surgical decision to trim or vent pulleys to aid in tendon repair or tenolysis. Closed injuries are frequently the result of forceful gripping, and are a common problem in rock climbers. Usually these are small (distal A2, isolated A3, or A4) and can be managed with taping and early return to sport (▶ Fig. 1.4). Even a complete A2 rupture, if isolated, can often be managed without surgery, using custom thermoplastic ring splints that allow some functional activity. Even in idealized cadaver models, a complete loss of A2 only results in a loss of around 20 degrees of motion, for a normal FDP excursion and normal joints. Such a loss is far smaller than the typical loss of motion, compared to normal, after a tendon repair in Zone 2. Ruptures of multiple pulleys, though, will require surgery. The situation is the same with open pulley injuries—short segments of loss can be left unrepaired or reconstructed, but longer segments will require surgical attention, because the consequence otherwise is marked bowstringing and, usually, a severe flexion contracture. As noted above, the length of pulley loss that can be tolerated without important functional impairment depends upon both patient needs and the mobility of the PIP joint, but there will be few patients who can tolerate combined loss of A2, A3, and A4 without substantial loss of function, usually due to a fixed flexion contracture, as the power of the

flexors, augmented by the leverage provided by the bowing, overcomes the ability of the extensors to counterbalance, and extend the joint.

1.2.2 Treatment

Nonoperative Treatment

As noted above, short segments of pulley loss (typically <1 cm), whether due to rupture, laceration, or surgical trimming, can be safely managed by fairly simple means. Even a loss of the entire A4 pulley can be managed in this way, provided that the A3 and A5 pulleys remain intact. Schoffl and Schoffl[7] have developed a useful classification of pulley injuries in climbers, which is relevant to all pulley injuries. Grade 1 is a sprain, with local tenderness but no loss of pulley integrity as demonstrated by either ultrasound or MR imaging. These can be managed symptomatically, and do not require immobilization. Taping the affected phalangeal segment and a graduated return to full function over the next few months is usually all that is required. Grade 2 injuries represent the shorter segment complete injuries (<1 cm) mentioned above, either partial A2, or A3, or A4, which can be managed similarly, with the addition of a few weeks of initial immobilization to rest the injured area. Grade 3 is basically a complete loss of the A2 pulley, which is around 15 mm long in the adult finger. Schoffl and Schoffl include also an isolated loss of A3 as a grade 3 injury, but we have not seen an isolated loss of A3 to cause clinical difficulties in my own experience, and again it is important to remember that A3 does not even come into play functionally until the PIP joint is flexed beyond 45 degrees. For isolated complete A2 injuries, taping is not sufficient to restrain bowstringing until the pulley heals, and in such cases a custom thermoplastic ring splint may be helpful. More prolonged protection is needed before returning to full use, usually 3 months or more, and the thermoplastic splint may be needed during activity for many months after that. Nonetheless, many such patients can function well without the need for pulley reconstruction.

Surgical Treatment

In contrast to short segments of pulley loss, grade 4 injuries, with complete loss of adjacent pulleys, will often require surgical reconstruction, tempered somewhat by the caveats mentioned above (▶ Fig. 1.5).

Acute repair of pulley injuries can be attempted in cases of open injury. Usually direct repair is not possible but a graft of extensor retinaculum can be used. However, results do not approach those of direct repair with pulley trimming, and so should only be considered if the extent of pulley loss is extensive, for example, complete loss of A2 and A3. In most cases, pulley reconstruction is typically the preferred option. When pulley reconstruction is needed, almost always it is the function of A2 that needs

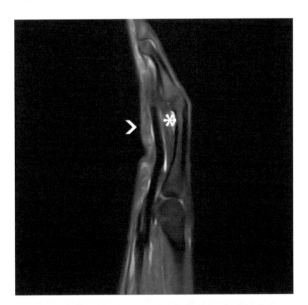

Fig. 1.4 A patient with rupture of the distal A2 pulley has a small but obvious amount of bowing (*arrow*). This amount of bowing is unlikely to require pulley reconstruction. Nonoperative methods are likely to suffice. Note however that the space posterior to the tendon (*star*) is not empty—it will fill with a wedge of scar, which must be excised before the tendon can be returned to its proper location adjacent to the phalanx, and an appropriate diameter pulley reconstruction performed.

1

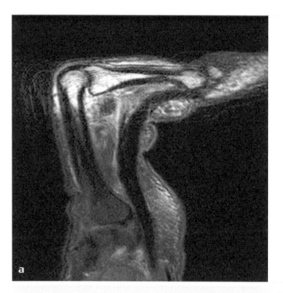

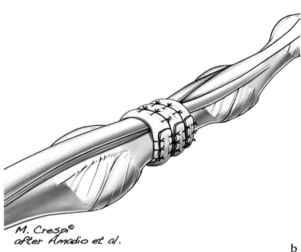

M. Crespi©
after Amadio et al.

Fig. 1.5 Loss of multiple pulleys is more likely to require reconstruction. **(a)** A patient with massive pulley loss, undergoing staged tendon and pulley reconstruction. **(b)** The most important pulley to reconstruct is the A2 pulley, and for this pulley, a tendon graft wrapped around the phalanx three times is the strongest construct. This also creates more pulley width. This is my preferred method of reconstruction at this level. A palmaris longus tendon is preferred, if available. Because pulley reconstruction is usually done in the context of tendon reconstruction, remnants of the flexor tendons can also be used, to preserve the palmaris longus for use as a later tendon graft.

to be restored, because it affects the ability of the PIP joint to move more normally.[8] In theory, A3 function can be restored, for example with the Karev "belt loop," using a portion of the volar plate, but this can only be done if the tendon is also being replaced with a tendon graft, and even then only if the graft is thin and narrow, for example, a palmaris longus tendon. Even then, usually if a tendon graft is being done it is because there is not only tendon loss but also joint contracture, so that any functional volar plate will have to be released to restore PIP extension. Sometimes, A4 reconstruction can be considered; it may help to avoid a distal interphalangeal (DIP) flexion contracture, which may be functionally limiting. An alternative, though, would be to consider DIP arthrodesis or capsulodesis, and concentrate motion on the PIP joint. In most digits that needed pulley reconstruction, it is not just the pulley that is the problem—aside from closed ruptures in climbers, where both A2 and A4 reconstruction over a normal tendon system may well be reasonable to consider, in nearly all cases of pulley reconstruction the pulley was injured along with, or as part of the initial repair, or tenolysis of, a flexor tendon or tendons. In such cases, goals are limited; a normal finger is not possible. Thus, most of the time, attention can rightly be focused on restoring A2.

There are several ways to recreate an A2 pulley, but we by far prefer the "around-bone" technique, using either a tendon graft, such as palmaris longus, or the remnant of a damaged and irreparable flexor tendon. This is the strongest construct. The main alternative is to weave a tendon graft through the "ever-present rim" of the pulley in a shoelace fashion, as popularized by Harold Kleinert. The

rim may indeed be "ever-present," but to us it seems quite narrow and we have had difficulty weaving a tendon graft through it. The main advantage of this latter technique is that it does not disturb the extensor mechanism, but we have not observed extensor difficulties with the around-bone technique, so long as the graft is truly on the bone and below the extensor mechanism, and the reconstruction is where the A2 pulley would normally be, away from both joints, roughly on the middle one-third of the proximal phalanx, and no more than 15 mm in width. Three loops, if possible, is the strongest configuration, and we do use the "ever-present rim" to anchor the loops so they don't spin or migrate, as well of course to suturing the loops to each other, after tensioning them around the underlying tendon or tendon spacer.

If A4 is to be reconstructed, the "ever-present rim" is even smaller, and typically just one loop is possible, and over the middle phalanx it is necessary to go around the extensor tendon. This causes inevitable adhesions and limits DIP motion, one reason why I do not typically reconstruct A4—capsulodesis or arthrodesis is easier.

Very commonly (again, aside from closed ruptures in climbers), when one is considering pulley reconstruction, the flexor tendons are also abnormal—at best, intact with loss of pulleys after tenolysis, but more commonly with either ruptured or badly frayed tendons as well as joint contractures and other soft tissue problems. In such cases, the pulley reconstruction is often combined with a staged tendon reconstruction, with the pulleys being reconstructed over a silicone tendon spacer, and coming back some months later when all has healed from stage 1, to do the stage 2 tendon graft. There is not enough room here to discuss all the intricacies of staged tendon reconstruction, but it is important that the implant be as large as whatever tendon is planned for the subsequent graft; otherwise there will be a fit mismatch at the time of grafting. If a large implant is chosen but the reconstruction is with a thin, flat palmaris longus, the tendon graft will bowstring within the too large pulley. On the other hand, if a Paneva-Holevich or other technique is planned, using a wide, round, profundus, or superficialis tendon, it will be important not to use a narrow, flat tendon spacer at stage 1.

Regardless of whether a pulley is being reconstructed over a tendon spacer or an actual tendon, it is imperative that smooth tendon gliding be verified intraoperatively. For a tendon spacer, this means that the implant, which is fixed distally and free proximally, can easily glide under the pulley, without buckling, with passive finger flexion. For an intact tendon (or if the surgeon is using an active tendon implant), it is important the tendon glide easily under the new pulley with active flexion, if this is at all possible.

1.2.3 Rehabilitation

Postoperative management of a reconstructed pulley is similar to that of a grade 3 closed pulley injury treated nonoperatively,[7] with variations depending on whether the underling tendons are intact, or have an underlying tendon spacer. If the tendons are intact, after an initial few days to allow for wound stabilization and to minimize the risk of stirring up bleeding, a gentle limited arc active motion program can begin, similar to what one would do after primary tendon repair. The initial rest period can include measures to reduce finger edema, including some gentle passive joint mobilization within a limited arc. Of course, uninvolved digits must be managed as well, lest they develop contractures from disuse. The pulley reconstruction should be protected with taping initially and, after the skin has healed, a ring splint can be considered. If a tendon spacer is present, then an initial period of rest will be followed by a passive mobilization program, as for any staged tendon reconstruction.

1.2.4 Tips and Tricks

The use of MRI to assess tendon bowstringing confirms what previously was a subtle clinical observation: the smooth dorsal gliding bed of a bowstrung tendon is usually not the palmar aspect of the phalanx, but rather a *wedge of scar holding the tendon away from the bone*, as shown in ▶ Fig. 1.4. This wedge must be excised before the tendon can be positioned appropriately against the bone, and a proper pulley reconstruction fashioned.

Another important point about pulley reconstruction is that sometimes it is better to "simplify" the finger rather than to reconstruct all the pulleys in a badly damaged digit. For example, while the loss of A4 is usually well tolerated, the loss of A3, A4, and A5 may cause a marked DIP flexion contracture. While reconstruction of the A4 pulley may correct the contracture, often the final active DIP motion is small. Thus, in a severely damaged finger with multiple distal pulley loss, consideration should be given to creation of a superficialis finger, and fusing the DIP joint. This is especially true if the FDP is damaged, while the FDS is intact, and one would otherwise be facing a staged tendon reconstruction. A one-stage DIP fusion may serve the patient better, and allow a faster return to function.

Finally, something less of a tip or trick than a strong recommendation—for any tendon surgery we strongly prefer the wide-awake approach popularized by Donald Lalonde, MD. This is the best way to be sure that the pulleys are strong and snug, while allowing good active tendon gliding without binding (the intraoperative forerunner of postoperative adhesions).

1.2.5 Conclusion

A thorough understanding of pulley function is necessary before the surgeon can adequately assess and manage tendon bowstringing, which is the consequence of pulley loss. In general, segmental pulley loss up to 1 cm in length can be tolerated, and need not be reconstructed, while defects more than 2 cm in length will often benefit from surgical reconstruction. For loss in between 1 and 2 cm, some judgment is necessary, and treatment will depend more on associated injuries and the exact location of the pulley loss. More distal pulley loss is better tolerated, for example. Pulley repair is usually not as reliable an option as reconstruction, but can be tried in acute injuries.

1.3 Rupture

1.3.1 The Problem

At the current time there is an interesting change in the philosophy of management of flexor tendon injuries. Since Harold Kleinert established the, then controversial, principle of primary flexor tendon repair, the main focus has been to preserve the anatomy of the gliding surfaces of tendon and pulleys. These central principles are being challenged by a new focus on strong repair[1] with sufficient release of the sheath to allow gliding of a bulky repair. There is not yet sufficient data to know if better outcomes are achieved but evolution is a constant feature in flexor tendon surgery.

Flexor tendon rupture after surgical repair is feared by surgeons as it is a sudden and dramatic event which may be seen by the patient as a failure of technique. In truth, it is a multifactorial event which has generally been a less common reason for poor repair outcomes than stiffness and adhesions.

1

Rupture abruptly interrupts the rehabilitation plan and the challenge for surgical repair and rehabilitation at this time is to restore and maintain mobility yet avoid re-rupture.

Why Do Tendon Repairs Rupture?

Three interacting factors are important in rupture: the complex tendon repair biology, factors attributed to the patient, and biomechanics of the surgical repair.

Tendon Repair Biology

Tendon healing and adhesions are essentially one wound, the morphology of which we try to focus by surgery and rehabilitation toward tensional load transmission while preserving marginal mobility. Inevitably the repair is initially very weak in comparison with intact tendon. Moreover, there is clear evidence that our repairs do further damage as each suture grasp creates an acellular necrotic zone[9] in areas of high strain gripped by the stitch.

Patient Factors in Tendon Rupture: Incidence and Causation

In a large series of 728 tendon divisions in 526 fingers published from David Elliot's carefully collected database, Harris et al[10] reported 28 ruptures in 23 fingers (4%.) Incidentally it is notable that this low percentage of rupture was achieved at that time using just a two-strand core suture. Rupture events were recorded in detail and were generally due to excessive loading as in a fall or unwise gripping. The rupture incidence in nonspecialist centers appears to be much higher.

Biomechanics of the Surgical Repair

The specter of tendon rupture has promoted a drive toward developing stronger repairs. In addition to traditional core sutures, a peripheral epitendinous stitch has generally been used to add to tensile strength by preventing the buckling which precedes failure. Recently there has been a tendency for some departments to omit this suture, relying entirely on a tight core suture.[11] Key steps in developing stronger repairs have been replacement of two-stranded suture techniques by multistranded configurations, a concept proposed and analyzed in detail by Savage[12] in 1985. This was a revolutionary concept which was the key step in heralding a generational step change toward stronger repairs. The concept of multiple strands was so strikingly innovative that the surgical community largely overlooked the other principle introduced by Savage of securing firm anchorage of the tendon suture through crisscross sutures encircling superficial fibers to prevent suture pull-out. The Adelaide technique is derived from this and in its current form

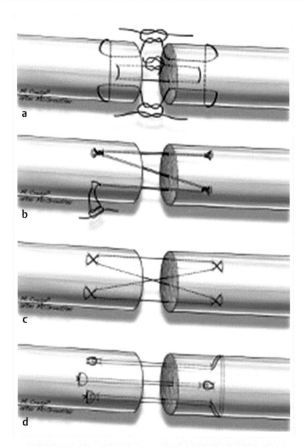

Fig. 1.6 Examples of multistranded repair techniques. **(a)** Strickland's tendon repair which is a modification of the Kessler two-strand suture which has four locking Pennington anchor points and an additional two core strands from a simple loop. As illustrated, this places much suture material between the tendon's ends. **(b)** This modification of the Lim Tsai technique uses a looped suture giving six strands with a single knot placed outside the contact zone of the tendon's ends.
(c) The Adelaide repair is a derivative of the Savage multistranded concept with four or six strands and a simpler criss-cross anchorage technique. **(d)** The M-Tang configuration uses three separate Tsuge-type looped sutures.

includes four strands and a simpler anchorage. Numerous multistranded configurations (▶ Fig. 1.6) aim to strike a balance between strength from increasing strand number and aggravation of the trauma to the tendon ends, four or six strands being popular compromise designs.

Suture Configurations and How They Fail

The two main modes of tendon repair rupture are pull-out of the intact suture or suture failure due to snapping or untying/slipping. Any of these possibilities may be responsible for rupture during the first week following repair when the initial strength is entirely due to the tendon suture. A tendon repair is weakest at 5 to 10 days following repair due to edema and enzymatic softening. By 5 to 7 days the repair gap has cellular infiltration and new but randomly aligned collagen deposition and from this point on failure by pull-out seems the more likely mechanism. The fibroblastic phase of tendon healing brings added strength to the repair site but also adhesions and it seems likely that the immobilized *tendon that fails to glide* due to adhesions will be particularly vulnerable to rupture from active or passive attempts to mobilize. A second cause of early failure to glide is impaction of a bulky tendon repair on an intact annular pulley such that the jammed repair is pulled apart during attempts at movement, whether active or passive.

A recent review of biomechanical cyclic testing protocols for flexor tendon repairs has emphasized the benefit of simulation of repetitive motion and force loading in developing tendon suture techniques and in demonstrating the mode of failure.[13] Skin sutures are not designed to bear the tensional forces traversing a tendon repair. Newer braided synthetic sutures such as Fiberwire have greater tensile strength but poor knot-holding properties, often requiring four throws to prevent slippage. This results in bulky knot material which can increase friction in the sheath or if tucked into the intertendon gap can block the fibroblastic repair line.

Factors leading to failure by pull out include patient overuse, tendon edema, or placement of the anchorage points too close to the tendon ends. Suture snapping can occur from high stress in the suture strands such as adjacent to knots or where one strand of a suture crosses another within the tendon substance. Use of an insufficiently strong suture is another factor or the suture may be damaged by handling with an instrument. Alternatively, knots may slip and untie.

The repair integrity can be checked prior to wound closure by repeated cycles of passive motion and surgical release of a sufficient length of the sheath (up to 20 mm) to allow gliding without impaction on the annular pulley margin. Wide-awake techniques allow visualization of free active tendon motion at the end of the operation to ensure there is no catching or triggering.

1.3.2 Management of Patient with Rupture Presenting Early after Tendon Repair

History

In managing tendon rupture the aim is to gather as much information as possible to predict whether re-repair is likely to be successful or whether another plan of action is appropriate.

Time points of injury, operation, and rupture may give clues as to the cause having assessed whether or not the patient has generally been compliant with treatment, the next area to assess is whether there were technical factors at the time of the primary repair that might predispose to rupture or impaired healing. Has there been infection at any stage? Are there comorbidities such as diabetes? Did the patient realize immediately that there had been a loss of mobility or was there a gradual deterioration, the latter suggesting that rupture may have followed a process of adhesion?

Examination

In the early period of the first 1 to 2 weeks, the digit or digits will be flail with full/near full passive but generally no active movement, although in a few cases there may be a small range of active motion due to an intact vinculum.

Imaging

An ultrasound examination is indispensable in defining the nature of the problem in a digit which has a limited range of motion following flexor tendon repair. The major benefit of ultrasound is that it provides an immediate and dynamic image. A gap between the ends will produce a hypoechoic defect. Adhesions can be seen as dragging of adjacent soft tissues on tendon movement. Bowstringing and its exact site can be visualized and measured. A complete rupture will show an empty and hypoechoic sheath, possibly unraveled suture material and a failure of active movement.

Informed Consent

In consenting the patient for re-repair, advice should make it clear that the chance of regaining full movement is less than that after a primary repair. The patient should also be advised that if wound conditions determine it a staged reconstruction by tendon (Hunter) rod and later tendon grafting may be the option with the highest chance of success.

Operative Plan

It is always difficult to predict the state of the tendon and sheath but some indication is possible from the condition of the hand tissues in general. The divided tendon ends may appear quite pristine but more usually they will be delaminated or shredded by suture pull-out. Early operative intervention will allow a "forensic examination" of the repair and hopefully point to the exact reasons for rupture. The condition of the sutures provides valuable clues. If loops of suture material are intact the likelihood is that the failure was by pull out, suggesting such possibilities as the tendon ends being softened by a delay in treatment or by infection. There is also the possibility of a technical failure in not placing the sutures far enough from the cut end, due to limited access—a minimum of 6 to 8 mm is recommended. Snapped sutures may suggest inappropriate choice of too flimsy a suture material or possibly damage to the suture by the cutting edge of a needle or crushing by a needle holder or other instrument. Where rupture occurs with minimal force and the suture is spiraling or with a long tapering end the knots may have untied. Surgeons are reluctant to conceive this possibility but any fisherman will know that monofilament, or even braided, synthetic polymer sutures cannot be held with a single reef knot as there is insufficient friction between the strands of material and the knots slip.

If the tendons and sheath are found to be inflamed and swollen, the surgeon must judge whether they have sufficient mechanical strength to hold sutures. The sheath should be assessed to see if it is likely that the repair has been disrupted by triggering on the edge of a pulley. It may be helpful to release the tourniquet, if there is one, to assess if the tendon ends have a blood supply. If the judgment is that conditions are suitable for a re-repair and if both tendons have ruptured, it may be best to excise either one slip or the whole of FDS but sparing any intact vincula and rely on repair of FDP alone as there will be considerable postoperative swelling after this second intervention with a risk of jamming of swollen tendons in the tendon sheath. It may be appropriate to incise or excise tendon sheath.

As with current trends in primary repair, the focus has moved from preservation of the entire sheath toward opening the sheath in its ventral midline over sufficient length to allow the tendon repair site to glide. Tang[14] has advised that sheath opening should be limited to 20 mm which would allow complete release of the A4 pulley for Zone 1 injuries or release of most of the A2. The maximum excursion of the intact FDP over the middle phalanx is 6 to 8 mm, proximal phalanx 15 mm, and palm 35 mm. It is important to map out the exact position of the tendon repair line and its excursion before planning the incision of the sheath to ensure that the appropriate part of the sheath is released. If there is sufficient access for the repair, the sheath incision can be left until the end of the procedure.

Where there has been little damage to the tendon ends as in situations of knot untying, then a re-repair may be feasible. There is no literature advice on which repair to use in such circumstances and the best advice is for the operator to use the one most familiar although attempting to obtain a longer grip on the tendon ends. If the tendon ends have a minor degree of disturbance, a minor degree of trimming may be acceptable for repairs in Zones 3, 4, 5 but any shortening in Zones 1 or 2 will significantly alter digital posture and the increased tension will predispose to a second rupture. Cellular analysis shows that the tendon stumps have the necessary cells and growth factors to allow healing and the main question in choosing re-repair is "will the suture have sufficient grip to prevent re-rupture?" Shortening due to trim-

ming in the thumb has been compensated by either step lengthening or intramuscular tendon lengthening.

More severe damage to the tendon ends but otherwise undamaged tendon may be managed by excision and a short interposition graft. Where both tendon and sheath are significantly damaged a two-stage reconstruction by tendon grafting offers the best chance of good function. If a re-repair becomes stuck by adhesion the digit is likely to develop flexion contractures at any or all of the joints and fixed flexion contracture is a very difficult condition to redeem, whereas embarking on the first stage of a two-stage reconstruction provides a flail digit where passive joint mobility can be easily maintained and converted to active joint mobility after the second stage.

Flexor Tendon Reconstruction by Tendon Grafting

As more and more primary repairs are successful, experience in tendon graft surgery becomes less. It is very rare today for the technique of primary tendon grafting to be performed as the uninflamed tissue bed is generally managed by secondary repair. For a two-stage reconstruction there are many variations in technique and many tips and tricks to get a good outcome. Many of these details are being lost in the mists of time and it seems appropriate to expand on technical details here (▶ Fig. 1.7). If there is any significant length of scarring in the wound bed (more than 2 cm in Zone 2), a two-stage reconstruction is a more predictable way to arrive at a good range of flexion and extension.

The first step is to identify the proximal motor tendons and to anchor these to the transverse intermetacarpal ligament by sutures to prevent them retracting proximally. It is my practice to anchor both FDS and FDP tendons. To accommodate the silicon rod it is necessary to remove the divided tendons from Zones 1 and 2. And this may require appropriate incisions. A silicon tendon rod is then inserted from the midpalm to the distal phalanx. The rod is sutured distally burrowing the rod deep to the tendon remnant overlying the distal phalanx and clearly distal to the dip joint as it is important to generate a new sheath beyond the DIP so that the later tendon graft will act as a flexor of both DIP and PIP joints. The proximal end of the rod must not be sutured and just lies loosely deep to the flexor tendons in the midpalmar space. The rod allows wound bed healing and regeneration of a synovial sheath which almost miraculously will develop within a few weeks. Although the rods are 3 or 4 mm in diameter, they encourage the development of a wider sheath which will later be suitable for a larger tendon. At this first reconstructive operation, it is necessary to define or create annular pulleys to retain the rod in its appropriate "anatomical" position.

The timing of the second operation is determined by achieving a suitable passive range of digital joint motion

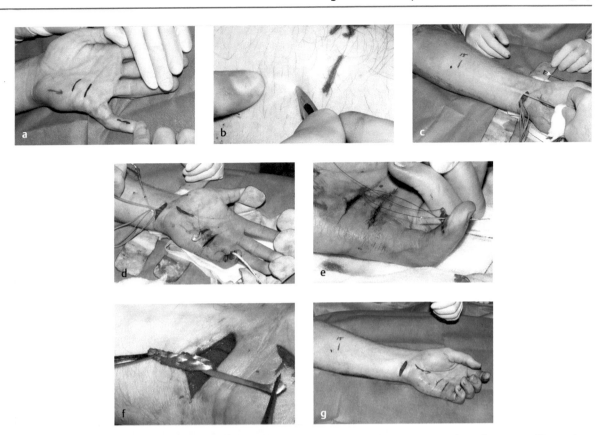

Fig. 1.7 The second stage of a two-stage tendon graft. **(a)** Following a failed primary repair, a 4-mm tendon rod was inserted from palm to distal phalanx. At 6 months despite a limited extension range, which is common, a second stage was planned. On exploration, the proximal FDS and FDP were found to be extensively scarred in the carpal canal and a decision was made to insert a graft above the wrist. **(b)** A 15-cm Palmaris Longus graft was required and the tendon was harvested by a transverse wrist crease and a proximal stab incision. **(c)** By applying strong traction to the distal Palmaris Longus, the tendon could be palpated at the 15 cm mark. The tendon was then stabbed with the point of a number 11 blade, which was moved backward and forward together with the surrounding skin thus dividing the tendon which was delivered by distal traction. **(d)** The tendon graft was sutured to the proximal end of the rod and pulled distally into the digital flexor sheath. The proximal end of the graft was sutured to a pediatric feeding tube introduced through the carpal canal for the purpose of delivering the graft to the wrist. **(e)** A strong suture was inserted in the distal end of the graft. Two green hypodermic needles were passed from proximal to distal from the tendon sheath around the waist of the distal phalanx and out through the nail. The needle hubs were broken off; the two sutures were passed through the needle shafts which were extracted distally leaving the sutures through the nail. Traction on the sutures ensured that the distal end of the tendon graft was now distal to the dip joint. The sutures were tied over the nail (no button required). **(f)** The proximal end of the graft was passed through the FDS tendon and initially secured with a single stitch. The cascade of finger posture was then checked by a wrist tenodesis test and the position of the one suture moved until the cascade was satisfactory. The Pulvertaft weave was completed (shown out of the wound for photographic purposes). **(g)** The final finger cascade.

and the general state of the tissues with inflammatory change resolved, generally around 6 months.

The two flexors are released from their anchorage and the excursion can be checked by traction. The FDP has the advantage of having a lumbrical and the FDS the advantage of independent motion without the quadriga. It is best to choose the one with the better excursion, after localized tenolysis. The ideal in the palm is 35 mm, but generally less has to be accepted.

For tendon grafts from palm to digit palmaris longus is the favorite donor. It is however absent in around 20% of the population and can leave an obvious volar wrist scar. The scarring can be minimized by employing a minimal transverse wrist crease scar 10 to 15 mm. By mobilizing the distal end of palmaris from the deep fascia and then gripping the divided tendon at the wrist crease and applying strong distal traction, the tendon can be palpated as a tight band in the middle third of the forearm and the desired length measured on the skin. The proximal wound and scar can be minimized by stabbing the skin with the point of a number 11 blade. By pinching the skin around the blade and slipping skin and blade together from side to side, the tip of the blade will cut the tensioned palmaris tendon. The skin wound is only the

1

size of the tip of the blade. It is important to have the tendon under strong traction tension from distally and to perform the stab maneuver as high as possible in the forearm to ensure that the median nerve is in a deep position. We first saw this done by Harold Kleinert and it leaves very minimal scarring.

Some surgeons prefer to do the proximal junction above the wrist in every case to capitalize on the greater excursion at that point. However palmaris longus is often not long enough to reach from wrist to digit and other tendons must be considered: plantaris (visible on ultrasound if present), toe extensors (very difficult to harvest), FDS, and others. There is also great variability in choosing whether to repair the proximal graft repair (Pulvertaft weave) first and adjust the graft length by the position of the distal repair. Our preferred method is to attach the distal end first by a Kirchmaier-Kessler suture inserted into the end of the graft and then passing the two suture ends around the neck of the distal phalanx using green needles. The sutures are passed through the nail and knotted. The proximal end is commenced by forming a Pulvertaft weave and holding with one interrupted suture. The length of the graft is then checked by a passive wrist tenodesis test to ensure the graft has the correct length by observing the digital cascade. When the correct tension on the tendon is decided, additional sutures are placed to lock the weave.

If, however, only the FDP has ruptured but FDS remains intact it may be better to leave the situation undisturbed as surgery may run a risk of losing the range of PIP motion that the patient has retained. This is particularly true in the case of the little finger where re-repair of FDP has shown disappointing results. Guy Pulvertaft described the reconstruction of an FDP in the presence of an intact FDS as "an operation for the patient determined to achieve perfection."

Management of Tendon Rupture Presenting Late after Repair

In cases of rupture presenting late after primary repair there is likely to be extensive scarring of tendon and sheath and joint contractures. A simple re-repair is rarely possible. Rupture in such circumstances is often secondary to adhesions and the diagnosis of rupture can be difficult if stiffness and fibrosis have been slowly progressive, ultrasound imaging is helpful in making this distinction. Several stages may be required to release joint contracture and replace the scarred tendon. In such circumstances it is virtually impossible to core out the tendon from the annular pulleys and retain the integrity of the pulleys which tend to rupture. It may be necessary to resect and reconstruct pulleys with the insertion of a tendon rod.

The aim is to establish a useful passive range of motion and await maturation of scar tissue which will remain contractile for several months. Rather than suggesting a fixed time limit it is better to observe the state of the healing digit and the amount of inflammatory swelling. Generally, the time chosen for a second stage is between 6 months and 1 year. After a year there is a possibility of the silicon rod snapping and the proximal part migrating with collapse of the neo-sheath. In the interim the patient may be able to return to work after skin healing and the flail finger can be buddy taped to a neighboring digit to prevent it "getting in the way." The patient may decide against further reconstruction and just request removal of the tendon rod, or arthrodesis of one or other joint.

1.3.3 Rehabilitation

An important factor in the management of a rupture re-repair is to decide on a careful and individual hand therapy regime depending on the confidence of both professionals. If the patient was tending to overdo the active mobility, then particular restraint and oversight would seem appropriate.

As primary tendon repair has evolved, the original focus of rupture prevention was on protection of the repair by postoperative protocols of passive mobilization. The Duran and Houser protocol of therapist-supervised passive mobilization of the repair site by 3 to 5 mm or the Kleinert system of active extension and passive rubber band flexion were popular techniques of achieving passive mobilization. Active mobilization is now the favored policy, although this must be limited to avoid power grip. Many different protocols of splintage are in use but the aim is generally to limit the joints proximal to the repair site, partly or completely. Active mobilization of joints distal to the repair will then produce an excursion at the repair site. Important components of this plan are to commence before the tendon is anchored by adhesions, generally around 5 to 7 days, and to gradually increase load and range of motion over an 8 weeks period. Serial ultrasound examination is helpful to ensure that an excursion at the repair site is achieved and maintained. Ruptures seem to be most common during the second week of mobilization. It is likely that many of the improvements that are thought to be from surgery are in fact due to better supervised rehabilitation and in particular early active motion.

1.3.4 Tips and Tricks

The whole sequence of two-stage tendon grafting is a sequence of tips and tricks as outlined above but a note on pulley reconstruction seems appropriate. Whereas reconstruction can be successful in highly motivated rock climbers, we have had little success with extensive pulley reconstruction in digits presenting late after tendon rupture and have preferred a salvage operation of excision of scarred tendon only between the A2 and A4 pulleys leaving the scarred tendon remnants within these pulleys in place and tunneling deep to the scarred tendon remnants and inserting a tendon rod. With this degree of pathology there is no certain way of guaranteeing a successful outcome and there is no published data on such salvage procedures. A colleague has independently evolved the same approach but no one has had the patient numbers, or courage, to report this technique, which has nevertheless been successful in restoring a useful range of movement in such cases, where the goals are necessarily limited, and the alternative is often amputation.

1.3.5 Conclusion

Experience shows that re-repair offers approximately equal chances of a good or excellent function versus a poor outcome or re-rupture. It is the author's practice to explore all, selectively re-repair the tendon if all factors are favorable but to opt for a two-stage reconstruction if there is anxiety about any of the conditions being unsatisfactory. Other options should be considered especially in the little finger such as arthrodesis/tenodesis.

Overall rupture of a flexor tendon repair is a serious complication. The incidence is low with long-established repair techniques and it remains to be seen if it can be further reduced by the newer trends focused on stronger repairs.

1.4 Infection after Flexor Tendon Repair

1.4.1 The Problem

This section will concentrate on the management of infection following flexor tendon repair or reconstruction, a challenging problem little discussed to date. As infection at this stage of treatment is often a consequence of earlier events it is appropriate to review relevant issues in relation to primary management of tendon injury and wound management in general.

With a confidence that antibiotics are available, primary repair of flexor tendon injuries has become the norm. However with the rise of antibiotic resistance, it is timely to reconsider the logic of the surgical principles of the preantibiotic era and how they can be applied to our new understanding of cellular mechanisms in infection. These management principles based on enormous experience from an era when infection was a condition managed almost entirely by surgeons have much to teach at this time when sepsis threatens to gain the upper hand.

Surgery in the era of Kanavel[15] was largely focused on drainage of collections using small incisions and dissection to reach collections by stretching tissue using blunt-nosed instruments, followed by the insertion of drains.

During World War I, Alexis Carrel irrigated wounds with Dakin's solution (dilute bleach). By the 1940s Frank Meleney,[16] Professor of Surgery and a renowned microbiology research scientist at Columbia University in New York, described delivery of antibacterial agents or antibiotics for flexor sheath irrigation via plastic tubing. Today we have a different concept of the benefit of catheter irrigations of flexor sheaths and other anatomical spaces with physiological solutions which are used to dilute not only bacteria and their virulence factors but also cytokines and other endogenous proinflammatory molecules. Meleney also described the benefit of tissue decompression in streptococcal sepsis realizing that the edema fluid from increased vascular permeability was important in spreading the infection. He advised making long incisions in streptococcal cellulitis to drain "dishwater pus."

Taking all of these techniques together the principles can be summarized as drainage, decompression, and dilution of exogenous toxins and endogenous inflammatory molecules.

Delivery of therapeutic antibacterial agents by catheter is currently largely out of fashion, antibiotics are administered intravenously.

Our routine practice employs many layers of protection against wound infection and when we encounter it in association with flexor tendon surgery it is often possible to identify factors that have predisposed to sepsis such as biological contamination, delay before treatment,[17] or patient comorbidities. Even with an apparently clean incised wound, sepsis remains an occasional cause of failure to restore tendon function. The risk of wound infection is higher when the wound is untidy with more injury to surrounding tissues or tissue loss. Controversies remain about the benefit of prophylactic antibiotics, as large reviews have not shown any benefit in either elective or trauma hand surgery operations lasting less than 2 hours. These studies have shown that the major factors predisposing to hand infection are longer operations, diabetes, and smoking. And these vulnerable patient groups, in particular, have not been protected from infection by prophylactic antibiotics. These studies remain controversial and may not be relevant to other patient populations or environmental or socioeconomic conditions. Antibiotics do have a clear role in treatment of infection and generally a prophylactic role in contaminated wounds such as bite injuries or major tissue trauma.

Infection after flexor tendon repair is not common in published outcomes of tendon repairs which tend to focus selectively on sharp divisions treated within a short time interval with exclusion of untidy or contaminated wounds. In the generality of hand surgery practice internationally, infection is more common than reported in literature. Infection after a tendon repair is likely to lead to rupture of the repair or the inflammatory response may aggravate adhesions and general stiffness.

1.4.2 Management

As in so many areas of surgery, prevention is better than cure and as the root of postoperative infection in tendon repair often arises from preoperative and operative factors, it is appropriate to identify these factors when a postoperative infection arises as this information may impact on treatment choices and prognosis.

Clinical Assessment of the Acute Tendon Injury

Flexor tendon injuries are almost invariably associated with open wounds and various degrees of contamination. In predicting the likelihood of infection, much can be revealed by the history. The cutting implement, potential contamination, delays, and previous management of the wound are all relevant.

Anatomy of the Wound

A conceptual image of the anatomy of the wound can be largely defined by the history and examination and confirmed on subsequent exploration. The flat edge of a blade drawn across a limb will allow the examiner to visualize which tendons are cut in their anatomical layers whereas the stabbing action of a knife or the irregularity of broken glass can produce deep injuries even when more superficial structures are spared. In relation to infection it is important to define whether the wound has been likely to injure tendons within a synovial sheath or in an extrasynovial zone. Tendons pass through defined connective tissue spaces as described by the ingenious cadaveric injection studies of Allen Kanavel.[15] Using a pump at low pressure Kanavel showed the extent of the flexor tendon synovial sheaths radiologically and by increasing pressure he noted that delicate membranes between compartments could rupture allowing infected exudate to travel proximally. If therefore a flexor tendon in Zone 2 is cut by a knife heavily contaminated by raw fish or raw meat, the tendon will retract proximally inoculating the synovial lining of its own sheath with whatever bacteria were on the knife and therefore contaminating the entire synovial sheath. Delay is likely to allow further spread proximally and any tissue space opened by the wound or by spread of infection will require copious irrigation.

Kanavel's understanding that pressure was important for spread and that spread was proximal was very insightful. An up-to-date appreciation of the mechanisms of spread is important. Some organisms produce virulence factors, e.g., enzymes such as streptokinase, hyaluronidase which facilitate enzymatic spread but a major spreading effect is due to increased vascular permeability building up edema pressure in the tissue which travels proximally in the direction of least resistance. In choosing incision lines for draining of collections, there needs to be

a concept not only of drainage but also an appreciation of the need for decompression.

Debridement

The next principle to discuss is debridement, a blanket term for removal of foreign material and possibly tissue, which is imprecise and can lead to removal of either too little or too much tissue. The amount of tissue excised requires considerable judgment taking into account the amount of actual or potential contamination but also the potential for unnecessarily creating a wound which can only be closed under tension or where wound closure is even prevented and some alternative skin cover is required. There is clear agreement that foreign material, dead tissue, and devascularized (dead) tissue should be removed. Ambiguous terms such as "devitalized" should be avoided and a decision should be made as to whether tissue is alive or dead at the time of assessment. There is no clear evidence-based support for the excision of inflamed tissue and all living tissues should be preserved unless heavily contaminated with harmful foreign material. Vascularized tissue should be preserved and it is a mistake to excise vascularized synovium or paratenon as stripping these layers will devitalize the tendon and render it vulnerable to both ischemia and infection. Moreover, exposed tendon will desiccate and necrose if skin excision prevents wound closure.

Tissue samples or wound swabs should be sent for culture and bearing in mind the likely organisms antibiotic treatment should be started, with the expectation that it will be continued postoperatively for 5 days. Cephalexin has a fairly broad spectrum and the addition of Metronidazole will be appropriate for anaerobic organisms.

Management of Infection in the Postoperative Period after Flexor Tendon Surgery

Infection arising in a wound after tendon surgery is a significant management challenge. Infection may be predisposed to by skin necrosis which in turn may be the outcome of hematoma formation or by poor design of skin flaps created in extending the original traumatic wound. The potential for skin devascularization should be appreciated by taking into account likely injuries to digital arteries and veins when planning incisions to extend wounds. No skin flap should be based on a side of the finger where there is a digital arterial injury, as advised by Bruner. His incision is popular but his advice is not always followed in extending an original transverse or oblique incision. He advised a short longitudinal extension of the traumatic wound before making any zigzag incision, thus avoiding flaps with acute angles at the tip which have a potential to necrose. Alternatively, longitudinal lateral neutral-line incisions may provide appropriate access. Untidy wounds with skin loss or ischemia may require elective skin flap cover at the outset to ensure sound wound healing.

It is likely that the patient who has had a flexor tendon repair will be managed as an outpatient in the community. The first indication of a postoperative infection developing is likely to be a rising pain level a few days after the primary surgery. Were antibiotics prescribed and has the patient been taking them? Are culture results available? What are the blood levels of inflammatory markers? Are there comorbid factors rendering the patient more liable to infection, such as diabetes or immunosuppression?

For any infection more than a mild cellulitis, it is better to pause the rehabilitation. On examination, the diagnosis of tenosynovitis is rarely in doubt if Kanavel's[15] four cardinal signs of infection are present: the digit held in slight flexion, fusiform swelling, tenderness on palpation, and acute pain on passive extension of the affected finger. There is likely to be some surrounding cellulitis and possibly lymphangitis. Although some surgeons prefer to commence with antibiotic therapy alone, and consider that this alone may resolve the infection in the mildest cases, it is a mistake to persist for too long with antibiot-ics alone in the presence of a significant pain level as infection will damage important and delicate structural layers around the tendon. By definition an infection in the postoperative period following flexor tendon surgery in Zones 1 or 2 is a septic tenosynovitis as the original surgery has widely opened the sheath and it should be treated by the same principles as for tenosynovitis in general. The problem of flexor sheath tenosynovitis was classified by Jacques Michon[18] in three stages. The most mild group he described as producing serous exudate ("Michon 1") and his cases were resolved by antibiotics and a single irrigation. The next severity, which we now call "Michon 2," had purulent collection and granulations, whereas the characteristic of group 3 was tendon necrosis and these patients progressed to radical excision or amputation. It is hard to classify cases until explored and currently all cases should be constantly irrigated until the tendon is clearly viable or necrotic (▶ Fig. 1.8).

Once infection is established, any collection of serosanguinous fluid or pus should be drained or it will facilitate tendon softening and suture pull-out. Tendons have a precarious blood supply through vincular arteries. And trauma generally disrupts the delicate vincula.

With a rising pain level following flexor tendon surgery, all sutures should be removed to allow inspection of the

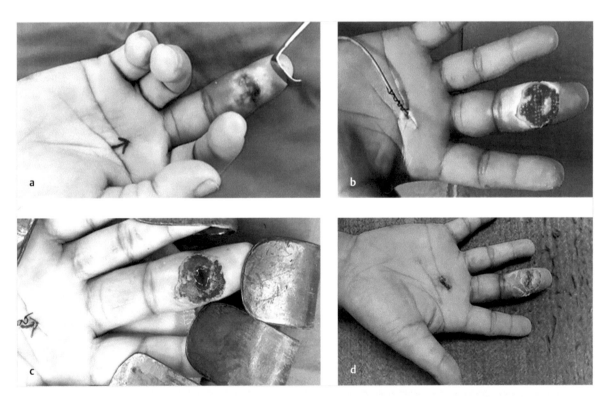

Fig. 1.8 Flexor sheath infection managed by catheter irrigation. (a) Late presentation of infected wound at distal digital crease with open flexor sheath injury and positive Kanavel's signs of tendon sheath infection. Intravenous antibiotics commenced.
(b) Catheter irrigation established using a pediatric feeding tube inserted proximal to A1 pulley and advanced to Zone 2.
(c) Irrigation fluid clear at 4 days.
(d) Wound healed at 20 days. No further surgery.

tendon. We advise catheter irrigation[19] of the sheath by making two small incisions, one over the A1 pulley and a second at the dip skin crease, or other traumatic wounds may be used. A pediatric feeding tube with additional side holes is then introduced into the synovial space. This is connected to a pump driver which delivers a continuous flow of 5 or 10 mL of normal saline per hour for 4 or 5 days. On occasions, the tendon is so swollen that there can be some difficulty in introducing the tube and a second tube can be introduced from distal to proximal either through an open wound or from the distal flexion crease. The logic of this therapy is not only drainage of pus or exudate but also dilution of endogenous cytokines and neutrophil-derived proinflammatory molecules and to a lesser extent dilution of the pathogens and their products. Much of the tissue damage is due to the vigorous inflammatory response and it is the inflammatory response of the host that is contributing to the tissue damage in addition to the pathogens. Having established the irrigation system, partial wound closure should be done to avoid exposure of the tendon repair area, leaving only enough open wound unsutured to allow egress of the irrigation fluid. The irrigation fluid is collected in a bulky cotton wool dressing changed daily. Frequently, the tubes can be removed in the ward or outpatient department without a need for further surgery to suture the wounds.

There are different situations where the tendon may be totally devascularized such as with FDP avulsion of the jersey injury type which frequently retracts to the palm after rupture of all vincula. Alternatively, a tendon originally perfused may suffer thrombosis of its vincula due to injury or thrombosis from infection. Whereas in a straightforward uninfected wound a devascularized tendon is capable of survival, presumably by revascularization, this will not happen in the presence of infection. The surgeon is best advised to accept this situation and excise the tendon as soon as an infected devascularized tendon is recognized. A silastic rod can be inserted in the sheath in the anticipation of returning months later to undertake a tendon graft. It is possible by catheter irrigation of the sheath for a few days and antibiotics for a few weeks to clear infection around a silicon rod.[5] Pressing on too long in the hopeless situation of a devascularized tendon will result in collagenolysis of the annular pulleys and all the structural tissues of the digit and no reconstruction will be feasible. With infection cleared around a tendon rod and all soft tissue inflammation cleared, the staged tendon reconstruction is as described for two-stage tendon grafting (see ▶ Fig. 1.7). Complex post infection soft tissue reconstructions are rarely done for a number of reasons. Many such patients have comorbidities and do not want to commit the time for surgery and rehabilitation. In addition, the infection is likely to promote widespread adhesions especially limiting the excursions of the intrinsic tendons and extensor apparatus. Some patients will opt for arthrodesis of interphalangeal joints especially if the little finger is involved. In the case of the thumb, despite its central role in the function of the hand, many patients choose arthrodesis of one or other joint, or even both as the intrinsic muscles provide some opposition function rather than the rehabilitation program required for extensive staged tendon reconstruction.

1.4.3 Rehabilitation

As with all hand surgery it is important to spend time assessing the individual requirements of the patient and their work and lifestyle and then provide a range of options with their respective advantages and disadvantages.

During the period of active infection it is important to continue a range of active mobilization unless the surgeon visualizes a high risk of rupture. Part of our protocol of catheter irrigation is to encourage active mobilization which helps with the circulation of irrigation fluid to all parts of the flexor sheath.

1.4.4 Tips and Tricks

Catheter irrigation has dramatically improved the outcomes from suppurative flexor tenosynovitis whether occurring after surgery or from other routes such as penetrating wounds or spread from pulp or paronychial infections.

1.5 Take-Home Message

All tendon repairs in adults develop *adhesions*. These can be minimized by contemporary repair and rehabilitation techniques, especially wide-awake surgery and judicious pulley trimming. *Pulley loss* does not necessarily equate to the need for pulley reconstruction. Most pulley loss can be managed nonoperatively. When reconstruction is necessary, usually the function of the A2 pulley is the most important to restore. Following *rupture* if tendon ends are sound and there is no pulley triggering, the tendon can be re-repaired. If tendon and sheath are inflamed or damaged, a two-stage reconstruction offers the best chance of recovery. For *infection*, early recognition, intravenous antibiotics, and continuous catheter irrigation with physiological solutions, together with continuing active mobilization throughout, offer the best chance of a successful outcome.

References

[1] Amadio PC, Hunter JM, Jaeger SH, Wehbe MA, Schneider LH. The effect of vincular injury on the results of flexor tendon surgery in zone 2. J Hand Surg Am. 1985; 10(5):626–632

[2] Tang JB. New developments are improving flexor tendon repair. Plast Reconstr Surg. 2018; 141(6):1427–1437

[3] Tang JB, Xie RG, Cao Y, Ke ZS, Xu Y. A2 pulley incision or one slip of the superficialis improves flexor tendon repairs. Clin Orthop Relat Res. 2007; 456(456):121–127

[4] Tang JB. Wide-awake primary flexor tendon repair, tenolysis, and tendon transfer. Clin Orthop Surg. 2015; 7(3):275–281

[5] Breton A, Jager T, Dap F, Dautel G. Effectiveness of flexor tenolysis in zone II: a retrospective series of 40 patients at 3 months postoperatively. Chir Main. 2015; 34(3):126–133

[6] Lin GT, Amadio PC, An KN, Cooney WP. Functional anatomy of the human digital flexor pulley system. J Hand Surg Am. 1989; 14 (6):949–956

[7] Schöffl VR, Schöffl I. Injuries to the finger flexor pulley system in rock climbers: current concepts. J Hand Surg Am. 2006; 31(4):647–654

[8] Lin GT, Amadio PC, An KN, Cooney WP, Chao EY. Biomechanical analysis of finger flexor pulley reconstruction. J Hand Surg [Br]. 1989; 14 (3):278–282

[9] Wong JK, Cerovac S, Ferguson MW, McGrouther DA. The cellular effect of a single interrupted suture on tendon. J Hand Surg [Br]. 2006; 31(4):358–367

[10] Harris SB, Harris D, Foster AJ, Elliot D. The aetiology of acute rupture of flexor tendon repairs in zones 1 and 2 of the fingers during early mobilization. J Hand Surg [Br]. 1999; 24(3):275–280

[11] Tang JB. Recent evolutions in flexor tendon repairs and rehabilitation. J Hand Surg Eur Vol. 2018; 43(5):469–473

[12] Savage R. In vitro studies of a new method of flexor tendon repair. J Hand Surg [Br]. 1985; 10(2):135–141

[13] Chang MK, Lim ZY, Wong YR, Tay SC. A review of cyclic testing protocols for flexor tendon repairs. Clin Biomech (Bristol, Avon). 2019; 62:42–49

[14] Tang JB. Release of the A4 pulley to facilitate zone II flexor tendon repair. J Hand Surg Am. 2014; 39(11):2300–2307

[15] Kanavel AB. Infections of the hand; a guide to the surgical treatment of acute and chronic suppurative processes in the fingers, hand, and forearm. 5th ed. Philadelphia and New York: Lea & Febiger; 1925

[16] Meleney FL. Clinical aspects and treatment of surgical infections. Philadelphia: W. B. Saunders Co.; 1949

[17] Reito A, Manninen M, Karjalainen T. The effect of delay to surgery on major complications after primary flexor tendon repair. J Hand Surg Asian Pac Vol. 2019; 24(2):161–168

[18] Michon J. Phlegmon of the tendon sheaths. Ann Chir. 1974; 28 (4):277–280

[19] Fujita M, Iwamoto T, Suzuki T, et al. Continuous catheter irrigation for the treatment of purulent tenosynovitis during two-stage flexor tendon reconstruction. J Hand Microsurg. 2019; 11(3):170–174

2 Management of Complications of Extensor Tendon Surgery

David Elliot and Thomas Giesen

Abstract

The complications following primary management of extensor injuries can be considered generally as (1) those relating to the anatomy and function of the tendons themselves, (2) their ability to glide within their immediate surrounds after trauma, and (3) the fact that the end result of treatment is rarely determined simply by the state of the extensor tendon as, taken in the wider perspective, dorsal injuries are frequently complex. Our basis of primary management of extensor tendon injuries, as with flexor tendon injuries, is early repair and early mobilization, with appropriate suture techniques and rehabilitation to protect the repairs. By virtue of anatomical and physiological variation along their length, and unlike the flexors, a single system of primary surgery and rehabilitation cannot be applied to extensor tendon injuries. Primary management must be tailored to the particular part of the extensor system injured, and each part of the extensor system from the proximal forearm to the tip of the digits is liable to different complications. Therefore, it is more practical to consider the likely complications which may ensue in each of Verdan's divisions of the extensor system separately (▶ Fig. 2.1).[1,2,3] Prophylaxis by appropriate primary management is often more effective than secondary treatment of an established complication, so this also needs to be considered.

Keywords: extensor tendon, extensor tendon repair, extensor tendon reconstruction, extensor tendon rehabilitation, extensor tendon secondary surgery, complications of extensor tendon repair

2.1 Introduction

When the hand evolved to become entirely an instrument of prehension, the extensor system proximal to the metacarpophalangeal (MCP) joints became simply a means of opening the hand sufficiently for the now dominant flexor system to start the next grasping activity, so the anatomy of this part of the extensor system is simple. At the same time, the extensor system in the finger was evolving very differently to become the mechanism controlling integration of the movements of the three joints of each finger. This required a complicated anatomy which included complex interaction of musculotendinous units both within the hand and more proximally, working through thin distal tendons compatible with the need for the fingers to remain slim. Two consequences arise from this. The first is that the extensor tendons are flimsy in the fingers so difficult to suture then mobilize early, and the second that success in regaining function is a difficult balance between rupture and adhesion, with the latter being the more common complication. The second problem arises from the mechanical complexity of the tendon

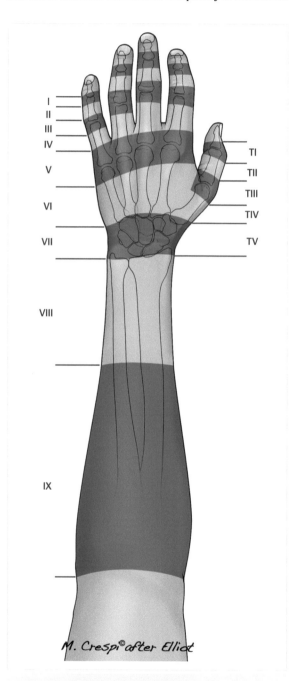

Fig. 2.1 Doyle's modification of the Verdan extensor tendon classification in which Zone 8 has been split into Zone 8, the tendons proximal to the wrist and Zone 9, the muscles proximally of all (Doyle, 1993).

anatomy in the finger. This becomes a headache if divided and not repaired immediately. When injured hands come to hand surgeons after considerable delay, the main complications of extensor tendon surgery requiring treatment are the set-piece deformities of the chronically injured extensor system, viz., mallet, boutonnière, and swan-neck fingers. These constituted a long-standing intellectual war for many of the greatest hand surgeons of the last century.

Unlike the flexors, the extensor system has no synovial tunnels but relies on the layers of interstitial connective tissue between the tendon and the skin and between the tendon and the bone to allow movement (▶ Fig. 2.2). A major problem after trauma or operations, as the body does not differentiate between the two, is the manner in which these layers accumulate edema in response to the trauma, with the sticky fibrin in the edema, described most aptly by Watson Jones as "physiological glue," preventing the extensor tendons from gliding. These adhesions and their effect on tendon gliding are, for today's hand surgeon, the commonest long-term disability resulting from trauma to, not only the extensor system, but all injuries to the hand, as the associated fibrin-edema migrates to the dorsum of the hand from whatever part is injured. Ninety percent of fluid normally returns from the tissues in the veins and 10% through the lymphatics. Unfortunately, large plasma proteins cannot get into the veins in an inflammatory site and they block the lymphatics, so the system of drainage is less efficient and the accumulation of fibrin can easily become pathological in the parts of the body which move continually. With adequate rehabilitation, the fluid component is removed through the lymphatics, but leaves a coating of fibrin in the interstitial layers around the extensor tendons. Preventing this from tethering the tendons to stop them

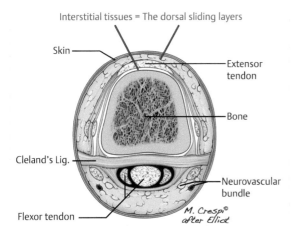

Interstitial tissues = The dorsal sliding layers

Skin

Extensor tendon

Bone

Cleland's Lig.

Neurovascular bundle

Flexor tendon

M. Crespi©
after Elliot

Fig. 2.2 Unlike the flexors, the extensor system has no synovial tunnels but relies on the layers of interstitial connective tissue between the tendon and the skin and between the tendon and the bone to allow movement.

gliding is aggravated by the fact that the distances being moved by the tendons to achieve movement of the joints are very small.[4] Much therapy thought and time is spent trying to keep extensors moving and, where the primary injury has been to the extensors, balancing this need against the need to protect tendon repairs from snapping. Later, over 6 to 12 months, this fibrin will form scar which is not amenable to mobilization by therapy but requires surgery (▶ Fig. 2.3a), followed once more by therapy to prevent the further fibrin-edema created by the secondary surgery from tethering the tendons again. The degree to which this process occurs varies with the degree of injury, between individuals and, possibly, between races, although all races will include individuals who exhibit florid fibrin-edema tethering of the extensor tendons. The problem of extensor tendon tethering is associated with tightening of the dorsal capsules and lateral ligaments of the finger joints to a variable degree, although this is not always present. Conversely, in some cases, the tendon tethering is minimal and the joint capsule changes predominate. As the joint problems are inseparable from that of the extensor tendons, etiologically, diagnostically, and in terms of hand therapy and surgical treatment, both can be considered as one entity.

The clinical effects of this are well recognized in severe cases, in whom the result is loss of both digital flexion and extension. However, it is mostly the loss of flexion of the fingers which impairs hand function. While lesser degrees of extensor tethering usually have little effect on the ability of the extensor tendon to straighten the fingers sufficiently, even slight tethering will impede distal gliding of the tendons enough to prevent adequate flexion of the fingers and affect hand function significantly. This manifests as a loss of full flexion of the fingers, with loss of ability to grip narrow objects, and pain on the dorsum of the fingers or hand at the sites of tethering of the extensor tendons which prevents strong or prolonged gripping and reduces grip strength.[5] This can be replicated by forced passive flexion of the fingers, when the patient will locate the pain to the site of tethering as distal movement of the tendon pulls on pain fibers in both the periosteum below and the subcutaneous fat superficially to which the tendon is tethering. If the radial digits are involved, clumsiness of pinch activity is experienced because of slowing of rapid small movements of these digits.

Where tethering of the extensor tendons cannot be reversed by therapy, whether only preventing pain-free and full, or near-full, flexion of the digits or complete arrest of digital movement in both directions, release of the scarred areas of the tendon(s) by "tenolysis" is necessary to restore adequate function. This must be followed by intensive, and often prolonged, therapy to keep the freed tendons moving as this surgery will stimulate further formation of fibrin-edema leading to further scar formation and the tendons sticking again. The timing of this surgery, whatever the Verdan zone of the tethering,

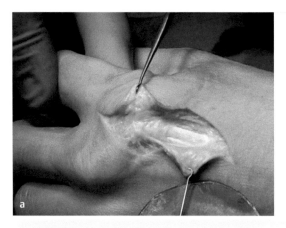
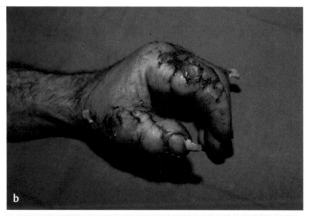

Fig. 2.3 **(a)** Scar tethering of a simple repair of the extensor tendons of the index finger in Zone 5 seen at tenolysis, performed for loss of index finger flexion and difficulty in pinching because of slowness of movement of this finger. **(b)** A severe injury of the left hand following trapping in a spinning industrial machine. The index finger suffered severe comminution of the proximal phalanx and shredding of the extensor tendon, although the tendon was intact longitudinally. This early postoperative view shows the fingers in maximum flexion with considerable fibrin-edema swelling. The loss of index finger flexion is a compound of the skeletal injury and fibrin tethering of the extensor tendon.

is important. If carried out too early after injury and/or previous surgery, the limb will still be in the active healing state and further (tenolysis) surgery can add to this with what seems to be an accentuated fibrin-edema response, resulting in the freed tendons tethering again rapidly despite all therapy efforts. While textbooks often advise waiting 3 or 4 months after previous injury/surgery before carrying out a tenolysis, many hands will still be "healing" from the previous insult at this time and arranging tenolysis on such a timed basis is unwise. Rather, the area of injury or surgery is inspected regularly in clinic until the inflammation of the overlying skin has disappeared completely, with the skin being supple and, in Caucasians, no longer red. While patients, keen to have hand function restored, will push for early tenolysis, this must be resisted: the author frequently tells these patients that if, personally, given the option of surgery at 3, 6, or 12 months after injury, the author would choose 12 months as the time most likely to give the best result as most hands will be quiescent in respect of the previous inflammatory response by this time. However, the timing of surgery should be determined by the state of the hand, not the calendar!

Taken in a wider perspective, 60% of extensor injuries have associated skeletal or skin injuries of significance and the end result of management is rarely determined simply by the state of the extensor tendon. At its worst, this may include a combination of extensor tendons which are shredded, or completely absent, overlying smashed, or absent, parts of the skeleton, with no overlying skin cover. In Europe, where most injured hands are seen within hours or days and much of the secondary work is secondary to our primary treatment and not the result of neglect of the primary injury, as it once was, these are now our "bread and butter." The primary surgical management of

these complex dorsal injuries, with any combination of skeletal, tendon, and skin damages, aims to create a stable skeleton with good skin cover and an intact extensor tendon to allow movement of the repaired tendon as early as possible. Over and above the problems caused by failures of primary management of the skeleton and skin, which are beyond the scope of this chapter, these complex injuries all accentuate the problem of fibrin-edema and tethering of the extensor tendon (▶ Fig. 2.3b). So, our concern today is more often tethered tendons, albeit sometimes with associated skin, skeletal, and nerve problems, than the boutonniere, swan-neck, and mallet deformities which fascinated earlier hand surgeons.

2.2 Complications after Extensor Tendon Lesion Zone 1 and Zone 2

Zone 1 is that part of the extensor of the finger overlying the distal interphalangeal (DIP) joint and Zone 2 that part over the middle phalanx. Our frequent failures and poor results in treating the mallet finger, and the varied primary treatments of this injury, highlight the difficulties of achieving healing of the paper-thin tendon at all, then achieving enough gliding of the tendon to achieve flexion, as well as extension, of the DIP joint. Because of the flimsy nature of the tendon, primary management here favors restoration of tendon union and full extension by enforced and lengthy immobility, by splinting or by surgical repair, after coapting the tendon ends. The long period of external splinting necessary to achieve healing is a major inconvenience to the patient, so compliance is poor. Other than failure to achieve tendon union, necessitating repeat of one or other method of achieving this, the common complications of treatment are those of fail-

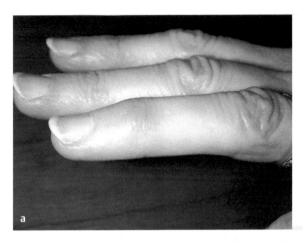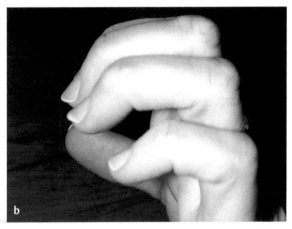

Fig. 2.4 Closed mallet injury seen several months after release from splinting. **(a)** As a consequence of healing with slight lengthening, there is the almost inevitable slight extensor lag typical for this injury but requiring no further treatment in this respect. **(b)** The joint has a loss of full flexion as a result of tethering of the extensor tendon to the middle phalanx as a consequence of 8 weeks of immobilization. This may improve with therapy. It is of note that other fingers are affected by the extensor tethering and also have loss of full distal interphalangeal (DIP) flexion.

ure to achieve full DIP extension, occasionally with pain, and tendon tethering with loss of DIP joint flexion (▶ Fig. 2.4). Rupture of the repair, or, more commonly, lengthening of the extensor tendon, by interposition of a small length of scar or bone at the site of original division, and incomplete extension may often require no treatment but may require resuture to shorten the tendon or, particularly where pain is a feature, or repeated attempts to achieve the desired degree of extension have failed, fusion of the DIP joint. The hidden consideration in the mallet injury is the flexion function of the DIP. Although this joint only contributes 15% of finger flexion when power gripping, we need a minimum of 30 to 40 degrees of motion of this joint, with the ability to move it back and forth quite rapidly, to carry out fine pinching and span gripping activities with the digital tips. After 6 or 8 weeks of splinting, it may take many weeks, with therapy help, to free a tethered extensor tendon and regain flexion. The primary option of not repairing the tendon and relying on automatic recoil of the joint to a position of a slight residual extensor lag may avoid the need for secondary tenolysis of a tendon stuck firmly to the middle phalanx and tenodesing the DIP in full extension. This, particularly, in complex situations such as replantation or severe middle phalangeal fractures, in which the degree of fibrin-edema production is greater relative to the small space between skeleton and skin at this level of the finger. Prophylaxis by calculated neglect in such cases is more likely to achieve long-term DIP flexion than secondary surgery. Tenolysis of tethered tendons at this level is liable to fail as the surgery heals with further fibrin-edema in the confined interstitial spaces around the tendon. Fowler's extensor tenotomy over the middle third of the middle phalanx, with release of the dorsal and lateral ligaments of the DIP joint, may regain flexion.[6] Because of

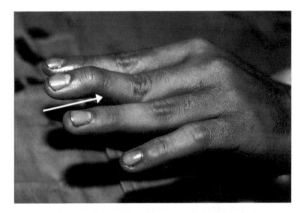

Fig. 2.5 The left hand of a patient from the Indian subcontinent showing normal racial swan-necking of the index and ring fingers which is accentuated in the middle finger following a mallet injury of this finger.

secondary ligament changes of the joint, a mallet rarely occurs. Rather, the problem is trying to get the DIP to flex even after extensive releasing surgery, sometimes followed by K-wiring the DIP in flexion for 4 to 6 weeks, or even placing a skin graft between the cut tendon ends.

The lengthening of the distal extensor after a mallet deformity throws a greater extension force onto the central slip and may cause pathological swan-necking (▶ Fig. 2.5). While correction of the mallet may correct the swan-necking, it sometimes does not, particularly in an individual in whom this problem is chronic and in those with congenital swan-necking. Elongation of the central slip by central slip tenotomy[6] alone, or carried out at the same time as distal tendon shortening and repair, or reconstruction of Landsmeer's spiral oblique retinacular ligament (SORL)[7,8] are alternative and useful approaches to this problem.

2.3 Complications after Extensor Tendon Lesion Zone 3 and Zone 4

Zone 3 is that part of the extensor of the finger overlying the proximal interphalangeal (PIP) joint and Zone 4 that part over the proximal phalanx. In these zones, the tendons are more substantial and rupture of primary repairs during early mobilization is less likely. Despite the emphasis on early movement, the main, and recurring, problem, as elsewhere in the extensor system, is scar tethering to the proximal phalanx and to the dorsum of the PIP, often associated with shortening of the dorsal capsule and collateral ligaments of the PIP, preventing the extensor gliding distally, to allow PIP and DIP flexion, when the flexors are activated. The principle of treatment, as in the other zones, is not the sudden forced movements used frequently by surgeons, whether done in clinic or as a manipulation under anesthetic (MUA). Rather, the gentle, repeated, small discomforts of forced passive flexion exercises by skilled therapists and the (instructed) patients themselves, regularly and frequently pushing these fingers just beyond the limit of flexion imposed by the setting edema/fibrin glue. Slow traction, either by repeatedly changed static splints or dynamic splints, is also useful. Failures of therapy need surgical release then further therapy to prevent further fibrin tethering: surgery alone will fail.

In Zone 3, primary management can be complicated by the tendon anatomy: the tendon is now splitting into a central slip and two lateral bands with the latter capable of moving away from the central slip on finger flexion. While division of one lateral band will not affect DIP extension, division of both requires repair and guarded postoperative mobilization, walking the tightrope between adhesion and rupture, to achieve DIP movement. Immediate central slip reconstruction is simple, and made simpler by the introduction of bone tags. Where there is delay in presentation, the lateral bands may extend the PIP joint for a short time. However, the tear then extends proximally between the central slip and the lateral bands and the lateral bands descend laterally off

the extensor surface of joint, such that they can no longer extend the joint (▶ Fig. 2.6). The end point for a very delayed presentation of a PIP joint without a central slip is what is called a "Boutonnière" deformity, with the head of the proximal phalanx pushing through between the lateral bands, now lying down the sides of the joint, like a button pushing through the buttonhole of a shirt. In the early stages, this injury may respond to extension splinting. However, as time passes, the lateral bands become fixed in their new position and splinting cannot reverse this. A secondary volar plate tightening may also develop. As the lateral bands move volarly, they tighten and pull the DIP into extension. With time, the ligament system of the DIP contracts to set this joint in a hyperextended position which is usually very difficult to correct. Few trauma patients present at this late stage. Many have a relatively mild PIP loss of extension and, sometimes, no DIP hyperextension. The loss of PIP extension usually causes little functional problem until is greater than 40 to 45 degrees, when moving the hand forward to grasp objects pushes the flexed finger(s) into the palm. Reconstruction of the central slip is then necessary. If the PIP joint has a limited range of motion, particularly if the DIP joint has no flexion, a compromise of half, not complete, correction of the PIP extensor deficit is carried out. If one tightens the extensor too much, the PIP joint will have limited flexion and the finger, with no DIP flexion either, cannot play a part in grasping (▶ Fig. 2.7). By contrast, loss of PIP full extension can often be compensated by either normal MCP hyperextension or wrist extension or a combination of both. Where there is a secondary volar plate contracture, this may require splinting, or, more occasionally, surgical release, to allow sufficient PIP extension. A staged approach, releasing the volar plate first surgically, then reconstructing the extensor system at a later operation is advised as combining the two operations usually creates such a swollen finger that loss of movement from extensor tethering occurs. There are almost as many ways of actually reconstructing the central slip after delayed presentation with an established "Boutonnière" deformity as there were famous hand surgeons in the 1950 to

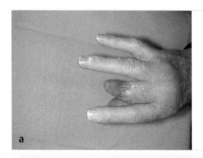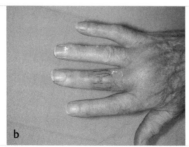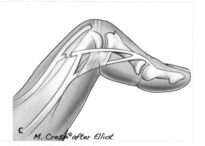

Fig. 2.6 Closed rupture of the central slip with early presentation. **(a)** Although the finger rests in a position of full proximal interphalangeal (PIP) flexion, **(b)** the PIP joint will remain extended once lifted into the extended position passively as the lateral bands can still ride onto the dorsum of the joint. **(c)** Diagram showing how, with time, the tear extends proximally between the central slip and the lateral bands and the lateral bands descend laterally off the extensor surface of joint, such that they can no longer extend the joint. The head of the proximal phalanx pushes through between the lateral bands to create the so-called "Boutonnière" or "Button-Hole" deformity.

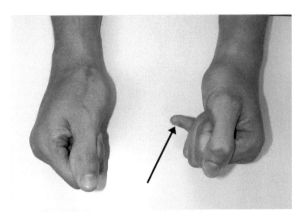

Fig. 2.7 A left hand with a long-established Boutonniere deformity of the little finger is shown in full flexion before central slip reconstruction. The distal interphalangeal (DIP) joint is hyperextended and it is unlikely that extensor tenotomy over the middle phalanx will achieve flexion of this joint. If the central slip reconstruction is set to fully extend the proximal interphalangeal (PIP) joint, limited PIP flexion is likely. With no DIP flexion either, the finger cannot then play a part in grasping. Therefore, a compromise of half, not complete, correction of the PIP extensor deficit is carried out.

1980 era. Particularly useful in cases with DIP hyperextension and very little DIP movement is making a distal (Fowler) tenotomy over the middle phalanx and rolling the entire lateral bands centrally to make a new central slip, which is then attached to the base of the middle phalanx.[9] If the DIP is working as a flexing joint, a split palmaris tendon graft attached to the base of the middle phalanx then woven into the proximal tendon as far back as the dorsum of the hand is arguably the most useful technique of central slip reconstruction. Both these techniques allow enthusiastic early active mobilization. Where the MCP joint is particularly mobile, temporary K-wire fixation of this joint in slight flexion, or a volar tethering procedure, may be necessary to avoid hyperextension of the MCP at the expense of restoring PIP extension.

Swan-necking of the PIP joint is rarely an extensor problem. A few are due to complete rupture of the volar plate of the PIP usually in teenagers. These sometimes present acutely, or as a chronic problem: in both it may be possible to suture the volar plate. If this is attenuated, the flexor digitorum superficialis (FDS) tendon, or half of it, can be divided about a centimeter and a half from its attachment to the middle phalanx, thinned longitudinally and sutured to the lateral part of the tendon sheath to hold the PIP in about 20 to 30 degrees of flexion. The joint is then splinted to avoid full extension for 4 weeks. The management of swan-necking secondary to a mallet deformity was discussed earlier. The principle of treatment of most other pathological swan-necking is the same as that used by horsemen to prevent a horse throwing its head back by placing a strap, known as a Martingale, from its chest to its bridle. In young and strong

hands, a distally based slip of FDS looped around the distal third of the A2 pulley and sutured back to itself is the strongest of these restraints. An alternative for use in older and more compliant patients, particularly if the lateral bands are sticking dorsally, is to release the lateral bands then move the ulnar lateral band volar to the axis of rotation of the PIP to achieve the Martingale effect.[7,10,11]

2.4 Complications after Extensor Tendon Lesion Zone 5 and Zone 6

Zone 5 is that part of the extensor of the finger overlying the MCP joint and Zone 6 that part over the dorsum of the hand. The tendons are now more substantial and many can be repaired with the techniques of suturing we use on the flexors. Early mobilization is now accepted as having better results than immobilization.[12] So, rupture of primary repairs is less of a problem. Where ruptures do occur and when segments of tendon are missing, tendon transfers become available in these zones as alternatives to tendon grafting. Unlike primary repairs, these tendon grafts and transfers are connected using Pulvertaft weaves, so can be moved, albeit still with splinting, with more confidence from very early after surgery. Argument continues over whether grafting should be carried out in a single or two stages. Use of vascularized replacement of these tendons with their surrounding layer of sliding tissue has largely disappeared. It has been recognized for many years that adequate hand function can be achieved without secondary extensor reconstruction after traumatic loss at this level,[13] the MCPs recoiling to about 30 degrees short of the neutral position when the flexors are relaxed, which is all of the extension needed to allow the fingers to start a further grasp maneuver.

2.4.1 Tethering of the Tendons: Tenolysis

Of the secondary problems we face in these zones, the overwhelming problem is tendon tethering with loss of flexion. All of these injuries heal too well and it could be argued that we overprotect our extensor tendon repairs and allow them to be "welded" to their surrounds by fibrin then scar. If therapy fails to release any tendon tethering, surgical tenolysis, with arthrolysis, viz. MCP dorsal capsulotomies and lateral ligament releases, if necessary, then early and persistent therapy is necessary. After releasing the tendons proximal to, and over the MCP joint(s), the need for arthrolysis of the MCP(s) becomes obvious by the inability of the joints to move into full flexion on passively flexing the fingers. One is sometimes faced with a need for tenolysis in all four rays, whether of Zones 3/4 or 5/6 only or anywhere from the forearm to the DIP joint. There is a balance between achieving free tendon movement on as many parts of the hand and fingers as possible at a single operation and (i) the increasing amount of fibrin-edema caused by this operation and subsequent tendency to tether again and (ii) the increasing level of pain as the dissection widens, bearing in mind that the patient often has this tendon problem because of a low pain threshold and/or reluctance to mobilize after a primary operation. Tourniquet time constraints may also limit the dissection. The questions arise as to (i) whether to do all four fingers at one operation or release only one or two at a time, (ii) and whether to free all three joints of each finger at one operation or concentrate on the MCPs first and the interphalangeal (IP) joints at a later operation. In recent cases, the author has tended to split the problem into proximal (forearm and hand) and distal (fingers beyond the MCPs) operating proximally first, as this is likely to achieve maximum gain. Where multiple fingers are involved, freeing only two fingers at a time may be necessary. In cases of very extensive extensor tendon scarring, usually after crush injuries, burns and, sometimes, after repeated surgery, it may be of more benefit to abandon tenolysis and divide the tendons proximal to the MCPs, as described above. Even if complete freeing of the tendons is possible in such cases, the degree of fibrin-edema reaction to the tenolysis surgery is likely to be such that maintaining tendon mobility in the long term is unlikely.

2.4.2 Tethering of the Nerves

At this level, tendon tethering may have an additional complicating factor of nerve pain from cut, or tethered, nerves. It is most common after crush injuries, infections in trauma wounds and, sometimes, after repeated surgery: essentially in any situation where the fibrin-edema reaction is considerable, or summates, and scarring not only tethers the tendons but also tethers the fine branches of the superficial radial or the dorsal branch of the ulnar nerve, or both. The clue to diagnosis is that the pain of trying to flex the joints distal to the scarring is much greater than normal and there is significant pain on Tinel testing the skin over the tethered tendons and nerves. Tenolysis alone is likely to fail as postoperative mobilization is impossible for the patient as it remains too painful. Relocation of the involved nerves is necessary before tenolysis.[14,15] A combined operation is impossible as the nerve relocation needs rest postoperatively, while the tenolysis requires early mobilization. Many of the other complications in these zones are those of failures of primary treatment of skeletal and skin problems as many of these injuries arise from significant trauma to the body of the hand (▶ Fig. 2.8).

2.4.3 Punch Injury: Risk of Infection

Two particular acute problems arise in Zone 5 which may lead to secondary complications. The first is the punch

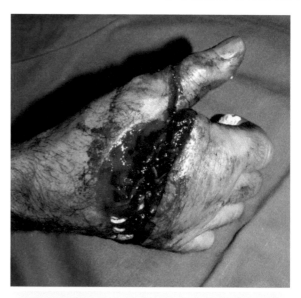

Fig. 2.8 Typical industrial injury in Zone 6 of the hand resulting from a heavy roller crush injury in a fish processing plant. All four metacarpals have sustained comminuted shaft fractures. All of the extensor tendons are shredded and most are also divided. The skin has a bursting laceration with division of the draining veins of a distally based flap, which is surviving on the Quaba perforating arteries feeding through from the palmar vessels. The hand is already swelling rapidly at this early stage and can be expected to swell further during the postoperative period. Even with the best of primary management, the overwhelming problem is likely to be tendon tethering with loss of flexion.

injury with infection driven into the metacarpal head by the teeth. As one repairs the tendon with the hand flat on the operating table and the tendon injury lies on the dorsum of the MCP, while the tooth penetrated the distal surface of the metacarpal head, the joint damage may be missed unless the entire surface of the metacarpal head is inspected before repair of the joint capsule and extensor tendon. As a result, osteomyelitis of the metacarpal may occur. In this situation, prophylaxis is more effective than secondary treatment. Attempts to pull the small fragments back in line from distally in the joint usually fail. A solution to the two problems is to cut a window in the dorsum of the metacarpal, push the broken surface out to its correct position and pack the medulla of the metacarpal with an antiseptic wick, which can be removed 2 to 3 days after surgery.

2.4.4 Sagittal Band Lesion

The second problem of Zone 5 is the so-called "fly flicking injury," rarely caused by flicking a fly and missing, which defunctions the normal sagittal band activity of holding the extensor on top of the MCP when this joint flexes. Sudden arrest of the extending joint by the finger catching on a hard object stops the tight extensor moving proximally, causing the sagittal bands, mostly on the radial side, to tear. This takes tension off the tendon by allowing it to fall off the dorsum of the joint into the (ulnar) gutter. The finger cannot then be lifted actively from the flexed position. If presenting late, which is the norm, primary repair is no longer possible. The simplest effective radial sagittal band reconstruction is to create a distally based strip of tendon by separating the radial third of the extensor tendon of the involved ray from the remainder of the tendon from the level of the dorsum of the wrist to the MCP, and passing this around the radial collateral ligament of the MCP to suture it back to itself.[16]

2.5 Complications after Extensor Tendon Lesion Zone 7–Zone 9

Zone 7 is that part of the extensors of the fingers under the extensor retinaculum, Zone 8 includes the extensor tendons within the dorsal compartment of the forearm and Zone 9 the actual extensor muscles further proximally. The long finger extensor tendons of Zones 7 and 8 are substantial and repair with the techniques of flexor surgery then early mobilization can be used. In respect of these tendons, many of the same problems occur in Zones 7, 8, and 9 as in Zones 5 and 6, with tendon adherence being the main secondary problem and treatment as described above. Whether repaired in isolation, or in conjunction with the digital extensors, postoperative management of the wrist tendons is by fixed wrist splinting in the 20 to 30 degrees of extension position for 4 weeks. Secondary rupture of tendons at this level is rare.

2.5.1 Zone 7

Zone 7 has the additional problem of the extensor retinaculum. Without the retinaculum pulley, bowstringing of the extensor tendons occurs on wrist extension, except in patients with little, or no, wrist movement. Fortunately, the retinaculum is several centimeters in depth and it is usually possible to preserve 1 cm of one part of the retinaculum while excising the remainder to allow tendon repairs to run through their full range of motion without catching on it. Which centimeter one needs to preserve needs to be considered as one enters the wrist and not after the repairs are completed. When bowstringing does occur, the retinaculum can usually be reconstructed using part of the remainder of the retinaculum. If need be, strips of any tendon can be used to reconstruct the extensor retinaculum (▶ Fig. 2.9).

2.5.2 Zone 9

Zone 9 has three specific problems. The first is the poor suture holding power of muscle. It is important to look for the extensions of the tendons back into the substance of the muscles as suture of these may give adequate

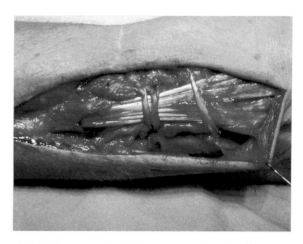

Fig. 2.9 Reconstruction of the extensor retinaculum with palmaris longus tendon to correct extensor bowstringing after previous exploration of a wrist laceration with complete division of the retinaculum.

strength to allow early mobilization, albeit more carefully, whereas muscle-to-muscle suture probably will not and requires delay of mobilization for 4 weeks (▶ Fig. 2.10). The second problem is the difficulty identifying individual muscles, then repairing them individually: this problem, and the tendency of the muscles to heal into one mass, often makes the result of primary suture poor and the fused muscle mass is not amenable to secondary separation by tenolysis. The third problem is that deeper cuts may divide the small terminal branches of the posterior interosseous nerve, so muscle repairs fail to result in muscle function. While it is sometimes possible to find these little nerves at primary operation, they are often too badly damaged to repair, or the distal ends simply cannot be found in the "mess" of cut muscles. They are also often impossible to find in the scar tissue at secondary surgery. When this situation arises, early posterior interosseous nerve palsy tendon transfers are necessary. Occasionally, a Zone 9 injury will divide the three branches of the posterior cutaneous nerve of the forearm, giving rise to three painful end-neuromas. These can be treated by nerve relocation.[17]

2.6 Complication of the Thumb Extensor Tendons

Secondary surgery of the thumb extensor tendons is largely needed to reconstitute the extensor pollicis longus (EPL) tendon and, as elsewhere, tendon tethering is the common problem. While the abductor pollicis longus (APL) and extensor pollicis brevis (EPB) tendons should be repaired or reconstructed whenever possible as their absence does reduce full thumb extension slightly; integrity of these tendons is not vital if all the other musculotendinous units of the thumb are intact

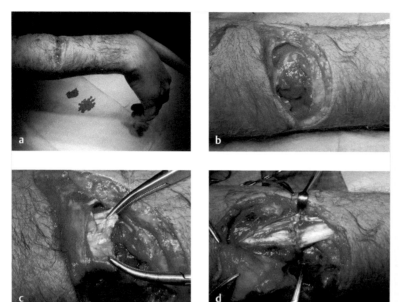

Fig. 2.10 (a) Lacerating injury at the level of Verdan's Zone 9. **(b)** Muscle division but no obvious tendon showing in the wound proximally. **(c)** Retracted proximal tendon pulled out from the muscle. **(d)** Strong tendon-to-tendon repair, allowing early active mobilization.

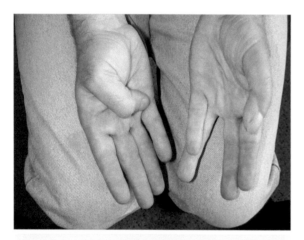

Fig. 2.11 A late postoperative view of a crush injury of the left thumb with fracture of the distal phalanx treated by K-wire fixation across the distal interphalangeal (DIP) joint for 6 weeks. Tethering of the extensor tendon to the proximal phalanx now prevents full flexion of the IP joint and pain over the proximal phalanx, not the IP joint, on prolonged or strong IP flexion to pinch.

ture internal fixation crosses the IP joint (▶ Fig. 2.11) and when Zone 1 repairs are treated like mallet injuries of the finger. The EPL tendon distally, as elsewhere, is a thick structure, capable of taking sutures of the kind used in flexor tendon repair and does not need the postoperative protective splinting or K-wiring necessary after repairing the distal extensors in Zones 1 and 2 in the fingers. Prophylaxis is, again, more successful than secondary treatment as secondary tenolysis rarely restores the essential IP joint function; tethering usually occurs again over ensuing months even with lengthy postoperative therapy. Where the EPL tendon has ruptured following trauma at the wrist level, probably as a result of disruption of the blood supply of the tendon, or presentation after division is late, transfer of the extensor indicis proprius muscle to the distal EPL tendon is more effective and involves less scarring of the forearm than grafting the gap in the tendon.

2.7 Take-Home Message

In 1944, Bunnell wrote "My first attempts at repair of tendons in the fingers resulted in immediate success, but as succeeding days went by motion became less and less, until at the end of a few weeks it was nil."[19] Although he included both the flexor and extensor tendons in this statement, it is fair to say that the common perception that the skill needed to treat flexor tendon injuries is not necessary for the extensor apparatus is false. As can be concluded from this chapter, the extensor system of the hand creates as many difficult problems in hand trauma practice as any other part of the specialty, except possibly the neuralgia of divided and tethered nerves.

and functional.[18] While active loss of thumb extension is rarely sufficient to cause a functional problem, the tethering may cause disability, either because of an absolute loss of flexion of the interphalangeal joint with pain on the dorsum of the thumb at the site of tendon tethering on maximum flexion or because of a loss of the rapid flexion-extension activity of the thumb IP joint essential to fine pinch function or a combination of both.[12] This is particularly likely if phalangeal frac-

References

[1] Doyle JR. Extensor tendons—acute injuries. In: Green DP, Hotchkiss RN, Pederson WC, eds. Green's operative hand surgery. 4th ed. New York: Churchill Livingstone; 1999:1950–1987

[2] Kleinert HE, Verdan C. Report of the committee on tendon injuries. J Hand Surg Am. 1983; 8(5 Pt 2):794–798

[3] Verdan CE. Primary and secondary repair of flexor and extensor tendon injuries. In: Flynn JE, ed. Hand surgery. Baltimore: Williams and Wilkins; 1966:20–75

[4] Elliot D, McGrouther DA. The excursions of the long extensor tendons of the hand. J Hand Surg [Br]. 1986; 11(1):77–80

[5] Kulkarni M, Harris SB, Elliot D. The significance of extensor tendon tethering and dorsal joint capsule tightening after injury to the hand. J Hand Surg [Br]. 2006; 31(1):52–60

[6] Fowler SB. The management of tendon injuries. J Bone Joint Surg Am. 1959; 41-A(4):579–580

[7] Littler JW. The finger extensor mechanism. Surg Clin North Am. 1967; 47(2):415–432

[8] Thompson JS, Littler JW, Upton J. The spiral oblique retinacular ligament (SORL). J Hand Surg Am. 1978; 3(5):482–487

[9] Littler JW, Eaton RG. Redistribution of forces in the correction of Boutonniere deformity. J Bone Joint Surg Am. 1967; 49(7):1267–1274

[10] Sirotakova M, Figus A, Jarrett P, Mishra A, Elliot D. Correction of swan neck deformity in rheumatoid arthritis using a new lateral extensor band technique. J Hand Surg Eur Vol. 2008; 33(6):712–716

[11] Zancolli EA. In: Lamb DW, ed. The paralysed hand. Edinburgh: Churchill Livingstone; 1987:163–167

[12] Khandwala AR, Webb J, Harris SB, Foster AJ, Elliot D. A comparison of dynamic extension splinting and controlled active mobilization of complete divisions of extensor tendons in zones 5 and 6. J Hand Surg Am. 2000; 25B:140–146

[13] Quaba AA, Elliot D, Sommerlad BC. Long term hand function without long finger extensors: a clinical study. J Hand Surg [Br]. 1988; 13(1):66–71

[14] Atherton DD, Leong JCS, Anand P, Elliot D. Relocation of painful end neuromas and scarred nerves from the zone II territory of the hand. J Hand Surg Eur Vol. 2007; 32(1):38–44

[15] Elliot D, Sierakowski A. The surgical management of painful nerves of the upper limb: a unit perspective. J Hand Surg Eur Vol. 2011; 36(9):760–770

[16] Carroll C, IV, Moore JR, Weiland AJ. Posttraumatic ulnar subluxation of the extensor tendons: a reconstructive technique. J Hand Surg Am. 1987; 12(2):227–231

[17] Atherton DD, Fabre J, Anand P, Elliot D. Relocation of painful neuromas in Zone III of the hand and forearm. J Hand Surg Eur Vol. 2008; 33(2):155–162

[18] Britto JA, Elliot D. Thumb function without the abductor pollicis longus and extensor pollicis brevis. J Hand Surg [Br]. 2002; 27(3):274–277

[19] Bunnell P. Surgery of the hand. Philadelphia: Lippincott; 1944:277

3 Treatment of Complications after Surgical Management of Tenosynovitis

Jin Bo Tang

Abstract

This chapter discusses and summarizes the common complications of trigger finger/thumb and de Quervain's disease, such as nerve injury, bowstringing, or subluxation of the tendons. The methods of preventing and treating the complications are presented and discussed.

Keywords: trigger finger, de Quervain's disease, surgical release, nerve injury, tendon bowstringing, infection, recurrence

3.1 Introduction

Tenosynovitis in the hand usually indicates either a trigger finger including trigger thumb (caused by constricting A1 pulley in the fingers or thumb) or de Quervain's disease (tenosynovitis of the first extensor tendon compartment at the wrist). Tenosynovitis is the inflammation of the fluid-filled sheath that surrounds a tendon, typically leading to joint pain, swelling, and stiffness, often after repetitive use of the hand. The disease can be self-resolving after rest or conservative treatment.[1,2,3,4]

Surgical release is indicated if conservative treatment is not effective for several weeks, and the surgical procedures are straightforward, with little risk of complications.[1,2,3] I have not encountered any cases of complications in my practice of 30 years. However, because of the proximity of the digital nerve to the A1 pulley in the distal palm, and the radial sensory nerve to the first extensor compartment in the wrist, risk of injuring these nerves can be a complication of surgery. I consider nerve injury an important complication of the surgical release of these sheaths. Reoccurrence is possible if the surgical sheath release is insufficient. Therefore, the nerve injuries and possible reoccurrence should be given sufficient attention, which are discussed in more details in this chapter.

Tendon bowstringing and subluxation after releasing the sheath are rarely possible when the surgery is correctly performed and risk of having surgical infection is rare. To provide a full picture of possible complications, I will include subluxation and bowstringing and infection into discussion.

3.2 Nerve Injury

3.2.1 A1 Pulley Release

The digital nerve to the finger including the distal part of the common digital nerve in the palm to the finger run close to the A1 pulley. By surgical incision to release the A1 pulley, when the skin incision is right over the A1 pulley and about 1 cm long, and the dissection is carried out directly to the A1 pulley without extending the tissue release to either side of the A1 pulley, the risk of cutting the digital nerve is little or low. On the contrary, if the surgical incision is large and the exploration of the A1 pulley involved tissue release on both sides of the A1 pulley, there is a risk of damaging the digital nerve. Such a wide incision and wide release is in fact unnecessary and incorrect.

The correct surgery is a narrow incision (1 cm) and directly reaching the volar aspect of the A1 pulley and releasing the A1 pulley through a longitudinal midline incision with a scissor. The A1 pulley may be tight in these cases, but a release in the sheath just proximal to the margin of the A1 pulley would allow access to the sheath cavity and the tip of the scissor can be inserted to carry out the release. The A1 pulley is about 1 cm, and trigger fingers rarely extend to the other pulleys or involve multiple pulleys; therefore, the release should be confined to the A1 pulley, not extending to the other pulleys. There is a rare chance of trigger fingers of the pulleys other than the A1; in that case only the pulley which causes the triggering as identified by clinical examination or ultrasound examination should be accessed and released.

The radial side digital nerve of the thumb runs across the flexor tendon proximal to the A1 pulley in the thumb (▶ Fig. 3.1). Therefore, the risk of injuring this digital nerve is higher. The key is to keep the surgical incision short and be alert to the course of this nerve and avoid cutting it. Proximal extension of the surgical incision of releasing the trigger thumb is rarely necessary; if this becomes necessary, the surgeon should be very careful to identify this digital nerve to avoid injury to it. If a digital nerve is cut, repair surgery should be performed.

3.2.2 First Extensor Compartment Release

The radial sensory nerve runs obliquely proximal to the first dorsal compartment of the wrist (▶ Fig. 3.2). In most cases, it is about 1 cm proximal to the proximal margin of this compartment. However, there is variation of the path of this nerve and extended proximal surgical incision should always be avoided. Before the surgery, the operator may also examine the course of the nerve in non-obese patients as this nerve can be visible in some patients. In obese patients, the operators should take care

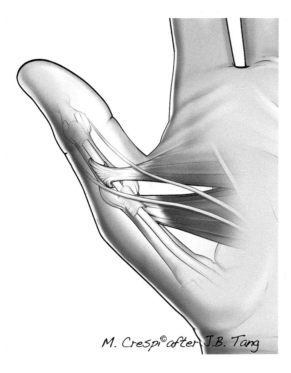

Fig. 3.1 Anatomy of the radial digital nerve of the thumb. This nerve passes just proximal to the A1 pulley, which can be damaged during the release of the A1 pulley in the thumb.

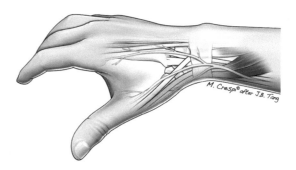

Fig. 3.2 Anatomical course of the radial sensory nerve dorsal to the first dorsal compartment of the wrist.

3.3.2 First Extensor Compartment Release

When the first dorsal compartment of the wrist was released, there is a risk of subluxation, rather than bowstringing. The subluxation occurs when the release is unnecessarily long, and the treatment is to reconstruct a part of released sheath including a Z-plasty of the first dorsal compartment[7] (▶ Fig. 3.5).

3.4 Infection

Trigger finger or thumb release surgeries and release of the first dorsal compartment of the wrist often are performed in office settings or in minor procedure rooms. There is a low chance of infection, though it is unclear whether the rate of infection is higher than those in more standard major operating theaters, which are unnecessary. I personally did not encounter a single case of infection. If there is infection, that is usually not severe. Oral antibiotic treatment should suffice in treating the infection. The key to prevent the infection is correct field sterilization of the surgical field. It is not necessary to conventionally take antibiotics to prevent infection as the rate of infection is very low.

3.5 Recurrence of the Triggering

3.5.1 A1 Pulley Release

This is not common. However, if the release of the trigger finger is incomplete, the triggering may occur. The treatment plan is to perform the release again and make sure the entire A1 pulley is released and the flexor tendons can be passively move very freely during surgery. If a wide-awake surgical setting is used, the patients should be asked to move the finger actively. The patients should be able to confirm free active motion and feel no resistance of the finger active motion once the A1 pulley is

to identify and protect this nerve if a longer surgical incision is made (which is often necessary in obese patients). I use a longitudinal incision right over the first dorsal compartment of 1 to 1.5 cm (▶ Fig. 3.3), which sufficiently exposes the tendon sheath and allows easy release of the sheath and any subsheath that separates the two tendons inside the first compartment (▶ Fig. 3.4).

3.3 Bowstringing and Subluxation

3.3.1 A1 Pulley Release

This cannot happen if the surgical release is confined to a single pulley which has caused triggering. However, if the surgery is improperly done with release to other pulleys, creating a long pulley deficiency, tendon bowstringing may occur. If the A1 pulley is released with only a part of the A2 pulley, no repair or reconstruction is necessary as bowstringing does not cause any clinical consequences.[5,6] However if the entire A1 and A2 pulleys are released, there will be bowstringing of the flexor tendons, and repair of the A2 pulley should be necessary, and the surgery should be done immediately after confirming the A2 pulley is inadvertently cut, or a subsequent surgical repair or reconstruction with a Z-plasty of the A2 pulley is planned after confirming the loss of both A1 and A2 pulleys after surgical release of the trigger finger.

1

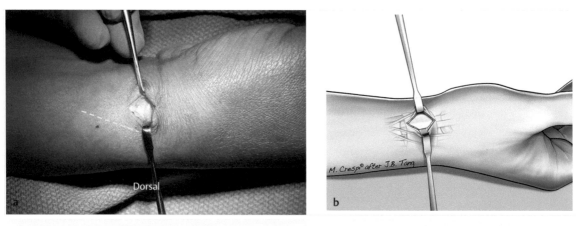

Fig. 3.3 (a, b) A longitudinal short surgical incision over the first dorsal compartment as shown can avoid the damage to the radial sensory nerve (its path shown in the yellow dash line).

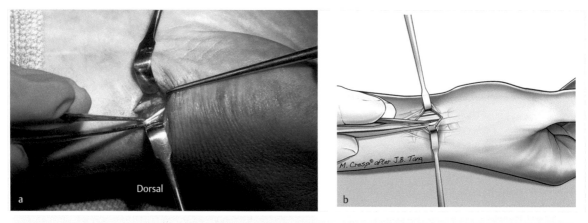

Fig. 3.4 (a, b) A subsheath is identified when the first dorsal compartment is completed release, which covers one tendon in the first compartment. This subsheath should be released as well to avoid reoccurrence of the tenosynovitis of the dorsal wrist.

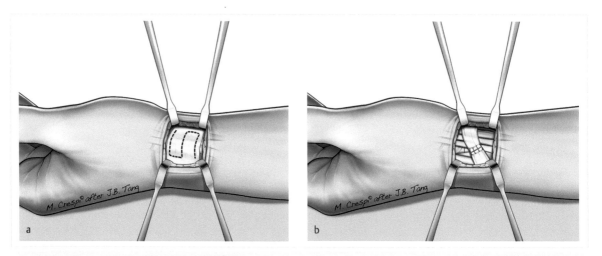

Fig. 3.5 (a, b) Drawings show the design of the Z incision in the first dorsal compartment sheath and completion of the Z-plasty after direct suture the two arms created from Z-plasty.

completely released. The changes that the patients feel during surgery are immediate and dramatic, which signal the complete release. The risk of forming adhesions after surgery is minimal as the flexor tendons are not damaged. The recurrence if occurring should mostly be caused in incomplete pulley release rather than tendon adhesions.

3.5.2 First Extensor Compartment Release

Recurrence of the tenosynovitis of the first dorsal compartment of the wrist usually relates to incomplete release or having not released the intracompartmental septum (subsheath) inside the first dorsal compartment.[8,9] Sato et al found that the prevalence of intracompartmental septum in patients with de Quervain's disease was 62% (69 of 112 wrists) with ultrasound examination. It should be a conventional part of the surgery to confirm there is no subsheath or the subsheath is released after releasing the first dorsal compartment.[9] Therefore, releasing the subsheath should be included as a necessary part of the surgery for De Quervain's disease.

3.6 Percutaneous Trigger Finger Release

More recently, some surgeons have used percutaneous or ultrasound-guided trigger finger release or release with a device.[10,11,12,13] It remains a question whether percutaneous release increases or decreases surgical complications.[12,13] The advantage of the percutaneous release is a smaller incision and less trauma to the site of surgery. However, percutaneous trigger finger release has a learning curve, which is a disadvantage, and injury to the digital nerve is more likely than that with an open surgery.

3.7 Discussion

Trigger finger and De Quervain's disease are commonly seen disorders of the hand in many parts of the world, though global statistics of incidence of these diseases are not available. Surgical release of the constricting part of the sheath through a small incision of 1 to 1.5 cm is a common office procedure or a procedure in minor procedure room. Complications after trigger finger or thumb release or surgical release for De Quervain's disease are much less common than complications after flexor or extensor tendon repair discussed in two earlier chapters. If the surgical release is properly done, there should be no complications. The complications of nerve injuries or bowstringing of the tendons relate to unnecessarily larger surgical incision and release of the pulleys/sheath. The reoccurrence relates to failure in complete release of the

A1 pulley in trigger finger, or in recognizing and releasing the subsheath of the first dorsal compartments. If above complications are found, proper surgical treatment should be given.

3.8 Take-Home Message

The release surgery for tenosynovitis is now popularly performed in office setting or minor procedure room with field sterility; therefore, field sterilization should be sufficient and properly carried out.[14,15] The patient who is operated in a wide-awake setting should be asked to actively move the fingers, thumb, or wrists during surgery to ascertain complete release of the constricting pulley or sheath. The authors advise any junior surgeons to review relevant anatomy before surgery and avoid any complications in surgical treatment of tenosynovitis as these complications are completely preventable if the surgeries are performed properly.

References

[1] Amirfeyz R, McNinch R, Watts A, et al. Evidence-based management of adult trigger digits. J Hand Surg Eur Vol. 2017; 42(5):473–480

[2] McAuliffe JA. Tendon disorders of the hand and wrist. J Hand Surg Am. 2010; 35(5):846–853, quiz 853

[3] Adams JE, Habbu R. Tendinopathies of the hand and wrist. J Am Acad Orthop Surg. 2015; 23(12):741–750

[4] Goel R, Abzug JM. de Quervain's tenosynovitis: a review of the rehabilitative options. Hand (N Y). 2015; 10(1):1–5

[5] Tang JB, Zhou X, Pan ZJ, Qing J, Gong KT, Chen J. Strong digital flexor tendon repair, extension-flexion test, and early active flexion: experience in 300 tendons. Hand Clin. 2017; 33(3):455–463

[6] Tang JB. Indications, methods, postoperative motion and outcome evaluation of primary flexor tendon repairs in Zone 2. J Hand Surg Eur Vol. 2007; 32(2):118–129

[7] Kim JY, Baek JH, Lee JH. Comparison between simple release and Z-plasty of retinaculum for de Quervain's disease: a retrospective study. J Hand Surg Eur Vol. 2019; 44(4):390–393

[8] Sato J, Ishii Y, Noguchi H. Clinical and ultrasound features in patients with intersection syndrome or de Quervain's disease. J Hand Surg Eur Vol. 2016; 41(2):220–225

[9] Bernstein DT, Gonzalez MA, Hendrick RG, Petersen NJ, Nolla JM, Netscher DT. Impact of septated first dorsal compartments on symptomatic de Quervain disease. Plast Reconstr Surg. 2019; 144(2):389–393

[10] Croutzet P, Guinand R, Mares O, Apard T, Candelier G, David I. Ultrasound-guided de Quervain's tendon release, feasibility, and first outcomes. J Wrist Surg. 2019; 8(6):513–519

[11] Werthel JD, Cortez M, Elhassan BT. Modified percutaneous trigger finger release. Hand Surg Rehab. 2016; 35(3):179–182

[12] Aksoy A, Sir E. Complications of Percutaneous release of the trigger finger. Cureus. 2019; 11(2):e4132

[13] Xie P, Zhang QH, Zheng GZ, et al. Stenosing tenosynovitis: evaluation of percutaneous release with a specially designed needle vs. open surgery. Orthopade. 2019; 48(3):202–206

[14] Lalonde DH. Conceptual origins, current practice, and views of wide awake hand surgery. J Hand Surg Eur Vol. 2017; 42(9):886–895

[15] Maliha SG, Cohen O, Jacoby A, Sharma S, Sharma, P. A cost and efficiency analysis of the WALANT technique for the management of trigger finger in a procedure room of a major city hospital. Plast Reconstr Surg Glob Open. 2019; 7(11):e2509

Section 2

Nerve Surgery

2

4 Management of Complications in Sensory Nerve Surgery

Pierluigi Tos, Alessandro Crosio, and Simona Odella

Abstract

Complications of nerve injuries repair or neurolysis in the hand or elsewhere include no recovery or incomplete sensory recovery, painful neuroma, painful scar neuropathy, and cold intolerance.

All of these can be summarized as painful neuropathy. It is important to identify this condition immediately. The longer the symptoms exist, the worse the resolution obtained is: the neuropathic pain becomes chronic. Furthermore, painful neuropathy can also lead to a complex regional pain syndrome II (CRPS II), a chronic (lasting greater than 6 mo) pain condition with burning pain and allodynia (pain to nonpainful stimuli).

In presence of a symptomatic neuroma or a scar neuropathy, surgical treatment can lead to a good result. But it is important to emphasize that surgical treatment has limited capacity in symptoms reduction when previous attempts have been performed.

Furthermore, in chronic neuropathic condition nonresponsive to surgery, a multidisciplinary approach is indicated.

The role of rehabilitation process following nerve injury and repair, a relearning process, is the key to preventing discomfort and pain after repair. The sensory re-education programs are very important for the recovery of functional sensibility and are essential before and after any surgical attempt in nerve surgery. Dysesthesia and disuse of the hand may occur, and are best treated with an aggressive desensitization and sensory re-education program under the supervision of a hand therapist.

Keywords: pain, neuroma, traction neuropathies, nerve injury, complications

4.1 No Recovery or Incomplete Sensory Recovery

4.1.1 Definition

About one-third of digital nerve repair results are stated as poor in adults. This is true both for primary and secondary, with or without a nerve graft/conduit repair, as reported in the meta-analysis by Paprottka et al.[1]

Nowadays, there is no surgical repair technique that can guarantee full recovery of tactile discrimination in the hand of an adult patient. In contrast, very young individuals usually reach a complete recovery.

4.1.2 Treatment

If no recovery occurs after nerve surgery, a secondary operation is always possible.[2] The lack of recovery is sometimes due to rupture of the suture site, sometimes due to a poor trimming of the nerve stumps to "healthy axons." In other cases, the cause is not clear.

Conduits or nerve grafts may give good results even after a long period.

The end organs of skin include Meissner and Pacinian corpuscles, Ruffini endings, Merkel cells, and free nerve endings. Pacinian and Meissner Corpuscle are quickly adapting fiber receptors that mediate moving touch and vibration. Merkel mediate slow adapting fibers for pressure and constant touch. The Ruffini endings play a role in vibration and proprioception. The free nerve endings are free unmyelinated fibers that are sensitive to touch, temperature, and pain. Pacinian corpuscle receives only one axon and normally do not reinnervate. All other sensory receptors are able to reinnervate.

Sensory reinnervation can occur, differently than motor reinnervation, many years after denervation. In this case, sensory organs may undergo changes that alter the ultimate quality of reinnervation. After a long-lasting period of denervation, the protective sensation can be achieved more by means of free nerve endings than receptors reinnervation.[3]

The technique indicated to restore the continuity of a sensory nerve depends on the length of the residual gap after the trimming of the two stumps. It is important to suture a proximal stump correctly trimmed without residual interfascicular scar. Furthermore, a direct suture should be performed without tension. It is demonstrated that an excessive tension at the suture site induces impaired activation of Schwann cells, and a higher amount of apoptotic Schwann cells, with a subsequent deteriorated axonal outgrowth and the well-known scarring across the nerve repair.[4,5,6] If the gap at the end of the nerve stumps resection is between 2 and 4 cm, a nerve conduit can be used to avoid a withdrawal of a healthy nerve as a graft, whereas if the gap is longer than 3 to 4 cm, a nerve graft should be indicated. It seems, without a clear evidence, that in sensory nerves the critical gap is 3 to 4 cm. It has been proven that there is no optimal surgical technique for digital nerve repair up to 3 to 4 cm.[1]

4.1.3 Rehabilitation

A specific rehabilitation program to enhance the residual sensibility should be started. MacKinnon and Dellon stated that up to S3 + results are classified as "poor," but we personally think that an S3 (discrimination between 7 and 15 mm, recovery of pain and touch sensibility without an over-response, as shown in ▶ Table 4.1) should be considered a good result.

Table 4.1 Sensory recovery outcome, the Highet classification, static two-point discrimination (s2PD), moving two-point discrimination (m2PD), and recovery of sensibility

Sensory recovery outcome	Highet	s2PD	m2PD	Recovery sensibility
Failure	S0			No recovery of sensibility in the autonomous zone of the nerve
Poor	S1			Recovery of deep cutaneous pain sensibility with the autonomous zone of the nerve
	S1 +			Recovery of superficial pain sensibility
	S2			Recovery of superficial pain and some touch sensibility
	S2 +			As in S2, but with over response
	S3	>15 mm	>7 mm	Recovery of pain and touch sensibility with disappearance of over response
Good	S3 +	7–15 mm	4–7 mm	As in S3, but with good localization of the stimuli and imperfect recovery of 2PD
Excellent	S4	2–6 mm	2–3 mm	Complete sensory recovery

Source: Modified from S. E. Mackinnon and A. L. Dellon. Surgery of the Peripheral Nerve. New York: Thieme Medical Publishers; 1988.

4.2 Neuropathy

Neuropathy is defined by the IASP (International Association for the Study of Pain) as "pain caused by a lesion or disease of the somatosensory system."[7]

Neuropathy is not a single disease with a single origin, but rather a group of symptoms caused by different pathologies ranging from diabetes to nerve compression and nerve injury, with the unifying cause that it is pain developed by a lesion or disease of the somatosensory system.

The core symptoms of neuropathic pain are temperature hyperesthesia (a painful stimulus perceived as more painful than normal), mechanical allodynia (a nonpainful stimulus, perceived as painful), and spontaneous burning pain also known as spikes.

For most of the underlying diseases the cause of the neuropathic component is still unclear, also because they are difficult to study in patients. Injury of the peripheral nerves is more clear in their pathology and a number of experimental animal models exist for the study of the development of neuropathic pain, like the "spared nerve injury model" and the "spinal nerve constriction injury model."[8]

It remains difficult to assess pain in animals directly, but these models provide indirect clues to the development of neuropathic pain. Using these models, it has been described that the cutaneous denervation following a nerve injury facilitates development of neuropathic pain. This is mediated by collateral sprouting fibers from adjacent uninjured nerves.[9,10,11]

This is probably why upper limb surgeons have maintained the thought of always repairing a nerve, as soon as possible, preventing a denervated area of the skin, diminishing the chances of developing neuropathic pain.

Clinically, the patient with neuropathic pain presents with brush pain, spontaneous burning pain, and severe temperature hyperalgesia. This usually means no garment can be worn on the afflicted area, a cool breeze can be excruciatingly painful, rain becomes a fearful event, and the area cannot be taken under a shower. Treatment of neuropathic pain remains difficult as long as we do not fully understand the mechanisms behind the origins of the pain. Pain medication is often trial and error, and usually neuropathic pain evolves in chronic neuropathic pain.[12] Grace et al demonstrated that prolonged pain is an unrealized and clinically concerning consequence of the abundant use of opioids in chronic pain.[13] Surgery for neuropathic pain is only successful if a specific cause for the pain is present, but most often it only partly resolves.

4.3 Hyperalgesia/Hyperesthesia

Hyperalgesia can be divided into primary and secondary. The distinction depends on how centralized the symptoms are.

The first case is a condition in which the primary afferent A-delta and C-nociceptors in the injured region begin to respond to normally non-noxious stimuli, respond to noxious stimuli in an amplified fashion, and may also develop spontaneous activity. This is due to genetic and molecular remodeling of the primary nociceptors as well as an "inflammatory soup" of chemicals present in the injured site.

Secondary hyperalgesia describes increased sensitivity in areas of the body that are outside the injured site and are therefore thought to reflect altered CNS function. Such situations indicate that the CNS is operating in a sensitized state. It responds in an amplified fashion resulting in pain evoked also by nonpainful stimuli. Both peripheral and CS play an important role in creating and maintaining neuropathic pain.

When the patient is affected by hyperalgesia or hyperesthesia, the treatment consists of desensitization programs and the use of plaster with local anesthetic drugs to reduce the symptoms.[14]

4.4 Cold Intolerance

Cold intolerance or sensitivity was initially thought of as a vascular problem[15] but is currently more viewed as one of the neuropathic symptoms (temperature hyperesthesia). It is frequently seen following hand injury and fractures (38%)[16] or for instance surgery for Dupuytren's disease, up to 63% of patients.[17] However, in approximately 80% of patients with nerve injury, cold intolerance will develop.[18] This mechanism is also seen in rodents.[19] Conditioned pain modulation seems to be reduced in patients with cold intolerance.[20] Classically cold intolerance is thought to diminish after a number of years, but recent studies have shown that the symptoms can last for longer periods. Fortunately, only one-fifth of these go on to develop severe or extreme symptoms, and of course this is more predominant in areas with colder climates. For many patients, treatment consists of adaptation and protective strategies when exposed to cold temperatures, like wearing heated gloves and raising the core temperature.[21]

4.5 Painful Neuropathies

4.5.1 Definition

This group of pathological conditions merges painful neuroma and painful scar neuropathy or traction neuropathy. These are the most important complications following peripheral nerve injury, seriously affecting patients' daily life. The true incidence of symptomatic neuroma is unknown and is estimated at approximately between 2 and 60% of patients involved in peripheral nerve injury.[22,23,24,25,26]

Interestingly, in digital amputations, only about 7% of the patients develop a painful neuroma.[27,28]

A neuroma is part of the normal biological process in a transected and unreconstructed nerve. The axons sprout and grow, but without direction and form the neuroma, if there is no connection to a distal part of the nerve. It is absolutely unclear why a neuroma becomes a painful neuroma.

Two processes are responsible for pain: (1) persistent mechanical or chemical irritation of the axons within the neuroma and (2) the development of spontaneous and disturbing sensory symptoms[29] caused by persistent stimulation of the axons within the neuroma and accompanied by the development of spontaneous activity of neurons within the dorsal root ganglion, dorsal horn of the spinal cord, or even more proximal level.[30] Neuromas are provoked by axons sprout into the surrounding scar tissue. It seems that an up-regulation of sodium channels, adrenergic, and nicotinic cholinergic receptors leads to abnormal sensitivity and spontaneous activity of injured axons.[31] During this time a central sensitization in the spinal cord and sensory cortex takes place.

The so-called "scarring neuritis" or "scar neuropathy," as defined by Elliot,[21] encompass all the conditions related to formation of perineural and intraneural fibrotic tissue involving neurological symptoms and induced by a nerve injury. Perineural scarring and consequently traction neuropathy has traditionally been associated to the complications of nerve decompression surgery. Nerve tethering in the surgical scar is still the main cause of symptoms related to perineural scarring. The problem of neuropathic pain can be present even only after surgery that "touches" the peripheral nerve, without interrupting the fibers, and causes a perineural scarring reaction. This problem can benefit from a new surgery with the application of antiadherent gels or adipofascial flaps. All these procedures aim to promote the normal sliding of the nerve on the surrounding tissues. It is absolutely not clear why certain patients are more susceptible to neuroma formation than others.

Spontaneous pain, allodynia, hyperalgesia, and cold intolerance are the main symptoms reported by the patient.

The neuroma can be:

- *Terminal without possibility to a distal reconnection* (i.e., a digital neuroma or the distal nerve trunk is not available for multiple surgery, loss of substance).
- *Terminal with the possibility to a connection* with a distal nerve stump (i.e., sensory radial nerve branch as a complication of surgery or traumatic transection of a nerve).
- *In continuity* (after a nerve suture or a trauma):
  Without residual function
  With a residual function

4.5.2 Diagnosis

The diagnosis of painful neuropathy is based on history and physical examination. The history of a nerve injury is accompanied by pain and typical symptoms with a defined neural anatomic distribution often with cold intolerance. History is crucial to establish the cause of symptoms: is it related to a simple nerve decompression, reconstruction, direct trauma, or posttraumatic scarring? Physical examination and pain type—at rest or elicited by movement or mechanical stimuli—may provide information on lesion type. Pain at rest commonly entails that the scar involves the deep nerve structure. Perineural scarring usually induces nerve tethering, which is exacerbated by movement. Another important information is the presence of a painful Tinel sign. A local anesthetic injection can be helpful to understand if the symptoms are related just to the neuroma or if they have already centralized. Furthermore, instrumental examination—US or magnetic resonance imaging (MRI)—can confirm the diagnosis. It is suggested to pair a simple assessment of pain, such as the visual analog scale (VAS), with a more detailed pain and function questionnaire, such as the DASH or PROMIS. Serial assessment with these forms facilitates tracking progress that is sometimes not apparent to the patients themselves.

Once you have completed the physical examination, diagnostic nerve blocks can be performed to determine what effect decompression or neurectomy might have in that region. Blocks provide patients with an idea of the potential area of altered sensation with nerve resection but do not guarantee operative success. On the other hand, if block doesn't relieve the pain, it means that no surgical procedure can solve the problem and surgery should be avoided.[32]

Ultrasound and dynamic US may also be used in experienced hands to diagnose the perineural scar neuropathy or an intraneural neuroma.

It remains unclear why the same pathological anatomy problem can cause pain in some patients and nothing in others.

4.5.3 Principles of Treatment

Every surgical procedure must be preceded by appropriate medical treatment and by pharmacological and physical therapy with dedicated operators for at least 6 months. There is no consensus on surgery timing.[33] As a general rule, surgery is indicated when medical and physical therapies have failed to bring benefit.

Different surgical treatments must be performed depending on the cause of pain. For the painful "scar neuropathy," treatment consists of a surgical exploration, neurolysis under magnification, and procedures aimed at preventing new scar formation such as flap coverage and application of antiadhesion devices. In case of a terminal neuroma or a neuroma without function, the procedure consists of resection of the neuroma and reconstruction of the nerve trunk with graft if it is possible. In other cases, the terminal nerve stump has to be transferred and covered with well-vascularized soft tissue.

Prevention and Treatment of Terminal Neuroma

Prevention of terminal neuroma formation should be attempted during revision amputation through some surgical precautions as avoiding tension, care in soft tissue management, and accurate debridement. Despite these precautions, a painful stump cannot be excluded because of the arise of a new neuroma in the apex of the cut nerve.[34] Actually just the targeted muscle reinnervation is the unique technique that limits the neuroma formation.[35] The prevention of neuroma formation in a nerve suture site due to "painful sprouting" can be obtained by "the vein conduit coverage" of the suture site as described by Alligand-Perrin et al.[36] This technique is useful for both the first nerve suture and the nerve grafting. We routinely apply this procedure in our department as shown in ▶ Fig. 4.1.

Many techniques have been advocated for the surgical treatment of terminal neuromas, but none have yet risen to the level of a gold standard treatment for this challenging problem. Most of the treatments are focused on containing regenerating axons or protecting them from exacerbating stimuli.

The simplest and easiest technique for a painful neuroma of a simple digital nerve is the shortening of the nerve and the implantation in adjacent, supple, and non-"touching" area. Some authors suggest electrical coagulation of the stump of the nerve (by slowly increasing the intensity of the current) as described by Gosset et al[37] and reproposed by Brunelli in 2002.[38] This procedure has been devised based on the fact that electrically burnt patients do not produce painful neuromas.

Centrocentral anastomosis[39] has been described to involve the coaptation of two nerve cords of central origin. The technique can also be applied for one nerve if it is split into two fascicles of equal size. A theory for the cessation of axonal growth is that there must be a continuous flow of axoplasm in both directions; if these newly formed axons are under pressure in the transplantation area, it results in a reduction of protein production and axoplasm flow in the neuron, acting to inhibit neuroma development. For connection of the two stumps of the same nerve or for two nerves of a digit, a vein can be used or a conduit (to avoid collateral sprouting).

For more proximal terminal neuromas, when a reconstruction is not feasible, it is described to perform a proximal crush, followed by transposition of the cut nerve end deep within a muscle, into bone, or to cover it with a vein cup or with synthetic cups composed by different materials. Also, epineural flap has been described to cover up the terminal end of the nerve, but no better results were achieved compared to resection alone.

Very few studies on the surgical treatment of neuromas include a control group. However, nerve transposition and implantation into muscle seems to be supported by the largest body of research among the techniques reported.

Nerve stripping is another technique described by Lanzetta and Nolli[40] for the treatment of palmar cutaneous nerve neuromas. Longitudinal traction along the direction of the nerve is then applied, until the nerve is disconnected from the main trunk without causing harm to the parent nerve.

2

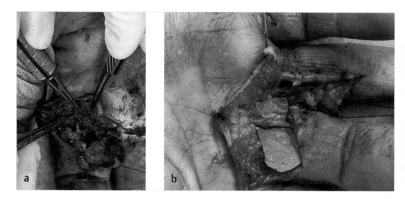

Fig. 4.1 (a, b) The nerve suture is routinely protected by a vein trying to avoid collateral painful sprouting.

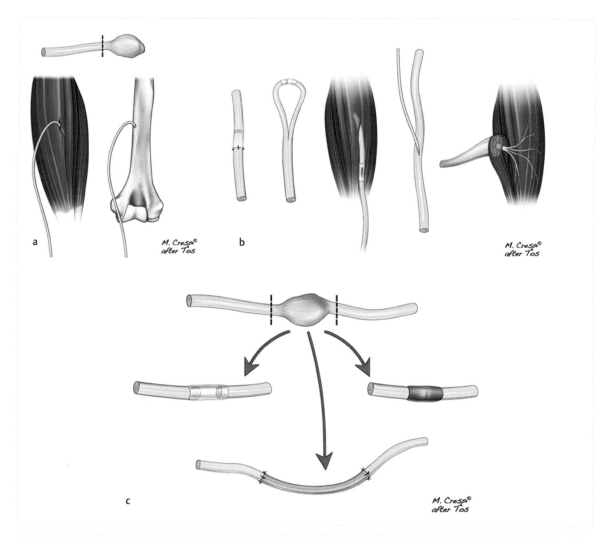

Fig. 4.2 (a–c) Different surgical options for terminal neuroma and neuroma with possible reconnection.

Following neuroma excision, the end of the nerve stump may be coapted to the side of an adjacent intact nerve by means of an epineural window in the recipient nerve. This was first described as "reverse end-to-side neurotization." This technique is designed to provide a pathway for regenerating axons like the centrocentral anastomosis. In ▶ Fig. 4.2, all possible techniques are shown schematically.

Prevention and Treatment of In-Continuity Neuroma and Scar Neuropathy

Neuroma Is in Continuity with a Residual Function (a Good Sensibility Has Been Recovered)

A relocation of the painful nerve in deeper tissue into an environment away from the original injury site is advised and this may need coverage with a flap or a vein. This should be the first attempt (protection from mechanical and thermal injury and with the possibility to avoid adherences around the nerve).

Antiadhesive Devices

After the neurolysis and relocation, hyaluronic acid (HA)–based antiadhesive devices have been proved to be effective. Initial preclinical studies have documented their antiadhesion properties and safety. HA is marketed alone as Hyaloglide(R) or associated to carboxymethylcellulose (CMC; Seprafilm(R)). However, there is no consensus on the actual effect of antiadhesion devices. According to some researchers they reduce collagen deposition by interfering with granulocyte diapedesis and blocking the synthesis of interleukin 1, which is crucial for fibroblast activation, whereas others deny an effect on cytokines and admit its action to only being a physical barrier.

Collagen-based products have recently been developed for wrapping around injured nerves.

Fat Graft

Some authors advocated to fat grafts, enriched with the stromal vascular fraction (SVF), the action of mechanic barrier with biological effects decreasing the resorption rate and boosting the graft's regenerative potential. They report good results in radial nerve sensory painful neuroma.[41]

Vein

The nerve wrapping in an "opened" vein segment provided satisfactory results in terms of both sensitivity improvement and reduction in recurrences.

Flaps

A variety of flaps, pedicled (local) or free, are used for coverage after neurolysis: synovial, fascial, adipofascial, muscle, and skin with subcutaneous tissue flaps. Compared to vein wraps, gels, and other antiadhesion devices, flaps have a dual function: to envelop the injured nerve in a highly vascular tissue to maximize nutrient supply, and to provide a bulk effect, i.e., protection against external mechanical insults. This approach is often used in patients where revision surgery has had poor outcomes or when the quality of local tissue does not allow per-

forming simpler procedures.[42] Typical local flaps raised in patients with recurrences or sequelae of carpal tunnel syndrome (CTS) include the hypothenar fat pad flap and the palmaris brevis flap. Their main advantage is that they provide a buffer of highly vascularized adipofascial or muscle tissue above the treated nerve. The synovial flap from the flexor tendons is still a very good option for recalcitrant CTS. Thicker flaps can be raised from the volar forearm: the dorsal ulnar artery adipofascial flap described by Becker and Gilbert can be used as an adipofascial flap to wrap the nerve or as a fasciocutaneous flap to provide greater protection; the adipofascial radial artery perforator flap and the adipofascial variant of the posterior interosseous flap raised from the dorsal portion of the forearm can be employed in the same way; the pronator quadratus muscle flap may be a useful solution when the injury is proximal to the wrist.

Treatment of Painful Neuroma without a Function

If the painful neuroma is *without a function* (i.e., insensibility distal to the site of injury or allodynia), a resection and reconstruction with a nerve graft or a tube is recommended. In our experience, it is always best to reconstruct a painful nerve injury if possible. Nerve reconstruction provides the nerve a biologic pathway through which to grow. In our experience, a tubulization with a "biological tube," "biological conduit" done by a muscle/nerve combined graft as described by Brunelli and coworkers many years ago could be the easiest solution. No other nerve withdrawal is necessary in patient potentially predisposed to the formation of painful neuromas. Vein alone or synthetic neurotubes are also advocated with same results. Allografts are being used in the United States and other parts of the world. However, we have no experience, as application of human tissue from a company is not permitted in Italy. We are studying an inexpensive way to decellularize a nerve.

Other Therapies for Painful Neuropathies

Radiofrequency Ablation

Pulsed radiofrequency (PRF), in particular, is a minimally destructive procedure; needles inserted through the skin near the painful area or adjacent to the nerve trunk deliver the radio waves to the targeted nerve; pulsed radiofrequency (PRF) and radiofrequency ablation (RFA) can be used in the management of chronic peripheral nerve pain.[43]

Pain Neuromodulation

Multiple surgical failures may provide an indication for direct peripheral nerve stimulation, to relieve chronic pain through preferential activation of myelinated fibers, inducing long-term depression of synaptic efficacy. Spinal cord stimulation (SCS), which is applied more often to treat Complex Regional Pain Syndrome I, may also be beneficial.

4.6 Rehabilitation—Sensory Desensitization

Different kinds of goals are searched during rehabilitation after a nerve injury. Treatments are directed to minimize the excessive response to cold intolerance, and all the programs are directed to treat the hyperesthesia (increased response to stimulus with or without pain), hyperalgesia (increased pain response from a pain stimulus), and allodynia (pain from a nonpainful stimulus) after nerve injury.

The term "hyperalgesia" is often used for all categories of increased pain sensitivity, including cold intolerance. Sensory desensitization approaches utilize progressive exercises to challenge the sensory responses in the reinnervated sensory distributions and essentially to relearn to interpret the tactile stimuli as nonpainful. Stimulation of the touch fibers via vibration can be used for desensitization and utilizes the Gate Control Theory to stimulate large A-Beta fibers and blocking the transmission of the nociceptive pathways. Mirror therapy with visual feedback has been widely used for treatment of chronic pain syndromes, and peripheral nerve injuries and amputations. The reflected image visualized as the uninjured limb activates the contralateral cortex of the brain to recognize the nonpainful stimuli.[44] Desensitization strategies include the use of different textures and cold exposure to visualize the image in the mirror as nonpainful. It is possible to use a sensory desensitization approach and to incorporate the cold stressors and responses in a progressive sensory reeducation/desensitization program.

4.7 Take-Home Message

Clinical practice demonstrates that neuropathic pain is difficult to treat and at times can only be partially solved.

In literature, the available studies cannot be compared due to different methodology and outcome measures. Therefore, it is difficult to definitively identify superior treatment options. Moreover, several studies failed to describe the length of their patient follow-up period.[45]

Patients should be warned that their condition is not easy to address, and that surgical treatment may have to be followed by a more aggressive approach if symptoms persist.

Patients with pain due to nerve entrapment in scar tissue require careful evaluation through history, assessment of pain type, and accurate US scanning, to establish the site of the scar tissue injury and whether the nerve presents internal damage.

Helping patients with these conditions requires a multidisciplinary approach and close collaboration of sur-

geon, pain clinician, physiotherapist, and psychologist, because for reasons that are still unclear, the patient is often the cause of the problem. Because there is a risk of nonimprovement or worsening, the pain symptoms should be clearly stated before surgery, given that any sort of intervention may induce symptom worsening in patients with complex pain syndromes.

If pain is not alleviated after the first procedure, subsequent operations are unlikely to be successful and further attempts may involve diminishing returns.

Overall, the diagnosis and treatment of scar neuritis and neuropathic pain still present significant problem areas. A clear injury classification correlating injury with the clinical problem and convincing evidences of the effectiveness of one treatment above the others would improve patient symptoms as well as clinical outcomes.

References

[1] Paprottka FJ, Wolf P, Harder Y, et al. Sensory recovery outcome after digital nerve repair in relation to different reconstructive techniques: meta-analysis and systematic review. Plast Surg Int. 2013; 2013:704589

[2] Mackinnon SE, Dvali LT. Basic pathology of the hand, wrist, and forearm: nerve. In: Berger RA, Weiss AC, eds. Hand surgery. Baltimore: Lippincott Williams & Wilkins; 2004

[3] Li XY, Chen SZ, Li YJ, Cheng B, Chen H, Qu H. Degeneration and regeneration of free nerve endings in denervated monkeys after implantation. Chin J Microsurg. 1998; 21:284: (In Chinese)

[4] Yi C, Dahlin LB. Impaired nerve regeneration and Schwann cell activation after repair with tension. Neuroreport. 2010; 21(14):958–962

[5] Goldberg SH, Jobin CM, Hayes AG, Gardner T, Rosenwasser MP, Strauch RJ. Biomechanics and histology of intact and repaired digital nerves: an in vitro study. J Hand Surg Am. 2007; 32(4):474–482

[6] Zhang F, Inserra M, Richards L, Terris DJ, Lineaweaver WC. Quantification of nerve tension after nerve repair: correlations with nerve defects and nerve regeneration. J Reconstr Microsurg. 2001; 17 (6):445–451

[7] Jensen TS, Baron R, Haanpää M, et al. A new definition of neuropathic pain. Pain. 2011; 152(10):2204–2205

[8] Decosterd I, Woolf CJ. Spared nerve injury: an animal model of persistent peripheral neuropathic pain. Pain. 2000; 87(2):149–158

[9] Duraku LS, Hossaini M, Schüttenhelm BN, et al. Re-innervation patterns by peptidergic Substance-P, non-peptidergic P2X3, and myelinated NF-200 nerve fibers in epidermis and dermis of rats with neuropathic pain. Exp Neurol. 2013; 241:13–24

[10] Leibovich H, Buzaglo N, Tsuriel S, et al. Abnormal reinnervation of denervated areas following nerve injury facilitates neuropathic pain. Cells. 2020; 9(4):1007–1028

[11] Duraku LS, Hossaini M, Hoendervangers S, et al. Spatiotemporal dynamics of re-innervation and hyperinnervation patterns by uninjured CGRP fibers in the rat foot sole epidermis after nerve injury. Mol Pain. 2012; 8:61

[12] Cooper TE, Chen J, Wiffen PJ, et al. Morphine for chronic neuropathic pain in adults. Cochrane Database Syst Rev. 2017; 5(5):CD011669

[13] Grace PM, Strand KA, Galer EL, et al. Morphine paradoxically prolongs neuropathic pain in rats by amplifying spinal NLRP3 inflammasome activation. Proc Natl Acad Sci U S A. 2016; 113(24):E3441–E3450

[14] Osborne NR, Anastakis DJ, Davis KD. Peripheral nerve injuries, pain, and neuroplasticity. J Hand Ther. 2018; 31(2):184–194

[15] Ruijs AC, Niehof SP, Hovius SE, Selles RW. Cold-induced vasodilatation following traumatic median or ulnar nerve injury. J Hand Surg Am. 2011; 36(6):986–993

[16] Smits ES, Nijhuis TH, Huygen FJ, Selles RW, Hovius SE, Niehof SP. Rewarming patterns in hand fracture patients with and without cold intolerance. J Hand Surg Am. 2011; 36(4):670–676

[17] Rodrigues JN, Zhang W, Scammell BE, et al. Functional outcome and complications following surgery for Dupuytren's disease: a multi-centre cross-sectional study. J Hand Surg Eur Vol. 2017; 42(1):7–17

[18] Stokvis A, Ruijs AC, van Neck JW, Coert JH. Cold intolerance in surgically treated neuroma patients: a prospective follow-up study. J Hand Surg Am. 2009; 34(9):1689–1695

[19] Smits ES, Duraku LS, Niehof SP, et al. Cold-induced vasodilatation in cold-intolerant rats after nerve injury. J Plast Reconstr Aesthet Surg. 2013; 66(9):1279–1286

[20] Vaksvik T, Kjeken I, Holm I. Self-management strategies used by patients who are hypersensitive to cold following a hand injury. A prospective study with two years follow-up. J Hand Ther. 2015; 28 (1):46–51, quiz 52

[21] Elliot D. Surgical management of painful peripheral nerves. Clin Plast Surg. 2014; 41(3):589–613

[22] Weng W, Zhao B, Lin D, Gao W, Li Z, Yan H. Significance of alpha smooth muscle actin expression in traumatic painful neuromas: a pilot study in rats. Sci Rep. 2016; 6:23828

[23] Atherton DD, Taherzadeh O, Facer P, Elliot D, Anand P. The potential role of nerve growth factor (NGF) in painful neuromas and the mechanism of pain relief by their relocation to muscle. J Hand Surg [Br]. 2006; 31(6):652–656

[24] Mavrogenis AF, Pavlakis K, Stamatoukou A, et al. Current treatment concepts for neuromas-in-continuity. Injury. 2008; 39 Suppl 3:S43–S48

[25] Campbell JN. Neuroma pain. In: Gebhart GF, Schmidt RF, eds. Encyclopedia of pain. 2nd ed. Berlin: Springer-Verlag; 2013:2056–2058

[26] Fisher GT, Boswick JA, Jr. Neuroma formation following digital amputations. J Trauma. 1983; 23(2):136–142

[27] Vlot MA, Wilkens SC, Chen NC, Eberlin KR. Symptomatic neuroma following initial amputation for traumatic digital amputation. J Hand Surg Am. 2018; 43(1):86.e1–86.e8

[28] van der Avoort DJ, Hovius SE, Selles RW, van Neck JW, Coert JH. The incidence of symptomatic neuroma in amputation and neurorrhaphy patients. J Plast Reconstr Aesthet Surg. 2013; 66(10):1330–1334

[29] Watson J, Gonzalez M, Romero A, Kerns J. Neuromas of the hand and upper extremity. J Hand Surg Am. 2010; 35(3):499–510

[30] Birch R. The peripheral neuroma. In: Green DP, Hotchkiss RN, Pederson WC, Wolfe P, eds. Green's operative hand surgery. 5th ed. New York: Churchill Livingstone; 2005:1102–1111

[31] Curtin C, Carroll I. Cutaneous neuroma physiology and its relationship to chronic pain. J Hand Surg Am. 2009; 34(7):1334–1336

[32] Stokvis A, van der Avoort DJ, van Neck JW, Hovius SE, Coert JH. Surgical management of neuroma pain: a prospective follow-up study. Pain. 2010; 151(3):862–869

[33] Lipinski LJ, Spinner RJ. Neurolysis, neurectomy, and nerve repair/reconstruction for chronic pain. Neurosurg Clin N Am. 2014; 25 (4):777–787

[34] Crosio A, Albo E, Marcoccio I, et al. Prevention of symptomatic neuroma in traumatic digital amputation: a RAND/UCLA appropriateness method consensus study. Injury. 2020; 9::S0020-1383(20)30240-0

[35] Souza JM, Cheesborough JE, Ko JH, Cho MS, Kuiken TA, Dumanian GA. Targeted muscle reinnervation: a novel approach to postamputation neuroma pain. Clin Orthop Relat Res. 2014; 472(10):2984–2990

[36] Alligand-Perrin P, Rabarin F, Jeudy J, et al. Vein conduit associated with microsurgical suture for complete collateral digital nerve severance. Orthop Traumatol Surg Res. 2011; 97(4) Suppl:S16–S20

[37] Gosset J, Andre P, Levame M. [The prevention of amputation neuromas of the fingers and of amputation neuromas in general]. Mem Acad Chir (Paris). 1962; 88:548–550

[38] Brunelli GA. Prevention of damage caused by sural nerve withdrawal for nerve grafting. Hand Surg. 2002; 7(2):163–166

[39] Belcher HJ, Pandya AN. Centro-central union for the prevention of neuroma formation after finger amputation. J Hand Surg [Br]. 2000; 25(2):154–159

[40] Lanzetta M, Nolli R. Nerve stripping: new treatment for neuromas of the palmar cutaneous branch of the median nerve. J Hand Surg [Br]. 2000; 25(2):151–153

[41] Calcagni M, Zimmermann S, Scaglioni MF, Giesen T, Giovanoli P, Fakin RM. The novel treatment of SVF-enriched fat grafting for painful end-neuromas of superficial radial nerve. Microsurgery. 2018; 38(3):264–269

[42] Tos P, Crosio A, Pugliese P, et al. Painful scar neuropathy: principles of diagnosis and treatment. Plast Aesthet Res. 2015; 2:4

[43] Racz GB, Ruiz-Lopez R. Radiofrequency procedures. Pain Pract. 2006; 6(1):46–50

[44] Novak CB. Cold intolerance after nerve injury. J Hand Ther. 2018; 31 (2):195–200

[45] Ives GC, Kung TA, Nghiem BT, et al. Current state of the surgical treatment of terminal neuromas. Neurosurgery. 2018; 83(3):354–364

5 Management of Complications of Surgery of the Median, Ulnar, and Radial Nerves in the Forearm

Erik Walbeehm and Dominic Power

Abstract

Following repair of the main nerve trunks in the forearm, complications may result in poor functional recovery, pain, and disability. Optimizing the primary procedure in terms of timing and technique may reduce the rate and severity of complications; however, the nature of these injuries and the requirement for successful axonal regeneration render the outcome unpredictable. Neuromas may form at the repair site, scar encasement and tether may result in neurostenalgia, delays to reinnervation leave muscles weak or paralyzed, trophic skin may ulcerate and rarely severe pain syndromes including complex regional pain syndrome type 2 may follow. Prompt recognition and treatment of these complications can salvage function, either by revision of the original repair or using adjunctive procedures to manage pain and improve function. Recognition that distal function may be poor due to the late presentation of the injury or its proximal location may enable the treating surgeon to introduce distal augmentation nerve transfers for key muscles into their primary algorithm.

Keywords: median nerve, ulnar nerve, radial nerve, nerve transfer, tendon transfer, neuroma, neuroma in continuity, neuropathic pain, neurolysis, paralysis

5.1 Introduction

Reconstruction following a traumatic peripheral nerve surgery is straightforward. Following a thorough physical examination and applying anatomical knowledge, most primary nerve pathologies in the forearm and hand can be diagnosed and treated. If a nerve is transected it can be repaired. Simple apposition of the two nerve ends with a number of microsurgical sutures and perhaps fibrin glue augmentation will suffice in most cases. If there is nerve tissue loss and too much tension, then consider a conduit as a bridging device or for longer gaps a nerve graft. This algorithm is easy to follow. However, unlike for a microvascular anastomosis, the final outcome following a nerve reconstruction must be awaited. The primary surgery must be well planned, promptly delivered, and performed with technical expertise. The local pathoanatomy dictates the potential for recovery and the expert clinician will be prepared for the challenges afforded by proximal nerve injuries, delayed presentation, long gaps, and poor surgical beds, offering adjunctive distal nerve or tendon transfers at the time of primary surgery or early in the recovery phase.

Failure of the repair can result in sensory loss, paralysis, and pain. Poor results may not be apparent for months and the opportunity for revision missed, leaving only salvage options. The clinician must anticipate recovery, monitor for any adverse signs, and be prepared to intervene if recovery is delayed.

5.2 Optimizing the Nerve Repair

An injured nerve should be recognized early and promptly explored. The management depends on the location and severity of the injury as well as associated injury. Debridement must be adequate, repairs should be tension free. Conduits may be used to de-tension repair sites or to leave short gaps up to 5 mm as a method of de-tensioning.[1] Theoretical advantages of adjunctive wrapping of the repair site or protecting a neurorrhaphy with a conduit to prevent axonal escape and extrinsic scar tether remain unproven. Longer gaps will generally require a nerve graft; however, a concomitant humeral fracture may be shortened and plated, avoiding the need for a graft. Avoiding two coaptation sites has obvious advantages in minimizing the risks of hold-up or misdirection of the regenerating axons. In the forearm, skeletal shortening is generally not advisable due to the loss of rotation; however, in a complex mangling injury, judicious use of this technique can assist with management of the soft tissues, including nerve reconstruction. Allograft reconstruction as an alternative is attractive, minimizing donor morbidity; however, the comparative efficacy to autologous graft in main trunk mixed nerve injuries is not known.

Recognizing the challenging injury perhaps due to a delay to diagnosis, proximal location, large gap, or poor surgical bed may allow the treating surgeon to introduce adjunctive primary tendon or nerve transfers into their primary treatment algorithm. Establishing that a repaired nerve is not progressing in line with expectation may enable prompt secondary interventions.

Following surgery, preparing your patient for a period of months before a return of function or sensation helps to manage patient expectations, prepares them for what is to come, mitigates the effects of neuropathic pain, and improves engagement, thereby preventing trophic complications.[2] This chapter focuses on problems and complications in the weeks to months following primary surgery, with the assumption that the primary surgery has been adequately performed.

5.3 Normal Recovery

Physiologically it is impossible to achieve accurate reconnection of all axons, even with acute repair of a sharp transection injury to a peripheral nerve. The mechanism of injury determines the survival of the axon population at the injury site. Proximal lesions are associated with more apoptosis, although surviving axons may have more vigorous axonal regeneration than distal injuries with a similar mechanism. Progressive loss of the sensory and motor neuron population in the proximal nerve trunk follows trauma, necessitating early intervention.

Following repair, regenerating axons may fail to cross the coaptation due to scar. Grafts provide two coaptation sites to navigate with less robust axonal regeneration to the distal stump than for a single repair site without tension. Each regenerating axon has multiple small exuberant projections that explore the local environment. Contact with surface proteoglycans in the endoneural tubes and neurotrophic gradients provide positive guidance signals. Axons failing to receive positive stimuli are pruned, allowing redistribution of regenerate efforts. In the absence of a strong positive signal, the multiple axon projections will form a disorganized microfascicular array, typical of a neuroma. The varied array of fiber types in a mixed nerve is a challenge. A mismatch of motor and sensory axons at the coaptation can cause fibers to enter the wrong type of Schwann cell sheath, failing to reach an appropriate target organ and eventually resulting in a nonfunctional recovery and subsequent cell death. Small fibers may regenerate more vigorously, with large fibers requiring mature myelin sheaths, taking longer to grow to the target and become functional. Brushart described preferential motor reinnervation.[3] Those axons that do reach their correct target organ will try to reconnect and regain function. Although the regenerated axons are fewer in number than the original pool, the human body has amazing adaptive physiology. Regenerated motor axons may innervate more muscle fibers than in the natural preinjury state, creating functional, albeit larger, motor units. This process of "adoption" of denervated muscle fibers by collateral sprouting from adjacent innervated muscle fibers was described by Brunelli[4] and explains the giant motor spikes measured by EMG following muscle reinnervation. Large motor units, coupled with loss of matched motor afferents, contribute to the loss of fine motor skills following recovery from injury to a motor nerve.[5]

Similarly, there is a resprouting of epidermal axons in the skin. Interestingly, this is a dynamic process. In rats following a sciatic nerve transection and reconstruction, collateral sprouts from adjacent intact fibers within the saphenous nerve spread to the denervated tibia nerve domain of the plantar foot. After 10 to 12 weeks, these fibers recede, when the regenerating tibial nerve fibers reach that area.[6,7,8,9] The adjacent collateral sprouting may reduce the impact of sensory loss after nerve injury, even without a complete recovery[10] and coupled with synaptic changes in the central nervous system, may contribute to the marginal hypersensitivity in cases where there is poor reinnervation in the injured nerve territory.

5.3.1 Timing of Normal Recovery

The rate of regeneration and functional recovery is dependent on a number of factors. Proximal injuries have faster initial axonal growth due to the proximity of the injury to the cell body. However, the long reinnervation distance to the distal targets leads to a prolonged period of denervation. Axonal growth is approximately 1 mm per day following a complete nerve injury transection and repair, although lower grades of axonopathy may recover more rapidly. Regeneration is less robust in more complex trauma when fewer cells survive the initial injury. Younger patients may have more resistance to apoptosis following injury, shorter limbs enable functional recovery more quickly than in adults, and the cortical plasticity potential in children enables better functional use when there is axonal misdirection following regeneration from a proximal injury. Clinical recovery may be monitored using the rate of progression of Tinel's sign after repair. The tender muscle sign may predate successful motor reinnervation and polyphasia may be detected on electromyography.[11]

5.4 Problems with Recovery

A surgical complication is any undesirable, unintended, and direct result of an operation affecting the patient which would not have occurred had the operation gone as well as could reasonably be hoped.[12] Nerve recovery after injury is frequently problematic, with neuropathic pain affecting the majority and trophic ulceration affecting denervated skin and stiff joints from disuse. Defining a complication is challenging. The Clavien-Dindo classification may be used to define variations from the planned postsurgery rehabilitation phase, with different degrees of severity indicated by unplanned therapy interventions, additional medication requirements, unplanned hospital admissions, or reoperations.[13,14]

5.4.1 Neuropathic Pain

Neuropathic pain follows disease or damage to the somatosensory nervous system. Pain is an inevitable consequence of peripheral nerve injury. There is normal nociceptive stimulation due to the injury and inflammatory response. However, disruption of both sensory and motor afferent signaling leads to modulation of the normal nociceptive pathways, increasing responsiveness to normal nociception. Maladaptive cortical plasticity leads to central sensitization, such that spontaneous pain may be experienced in the absence of nociceptive stimulation. Peripheral sensitization is associated with repair site neuromas and the abundant axonal sprouting results in chaotic immature microfascicles that are a source of both spontaneous pain and evoked pain from mechanical stimulation.[15] Marginal hypersensitivity results from collateral sprouting of intact cutaneous nerve ends in adjacent innervated skin in addition to modulation of normal sensory responses within the central nervous system. Scar tether of the repaired nerve may lead to neuropathic pain triggered by movement, known as neurostenalgia.

Neuropathic pain usually subsides as the axonal regeneration progresses and normal efferent and afferent signals are restored. Persistence of pain beyond the normal expected reinnervation window, especially when severe, may fulfill the criteria for a diagnosis of type 2 complex regional pain syndrome. This chronic pain condition has features of severe pain with over-responsiveness to painful (hyperalgesia) and nonpainful (allodynia) stimuli, hyperpathia, trophism, and autonomic disturbance.

Chronic pain is associated with a significant emotional impact with high rates of anxiety and depression. Coupled with the physical impact of the nerve injury, the socioeconomic impact of a nerve injury is profound. In a group of 31 patients, followed for 12 months following median and/or ulnar nerve repair, 21 patients were pain free. The remainder, with neuropathic pain, demonstrated greater impairment on tests of sensorimotor nerve conduction, worse sensory and motor recovery, as well as different personality structures and belief structures.[16] In a rodent peripheral nerve injury model, an unrepaired tibial nerve leads to the development of neuropathic pain characteristics. Delayed nerve repair is associated with neuropathic pain chronicity and poorer outcomes in humans. Undoubtedly, pain has a strong association with poor quality of life measures and also impedes functional recovery.[17] Davis and Curtin provide an overview of management of pain in complex nerve injuries.[15]

5.4.2 Scar

Scar is a normal consequence of injury and surgery. Scar within the nerve may follow under debridement, poor coaptation technique, excessive tension across the repair site or dehiscence of the repair site. Intraneural scar blocks axon regeneration resulting in a neuroma-in-continuity. Rupture of the repair may result in an end neuroma at the proximal stump. Nerves rely on a delicate paraneurium to allow physiological glide during functional movement. Nerves are flexible and can lengthen up to 8% strain before onset of irreversible changes to function. Following injury the nerve may scar within the surgery bed. Scar is more common in complex trauma with extensive tissue damage, poor vascularity, contamination, or following infection. Scar may constrict the nerve, resulting in ischemia, impaired conduction, and pain.[18,19,20] Scar may tether the nerve, preventing glide and producing neurostenalgia (neuropathic pain on passive stretch). Controlling scar at the site of nerve repair is a focus of contemporary research. Pharmacological manipulation of the intraneural milieu has demonstrated

promise in preclinical studies. Atkins et al demonstrated in M6PR/IGF2 null mice, which produce significantly less scar, that collagen staining decreased, compound action potentials increased, conduction velocities increased, and fiber counts distal to the repair site increased. This was in contrast to normal operated control mice and IL-4/IL-10 null mice, which produce increased scar.[21] To date, minimizing scarring, with anti-TGF β, has shown promise in rats. Tacrolimus administration has demonstrated enhanced axonal regeneration and reduced collagen formation. These results have not been translated to nerve repair protocols in humans, although studies evaluating the use with local delivery to minimize systemic side effects are gaining momentum. The effect of scar on the injured nerve has attracted attention from the biomedical device industry and innovation has resulted in the marketing of nerve connectors, using conduits as adjunctive detensioning devices for suture coaptation, entubulation of repair with suture-less coaptation,[22,23,24] and the use of biological and synthetic antiadhesion barriers.[25] Following re-exploration for neurolysis for repair site scar, autologous adipofascial tissues may be raised as vascularized pedicled flaps to resurface or even wrap a section of scarred nerve. Harvest site morbidity may be avoided by using commercially available wraps. Biological wraps are available with bovine, porcine, or equine origins and synthetic bioresorbable polymers provide alternative solutions. A porcine extracellular collagen-layered matrix from bowel submucosa has demonstrated increased vascularity in the nerve environment, allowing restoration of the normal mesoneurium. Antiadhesion gels containing carbohydrates or hyaluronic acid are commercially available, although there is no robust evidence to support their use currently.

5.4.3 Neuroma Formation

Following a transection of a peripheral nerve, damaged axons will repair their damaged cell membranes protecting them from further damage. Upregulation in the cell body prepares for regeneration. Axoplasmic transport carries new materials to the injury site. Surviving axons will expand and commence sprouting with multiple small filopodia. The growth cone represents this regenerative front, exploring the local microenvironment and responding to contact stimulation and neurotrophic feedback. Successful biofeedback will guide and strengthen regeneration. Without feedback, uncontrolled and disorganized proliferation of axons in scar creates a neuroma with histologically an array of microfascicles containing small and unmyelinated axons. Green's definition of a neuroma is "the inevitable, unavoidable, and biologic response of the proximal stump after it has been divided in situations where regenerating axons are impeded from re-entering the distal stump."[26] Therefore in every transected nerve, which is not reconstructed, there will be a fusiform swelling, or a neuroma, at the end of the proximal stump of a nerve. Every transected and unreconstructed nerve will form a neuroma, but this does not automatically follow that it will be symptomatic. Following a partial nerve injury with transection of some fascicles or a traction injury with some preservation of the nerve sheath, a neuroma-in-continuity may form at the site of injury. Following a repair, aberrant axon sprouting and scar will create a repair site neuroma. Typically, some axons will successfully populate the distal nerve segment and the recovery is incomplete. The need for secondary intervention on the postrepair neuroma-in-continuity will be determined by the proportion of axons reaching their targets, the site of the neuroma, and any scar tether. Superficially located neuromas are more commonly symptomatic due to their susceptibility to mechanical stimulation.

Symptomatic Neuroma

A clinically symptomatic neuroma is determined by spontaneous (basal and spikes) and evoked pain with a positive Tinel's sign at the site of injury. The pain is frequently described as having burning, shooting, electric shocks, pins and needles, crushing, or pressure characteristics. Local contact will evoke pain and this forms the basis of the Tinel's sign, reproducing unpleasant sensory perceptions in the territory of the injured nerve when tapping gently at the site of the suspected neuroma. Hyperalgesia and allodynia may be present with partial recovery through a neuroma-in-continuity; however, in an end-neuroma, the presence of these features in the distal cutaneous territory may be a sign of marginal hypersensitivity. There may be additional features typical of any nerve injury including cold sensitivity and a basal aching pain. Confirmation of the diagnosis is through pain reduction following a diagnostic local anesthetic nerve block.[27] Imaging with ultrasound or magnetic resonance neurography may have a limited role in confirming the site of neuroma; however, symptomatic neuroma remains a primarily clinical diagnosis.

Van den Avoort et al demonstrated that in only 7% of digital amputations neuromas become painful[28] and the rate of repair site neuroma in repaired digital nerves is approximately 5%.[29] Every neuroma may have the potential to produce pain. Perhaps the resilience of the individual has a role, or the reconfiguration of the spinal synaptic connections that rapidly follow nerve injury acts to suppress the pain successfully in the majority of cases. Smits et al identified that patients reporting cold intolerance demonstrated a disordered conditioned pain modulation (CPM) system[30] which is an inherent mechanism for pain suppression at the spinal cord level, tested by assessing whether a pain stimulus remains painful on provision of a strong contralateral limb pain stimulus. Neuromodulation therapy may reduce the pain severity and impact of a neuroma in some cases. Coupled with cognitive pain management strategies during the rein-

nervation phase and neurorehabilitation with mirror therapy, patients may avoid surgery.

5.4.4 Surgical Management of Symptomatic Neuromas

The surgical management of the painful neuroma depends on whether it is an end neuroma, a neuroma-in-continuity without useful distal function, or a neuroma-in-continuity with useful intact or recovered distal function.

Active Reconstruction Techniques

This term defines restoration of the original nerve gap allowing effective axonal regeneration to the original targets with the expectation of return or sensory and motor function.

Autologous Nerve Grafts

End neuromas, neuromas-in-continuity without function, and failed neurolysis for a neuroma-in-continuity require excision and reconstruction. The ideal technique is an active reconstruction procedure restoring physical continuity of the original nerve, reinnervating the distal targets, and restoring afferent signaling along the original neural pathway. Nerve autografts or allografts may be used in such cases. Typically, the resection gap is too long for bridging with a conduit in such salvage cases. The recipient site must be debrided to demonstrate fascicular structure, vascularity, and absence of intraneural scar to expose a cut nerve face capable of regeneration. There is no gold standard for debridement; however, neurotomes allow the nerve to be grasped without injury and the guillotine blade may be used to cut the nerve without crushing. Serrated microsurgical scissors are adequate for small diameter nerves; however, the main trunk nerves with dense scar are best managed with a blade. The nerve gap between the proximal and distal stumps must be measured in the anatomical position. Autograft requires harvest of an expendable cutaneous nerve to reconstruct the missing or damaged segment. There is a diameter mismatch and several cables of autograft will be used to build up the nerve gap to match the volume of the missing nerve. As such the length of autograft is often considerable and one or both sural nerves may need to be harvested from the lower limbs. The autologous graft cables are sutured into position and augmented with a fibrin glue. Coaptation sites may be wrapped; however, there is no evidence of additional efficacy to date in this type of reconstruction. The nerve graft must revascularize from the ends and additionally from the surgery bed. The high surface area conferred by the cable technique may aid this process. Animal studies have demonstrated that the main route of revascularization is through longitudinal growth from the proximal stump.

Nerve Allografts

Processed nerve allografts offer an attractive proposition for reconstruction of the failed nerve repair with a neuroma in continuity.[31] In a patient with established pain sensitization, the risk of donor site complications and symptomatic neuroma formation is considerable. There is no doubt that the published evidence supports the use of allograft in the management of symptomatic sensory nerve neuromas. However, to date, the evidence to support allograft for motor and mixed nerve reconstruction is limited. Allograft can be offered subject to appropriate consent and may have additional value in cases where lower limb surgery and general anesthesia is contraindicated. At this stage, it is recommended that allograft is used when functional reconstruction is not anticipated such as the longstanding lesion or in cases where an adjunctive distal motor reconstruction is planned with nerve/tendon transfer and therefore the prime objective of the allograft reconstruction is pain resolution and protective sensation. The current upper limit of gap length for allografts is 70 mm, although for sensory nerve reconstruction the robust evidence remains in gaps up to 50 mm only. In large nerve trunks, allograft can be used in a cabled configuration with individual allografts available in diameters between 1 and 5 mm.

Extra-anatomic Reconstruction Techniques

Nerve grafts provide an anatomical and functional reconstruction. In selected cases, using a nerve graft in combination with a distal nerve transfer for a key motor target or combining with tendon transfers allows pain management and sensory reconstruction through the original nerve with extra-anatomic motor function.

Passive Ablative Techniques

In rare cases for a main trunk nerve injury, particularly where the nerve gap is long, the nerve injury is longstanding and proximal so that useful functional recovery is unlikely, passive ablative procedures involving proximal nerve stump relocation or capping may be combined with a distal sensory nerve transfer as well as a motor reconstruction using nerve or tendon transfers, rather than reconstruction of a complex nerve gap that is likely to be unsuccessful.

Containment and shielding of the proximal nerve stump prevents mechanical stimulation, scar tether, and exposure to the biological stimulation afforded by nerve growth factor (NGF) in the vicinity of the nerve injury.

Active Ablation Techniques

Active ablative procedures are preferable to passive ablation of the proximal stump. An active procedure requires physiological axon regeneration without reinnervation of the original target. A nerve loop or graft to nowhere is an option; however, the use of targeted muscle reinnervation (TMR) or development of a reconstructive peripheral nerve interface (RPNI) are demonstrating superior efficacy in such cases. These can be combined with distal sensory and motor nerve/tendon transfers for functional restoration. TMR connects the proximal nerve stump, after neuroma resection, to a motor branch of a more proximal muscle.[32] Reinnervation from the mixed nerve stump to freshly denervated motor target may affect a functional recovery of that muscle with the additional benefit that normal efferent motor stimulation modulates the previously amplified sensory response. Some of the sensory axons will populate the intramuscular neural plexus, albeit without function, but the net benefit is a reduction in nerve pain. There is typically a size mismatch between the proximal and distal nerves. Additional wrapping with a denervated muscle flap (RPNI) potentially confers additional benefit, although it can be used in isolation where no expendable proximal motor branch exists.[33]

5.5 Sensory Recovery

Following proximal injury to the median and/or ulnar nerve, the loss of both functional and protective cutaneous sensibility causes considerable disability. All modalities of sensory innervation are lost, including somatic sensation and autonomic function. The loss of large diameter myelinated fibers which carry fast pain, temperature, and light touch sensation results in removal of protective feeling and the hand becomes vulnerable to trauma. Autonomic sudomotor loss results in absent sweating with dry skin that is prone to injury. The loss of vasomotor innervation results in erythema and altered temperature regulation. Patients must be educated so that they understand the risk of injury and maintain skin quality with emollients. Recovery of sensation is anticipated after nerve repair; however, the reinnervation window is dependent on the distance between the site of injury and the distal targets. Proximal injuries will take longer to regenerate distally. The final outcome is not easy to predict and there is a range of functional recovery, partly dependent on the number of axons reaching the hand, partly on the quality of the reinnervation, but importantly dependent on the injured nerve and the extent of relearning and cortical plasticity for an individual patient.

Recovering sensation can be estimated using quantitative sensory testing. Semmes-Weinstein monofilaments measure innervation density through pressure thresholds, 2-point discrimination (2PD), or moving 2-point discrimination (m2PD) measure innervation density as well as plasticity and may improve without further innervation due to learning. Both are practical tests to perform in the clinic and comparison is made with the contralateral uninjured hand.[34,35] The other sensory modalities may be tested using vibrometry, temperature perception, and skin capacitance (sweating); however, due to the complex testing protocols, they are generally reserved as a research tool.[36] Thermographic imaging demonstrates promise in measuring return of normal small fiber vasomotor tone. Small fibers regenerate rapidly and may predate large myelinated fiber functional innervation by some months. Perhaps the restoration of normal thermal responsiveness predicts further recovery of a repair or reconstruction.

5.5.1 Sensory Nerve Transfer

In a primary nerve injury case where there is extensive loss of a main nerve trunk, a poor surgical bed, and unlikely recovery through a graft, distal nerve transfers can be used as a primary reconstruction option. More often they are considered in the setting of a failed primary nerve repair, or in a situation where a proximal nerve repair has partial recovery. Excision and grafting of the primary lesion may confer no advantage and even pose a risk of further loss. In these situations, distal nerve transfer using an intact sensory nerve is potentially expendable to reinnervate the more important area of sensory loss. The donor is sectioned distally and rerouted proximally to the critical sensory nerve and an end-to-end coaptation is performed. This is useful when the patient has a risk of contact injury on the border hand areas due to trophic changes. An example would be using the third web space nerve from the median to transfer to the ulnar digital nerve of the small finger. The transfer can be performed distally in the hand to reduce reinnervation distances; however, if performed at the level of the carpal tunnel, the superficial branch of the ulnar nerve can be reinnervated in its entirety, providing sensory protection to the hypothenar area as well as the ulnar two digits. The scar from surgery is shorter and does not impact on finger mobility.

Reverse end-to-side suture of the recipient proximal cut end to a perineurial window in the otherwise intact donor is another option for restoration of some protective sensory; however, the quality is generally poor. The two techniques may be combined with a formal end-to-end coaptation for reinnervation of the primary target and an end-to-side to try and provide some recovery to the distal component of the donor sensory nerve.

5.6 Motor Recovery

Motor functional recovery is one of the primary objectives for acute repair or reconstruction of a main mixed motor nerve trunk within the forearm segment. Successful reinnervation is dependent on the severity of the original injury, the timing of the surgery, the quality of the repair, the distance to the target, and, for grafts, the length of the reconstruction gap. The majority of the fiber types in a mixed nerve are sensory and the relatively small population of motor axons must negotiate the repair site and successfully populate distal endoneural tubes to reach the intramuscular neural plexus of the correct target. Here they must restore the physiological coupling of the nerve and muscle at the motor end plate. The intramuscular neural plexus, the integrity of the motor end plate, and the receptiveness of the muscle to returning axons all decline with duration of denervation.[37,38,39] In time the progressive muscle atrophy is followed by fatty infiltration and fibrosis. The time limit for successful reinnervation is not fully understood. Optimum function is from early reinnervation; however, in the setting of a complete nerve injury, it appears that the failure to reinnervate by 9 to 12 months is associated with a high rate of failure. Even when a nerve is repaired acutely, the reinnervation distance can be too great for successful reinnervation of the most distally placed muscles in the reinnervation sequence. A high ulnar lesion at the level of the elbow remains a particular challenge because despite successful reinnervation of the proximal flexor carpi ulnaris and the ulnar innervated flexor digitorum profundus (FDP) to the ring and small fingers, the chances of reinnervation of the more distal intrinsic hand muscles is low. The hand will start to claw as the proximal muscles strengthen. The hand can be managed in a splint to control metacarpophalangeal hyperextension and later anticlaw tendon procedures can be completed. However, recognizing that the final outcome may be compromised can guide the treating clinician to consider augmentation of the primary reconstruction with a distal motor nerve transfer, or in the recovery phase, offering the patient a nerve transfer if the recovery rate is slower than predicted.

5.6.1 Motor Nerve Transfer

Nerve transfer is a rewiring of the nervous system. An expendable motor nerve branch or fascicle from within a mixed nerve is harvested distally and redirected into the proximally sectioned recipient motor nerve to a more important muscle or muscle group. The principle is that useful reinnervation of the denervated critical distal muscles can be accomplished more rapidly than from a proximal main trunk repair or reconstruction. When no recovery in the original nerve is to be expected due to the time-distance phenomenon, the coaptation of the nerve transfer can be as an end-to-end transfer, providing recovery potential only through the extra-anatomic pathway.

There is emerging interest in the role of either "babysitter" procedures, where some local neural support is provided to the distal nerve and muscle, to prevent complete atrophy while proximal regeneration proceeds distally.[40] The supercharging end-to-side (SETS) transfer has been popularized for use in the distal motor component of the ulnar nerve using the motor innervation of pronator quadratus from the anterior interosseous nerve coapted through a perineurial window in the fascicles supplying the deep motor branch of the ulnar nerve in the distal forearm.[41] Nerve transfer may be used as a component of the primary repair strategy, but is often considered when the rate of Tinel's progression from the proximal repair is slow. In such situations the nerve transfer is a salvage procedure and aims to bring motor axon innervation to denervated muscles between 6 and 9 months.

5.6.2 Tendon Transfers for Paralysis Reconstruction

Tendon transfers are the main reconstruction option for the management of longstanding paralysis. Early tendon transfer can be considered rarely in the setting of acute complex nerve trauma. For a high radial nerve injury requiring a nerve graft, an early distal pronator teres to extensor carpi radialis brevis (ECRB) tendon transfer allows functional use of the hand with active wrist extension and passive tenodesis digit extension. Typically tendon transfers are used as salvage when the primary nerve reconstruction has failed, or there is imbalance due to good innervation of proximal muscles and poor distal reinnervation, such as development of clawing in the hand after a high ulnar nerve repair. There is no upper limit after which tendon transfer cannot be performed, as long as the principles are adhered to and the donor muscle is strong and expendable and the recipient joints are flexible and stable. Due to the change of vector of pull and failure to restore the original sarcomere resting length after tenotomy and transfer, muscles used for tendon transfer will inevitably lose peak strength. One of the advantages of nerve transfer is the restoration of innervation to the original muscle, in its original bed without alteration of fiber length. However in the setting of a lower motor neuron injury, the time critical nature of motor nerve transfer renders this technique less useful in the context of salvage for a failed primary nerve repair. Motor nerve transfer is considered an adjunct to a primary nerve reconstruction when poor function is the probable outcome.

5.7 Distal Entrapment Following Proximal Repair

Following repair, the growth cone is the distal end of the regenerating axonal front where each axon has numerous filopodia searching for contact feedback and neurotrophic stimulation to enable potentiation and guidance of the axon. The distal nerve requires structural components and organelles for function and these must be assembled in the proximal nerve cell and transported to the site of injury along the cytoskeleton. Axoplasmic streaming is critical to this outward growth. Eventually, the large fibers will become invested in a mature myelin sheath to provide mechanical support, protection, and enable restoration of mature action potential transmission using saltatory conduction. Prior to these events, the regenerating axon is swollen and vulnerable to compression with impaired action potential transmission. The nerve as a whole is vulnerable to extrinsic compression. Less well described is the concept of distal entrapment remote from the injury repair site at a point of natural compression. Perhaps the presence of scar at the proximal site further renders the nerve susceptible to distal entrapment, as a "double crush." The clinical presentation is a slowing of the rate of Tinel's progression, a delay in further motor and sensory recovery, and strong Tinel's signs at compression points that persist on sequential visits. In this situation, distal entrapment release confers advantages, although there are few reports in the literature. Our experience is that distal decompression reduces pain, and improves conduction in regenerated nerves with demonstrable motor and sensory upgrading in a timeframe that cannot be explained by further regeneration.[41,42,43,44]

5.8 Follow-Up after Nerve Repair and Clinical Decision-Making

The peripheral nerve surgeon must be familiar with the anatomy of the peripheral nerves and the pathophysiology of injury and regeneration. Following proximal nerve repair or reconstruction with grafts, the rate of regeneration can be anticipated and monitored using simple clinical observations in the clinic. Tinel's points moving distally at a rate of at least 1 mm per day with gradual reduction of intensity at the repair site is a positive sign. Tenderness on muscle squeeze may be a sign of early motor reinnervation. Restoration of sweating in the target cutaneous area predates useful sensory reinnervation. Resolution of neuropathic pain with functional regeneration is to be expected. The problem is that there is often a delay between repair and the ability to measure useful distal functional recovery, and so monitoring the progression is key to determining whether an outcome is likely to be positive.

Worsening pain is concerning. Pain at the repair site with a poorly or nonadvancing Tinel's sign may predict a neuroma. Poor recovery with nerve tether on passive stretch producing pain may necessitate neurolysis; static Tinel's at distal entrapment sites, increasing pain, and slowing of recovery progression may diagnose distal entrapment. The nerve surgeon must be able to interpret these signs and be prepared to personally review the patient regularly and monitor progression at sequential clinic visits. The decision to re-explore the area of injury and consider revision of the primary repair with grafts must not be taken lightly. However, without close observation and prompt action when needed, the outcome will be compromised and salvage options for pain, sensory restoration, and motor recovery may be inferior to an early revision with distal nerve transfers if warranted. Imaging and neurophysiology testing have little role in the monitoring of recovery. A targeted electromyographic (EMG) sampling of a key muscle in the regenerating sequence can be helpful when motor recovery is delayed to determine whether there is any preclinical recovery that would defer re-exploration. It should be noted that EMG findings cannot predict the quality of the motor recovery and a clinical judgment is always required.[10,45]

5.9 Management of Nerve Specific Problems

5.9.1 Median Nerve

The median nerve sensory function is key to functional use of the hand. Repair site pain with no advancing Tinel's sign raises suspicion of a neuroma. Revision of the repair with debridement to healthy nerve stumps and autologous-cabled nerve grafting is the recommended treatment.[46] If there is pain from tether and some distal recovery, consideration should be given to neurolysis and wrapping to prevent further scar encasement and tether. Failure to resolve pain is a possibility and the patient should be aware that the next option is excision and grafting with consequent loss of any regenerated function. As a prelude, a diagnostic local anesthetic nerve block can demonstrate the likely effects of nerve resection and prepare them for surgery. When the bed is poor, consideration should be given to autologous flap resurfacing to ensure an optimized environment for nerve grafting. If the bed is likely to remain compromised due to the severity of the original trauma and the gap is likely to be longer than 70 mm, the option of salvage distal sensory transfers can be discussed. Superficial radial nerve branches can be sutured to the ulnar digital nerve of the thumb and to the radial digital nerve of the index to provide some contact sensation for precision grips. Alternatively, the fourth webspace common digital nerve can be sacrificed and directed to the first webspace branches of the median nerve at the level of the carpal tunnel.

In the setting of a high-median nerve injury at the level of the elbow, primary repair or if needed a graft should achieve functional recovery in the proximal forearm muscles. An augmentation distal nerve transfer to the motor branch of the median nerve may be considered as a distal augmentation. Donor motor nerves have been described from the palmar interossei (ulnar), from the abductor digiti minimi (ulnar),[47] from the distal PIN, and for median nerve injury with AIN preservation, the nerve to pronator quadratus (AIN) can be transferred to the motor fascicles of the median nerve in the distal forearm. In the setting of a distal median nerve injury, the AIN to thenar motor branch nerve transfer can be performed; however, an interposition nerve graft is required.[48]

The functional gains from a tendon transfer for restoring palmar abduction and opposition are predictable and an extensor indicis proprius tendon transfer to abductor pollicis brevis remains a useful strategy. Generally, this is reserved for later in the rehabilitation pathway when there is clear evidence of progressive recovery from the proximal recovery and no secondary surgery is predicted at the original site.

Soldado et al suggested the use of nerve transfers to improve function in high-median nerve lesions.[49] These techniques may be applied to the complex high-median nerve lesion as a hybrid reconstruction in combination with a nerve autograft for sensory function, or in combination with a distal sensory nerve transfer when the primary injury is not deemed suitable for an anatomical reconstruction. The transfers may also be offered in the setting of a failed primary repair in the upper arm presenting after 6 months when a revision of the primary repair to a graft is possible for sensory restoration and pain resolution, but useful motor recovery from a salvage nerve autologous graft is unlikely to be successful. Supinator nerve branches from the PIN may be transferred to the nerve to flexor digitorum superficialis, and the nerve to ECRB may be transferred to the AIN. These transfers can be combined with a distal transfer to the recurrent motor branch of the median nerve using the ADQ or with an opposition tendon transfer.[49]

In late salvage beyond 9 months, tendon transfers may be used for motor reconstruction of high-median nerve paralysis. Brachioradialis tendon transfer to flexor pollicis longus may be combined with buddying of the median innervated FDP tendons to the functioning ulnar innervated FDPs to the ring and small fingers in the distal forearm. The alternative is to use ECRL as a tendon transfer to the FDPs to the index and middle fingers. Opposition reconstruction can be accomplished using the EIP tendon transfer, or in distal median nerve injuries at the wrist, the FDS from the ring provides a useful opposition tendon transfer with an ulnar-sided pulley at FCU to redirect the pull. The FDS may not be available if the original median nerve injury also damaged the FDS tendons. Pedicled transfer of the ADQ muscle to the thumb is another option for restoring opposition and abduction function in the thumb.[50]

5.9.2 Ulnar Nerve

In the hand the ulnar nerve innervation of intrinsic muscles provides initiation of MCPJ flexion and fine motor control and balance to the long digital flexor and extensor function. The terminal deep motor branch of the ulnar nerve controls precision grips with the thumb and index finger. The sensory innervation to the ulnar two digits and the ulnar border of the hand provides sensory feedback to protect from injury. The proximal ulnar nerve supplies FCU for wrist control and the ulnar FDPs for power grip. The dorsal branch of the ulnar nerve, in the distal third of the forearm provides protective sensation to the dorsoulnar hand.

Injury to the ulnar nerve in the distal forearm results in loss of the distal sensation and the hand intrinsic function with preservation of the extrinsic digital flexion and FCU function. Failed primary repair, or late presentation of a transection injury, may be salvaged by exploration and debridement of any neuroma and autologous cable nerve grafts. Due to the distal location of the injury, revision surgery up to 6 months may successfully restore distal motor function and sensory improvements can be achieved up to 24 months. Generally, as in all anatomic nerve reconstruction, the best results are from early surgery. During autologous grafting, attention should be given to the topography of the ulnar nerve above the wrist. In the distal third of the forearm there is well-defined distribution of the motor fascicle groups in the central fascicles, between the superficial and radially placed superficial ulnar nerve and the deep and ulnarly positioned dorsal branch of the ulnar nerve.[51] Failing to direct the cabled grafts appropriately can result in no functional recovery. Non-reconstructable primary lesions and failed salvage with autologous grafts may be treated with sensory nerve transfer from the third webspace (median) to the superficial ulna nerve in Guyon's canal.

Persistence of clawing with failed distal motor recovery may be salvaged with anticlaw procedures, including static anticlaw from MCPJ volar plate advancement, FDS loops to provide a restraint to MCPJ hyperextension, or active transfer with FDS looped through the flexor sheath at the base of the digit or an intrinsic reconstruction with transfer of a split FDS transfer to the lumbrical or its insertion on the lateral band. Often in an ulnar nerve lesion, transfer is required only to the ring and small fingers. Thumb adduction and first dorsal interosseous (DIO) reconstruction can be achieved with transfer of the EIP to the adductor pollicis and transfer of a slip of APL, lengthened with a palmaris longus graft to the first DI.

High ulnar nerve lesions in the proximal forearm or above have the previously mentioned distal motor and sensory deficits in addition to the loss of the FCU and the FDP to the ring and small.[52,53]

Acute proximal UN repair at or distal to the midhumerus level should achieve innervation of the ulnar innervated FDPs; however, distal restoration of motor function to the ulnar innervated intrinsic muscles is unlikely in adults due to the time-distance phenomenon. Augmentation of distal motor function with transfer of the AIN innervation to PQ to the motor fascicles to the deep branch of the ulnar nerve above the wrist may provide an alternative pathway for some ulnar intrinsic reinnervation.[54] The transfer can be completed using the SETS, end-to-end, or hemi end-to-end onto a part sectioned deep ulnar motor fascicle. The evidence to support these techniques is limited; however, functional recovery has been demonstrated in small case series. The theory is that even partial nonfunctional innervation of the ulnar intrinsics may provide a longer reinnervation window for advancing motor axons from the proximal injury and repair in SETS and hemi end-to-end transfer. The completed end-to-end nerve transfer is recommended when there is no attempt at proximal repair or reconstruction. Transferring the motor branch of the opponens (median) to the deep branch of the ulnar nerve while leaving the branch to the abductor pollicis brevis intact is also an option.[55] Ulnar intrinsic reconstruction is also an option that can be used as salvage in a nonrecovering ulnar nerve repair within the forearm.

The advancing Tinel's sign is the only way to effectively monitor the rate of axonal regeneration from a proximal repair of the ulnar nerve, and the tender muscle squeeze sign in the FCU and FDP muscle mass may reassure that recovery is proceeding in line with expectation. A static Tinel's sign and neuropathic pain is suggestive of a neuroma. Re-exploration within 6 months and neuroma resection stump debridement and cabled autograft interposition may salvage proximal motor function and distal sensation. Presenting after 6 months, anatomical reconstruction at the primary site of injury is unlikely to achieve any motor recovery and is a strategy only for pain management and sensory restoration. TMR of the ulnar nerve to the motor branch to brachialis is an alternative strategy for neuroma pain and can be coupled with extra-anatomic distal motor and/or tendon transfer plus a distal sensory nerve transfer for functional recovery.

Motor reconstruction of proximal ulnar nerve function can be achieved with nerve to ECRB transfer to the FDP to the ulnar digits in the proximal forearm, and the brachialis fascicle can be transferred to the ulnar nerve as long as the primary lesion is above this coaptation. These are salvage nerve transfer options with severe proximal ulnar nerve avulsion injuries with long gaps and uncertain quality of the axon population of the proximal nerve stump. These transfers may be combined with the AIN to deep ulnar nerve motor transfer and sensory transfers using the third web (median) to superficial ulnar nerve and palmar branch median nerve or superficial radial nerve (SRN) branch to dorsal branch of the ulnar nerve for cutaneous protective sensation in the dorsoulnar hand.

Tendon transfer reconstruction of motor paralysis in the ulnar nerve is well documented.[52,53] Tendon transfers may be combined with nerve transfers and anatomical reconstruction of the primary nerve gap; however, typically they are reserved for the failed primary repair with no functional recovery or incomplete functional recovery with claw posture in the hand and absence of thumb adduction following successful proximal innervation. In such cases the aim is to rebalance the hand and improve function. Proximal reconstruction for the ulnar FDPs may be achieved through buddying to the median innervated FDPs to the index and middle in the distal forearm, or through transfer of the extensor carpi radialis longus (ECRL) tendon to the FDP ring and small. The loss of the radial deviating force at the wrist is a useful additional benefit due to the absent FCU function. For hand function the losses are thumb adduction, first DIO, the ADQ, the palmar and dorsal interossei, and the ulnar two lumbrical muscles.

Tendon transfers for the adductor of the thumb include EIP transfer to the adductor pollicis or ECRB to adductor pollicis with a lengthening tendon graft. These help to restore key and pinch grip for the thumb and can be combined with the transfer of the EPB to the first DIO with a graft described earlier. If a claw is present, this needs to be examined carefully. The most important test is the Bouvier maneuver.[52] If the IP-joint extends on passive flexion of the MP-joint, only a Zancolli lasso is necessary. In this procedure the FDS is fixed around the A1-pulley and this pulls the MP-joint in flexion, which corrects the IP-joint. If the IP-joint does not extend on MP-joint flexion different transfer is necessary, and a transfer needs to be attached to the lateral slips. The FDS can be transferred to the lateral bands. If the FDS is not available, for instance in a high ulnar nerve lesion, this can be corrected with an ECRB transfer to the intrinsics (a Brand procedure, for which two versions exist, Brand 1 and 2).[53] In that case the brachioradialis can be used for adductor-plasty. If no clawing is present, the addition slip of the APL to the first dorsal interosseous provides a counter force for the thumb.

5.9.3 Radial Nerve

The most common site of trauma to the radial nerve is in the upper arm, often associated with fractures of the humerus. Low injury may affect the PIN and the SRN. Early repair and, if necessary, nerve grafting are still considered the gold standard due to the anticipated success of the procedure. In severe lesions, a distal pronator teres to ECRB tendon transfer provides a useful internal splint for wrist extension and digital extension through tenodesis while recovery from the proximal repair is awaited.

Radial nerve neuromas at the site of previous repair may be suspected if there is no reinnervation of the brachioradialis (BR) in the expected time frame, neuropathic pain, and a static Tinel's sign at the site of repair.[27] In such cases, re-exploration within 6 months may enable excision of the neuroma, debridement to health nerve stumps, and cabled autograft reconstruction. Recovery of the BR, ECRL, and ECRB can be expected with sensory recovery to the SRN within 6 to 12 months. Recovery of the PIN innervated muscles is less predictable with salvage surgery at 6 months and there are different reconstructive strategies that may be employed. The radial nerve graft can be augmented with distal nerve transfers using flexor carpi radialis and palmaris longus fascicles from the median nerve to the PIN excluding the supinator branches and a PT tendon transfer to the ECRB end-to-side to provide an internal splint. Alternatively, the radial nerve can be grafted for pain management, sensory recovery, and functional recovery in BR and ECRL and a double nerve transfer using the FDS (median) to the ECRB and the FCR/PL to the PIN.[56] The PT to ECRB tendon transfer can be added for the early tenodesis and functional wrist extension. Finally, the patient can be observed to establish whether there is any recovery from the nerve graft, and if not a set of triple tendon transfers for high radial nerve palsy, or if there is functional wrist extension, low radial tendon transfers for PIN palsy can be performed at this late stage. There are several descriptions for triple transfer and the PT to ECRB, FCR to EDC, and PL to EPL are reliable. The latter two are used for PIN palsy alone. There is no consensus to date on the role of nerve transfers in the management of radial nerve palsy and proponents of tendon transfer express concern that using the FCR/PL fascicles for an early nerve transfer may exclude the option of a later tendon transfer should the nerve transfer prove unsuccessful. Bertelli compared nerve transfers and tendon transfers for radial nerve palsy.[57] AIN to ECRB and FCR branch to PIN and an FCU transfer to EDC, PT to ECRB, and PL to EPL found better results in the nerve transfers. Both groups had an extension lag of the thumb of 30 degrees. In the tendon transfers half of the group could not extend the fingers on wrist extension, which was possible in all nerve transfer patients. Drawbacks of tendon transfers include loss of terminal wrist flexion due to the tendon transfer to EDC crossing the wrist and the loss of some independence of MCPJ extension due to the mass effect of the transfer to all four digits.

In partial recovery through a radial nerve repair or graft, exploration and neurolysis with nerve wrapping may salvage additional function, with distal nerve and tendon transfers available for salvage.

In a severe injury with no recovery and neuroma pain, TMR of the proximal radial nerve stump to one of the triceps branches or brachialis may help manage the neuropathic pain and the motor reconstruction can be done using the distal nerve and tendon transfers discussed earlier.

The sensory loss from the SRN in such cases is usually not of a functional consequence; however, it is possible to reinnervate the SRN territory with a reverse end-to-side coaptation of the distal nerve to the median nerve in the forearm, albeit at some risk of inducing sensitivity in the median nerve territory. Other donor nerves may pose a lesser risk, and end-to-end transfer from the lateral cutaneous nerve of the forearm is an attractive option.

5.9.4 Combined Nerve Injury

Rarely there is injury to more than one of the main nerve trunks in the upper limb. In such cases, all efforts should be made to repair or reconstruct the primary nerve injury due to the uncertainty of recovery and the greater numbers of important functions to reconstruct with a limited number of donors for nerve or tendon transfer. In all such cases the salvage procedures offered will be dependent on the specific deficits and the availability of donors. Decision making is challenging. A functional assessment with a hand therapist will help guide reconstruction for an individual based on their specific needs. The use of wrist arthrodesis to free up additional tendons for transfer can be considered; however, the tenodesis action of wrist motion on digit position will be lost. Wrist tenodesis is valuable in augmenting the function of weak donor muscles for tendon transfer or poorly tensioned tendon transfers, improving excursion and function.

5.10 Failed Salvage Surgery

The prime objective of any surgery is to provide the greatest chance of functional recovery for a given injury. The first procedure must be performed well. Knowledge of the anticipated outcome and the need for later salvage can guide the primary treatment with introduction of augmentation nerve and tendon transfers to the primary algorithm, especially in cases of late presentation and with large gaps. The secondary surgery will be for pain management, reconstruction of paralysis, or recovery of protective sensation, or combinations of all three. Prior to any planned secondary intervention, the peripheral nerve surgeon should first attempt to ascertain the reasons for the failure of the primary procedure to achieve the planned objectives. Failure of secondary procedures leaves few options for salvage. Neuropathic pain may be managed by TMR, ignoring further attempts at functional recovery through the nerve and using extra-anatomic reconstruction techniques with nerve and/or tendon transfers.

5.11 Take-Home Message

Following primary surgery on a main nerve trunk in the upper limb, the common problems that the peripheral nerve surgeon must face include symptomatic neuroma formation with no functional recovery, partial recovery with nerve tether at the repair site, recovery with distal entrapment compromising the functional recovery, poor motor and/or sensory recovery, and rarely a neuropathic pain syndrome that is related to the peripheral and/or central reorganization of neuropathic pain pathways with pain modulation and sensitization.

Instigating the correct primary treatment, and recognizing the limitations of nerve repair at a given anatomical location, is key. Prompt intervention for the failed or faltering regeneration with secondary reconstruction and augmentation distal reconstruction may salvage the situation. Persistence of pain and recurrent neuromas may require neurolysis, nerve wrapping, and TMR. Poor recovery may be improved with distal decompression or distal nerve or tendon transfers for motor function. Poor sensory recovery can be treated with further attempts at nerve reconstruction, or rarely distal sensory nerve transfers. Key to success is early, appropriate surgery and regular clinical follow-up monitoring for critical signs of reinnervation.

References

[1] Boeckstyns MEH, Sørensen AI, Viñeta JF, et al. Collagen conduit versus microsurgical neurorrhaphy: 2-year follow-up of a prospective, blinded clinical and electrophysiological multicenter randomized, controlled trial. J Hand Surg Am. 2013; 38(12):2405–2411

[2] Kirsch M, Brown S, Smith BW, Chang KWC, Koduri S, Yang LJS. The presence and persistence of unrealistic expectations in patients undergoing nerve surgery. Neurosurgery. 2020; 86(6):778–782

[3] Brushart TM. Motor axons preferentially reinnervate motor pathways. J Neurosci. 1993; 13(6):2730–2738

[4] Brunelli G, Brunelli F. Partial selective denervation in spastic palsies (hyponeurotization). Microsurgery. 1983; 4(4):221–224

[5] Gordon T. Nerve regeneration: understanding biology and its influence on return of function after nerve transfers. Hand Clin. 2016; 32 (2):103–117

[6] Duraku LS, Hossaini M, Hoendervangers S, et al. Spatiotemporal dynamics of re-innervation and hyperinnervation patterns by uninjured CGRP fibers in the rat foot sole epidermis after nerve injury. Mol Pain. 2012; 8:61

[7] Duraku LS, Hossaini M, Schüttenhelm BN, et al. Re-innervation patterns by peptidergic Substance-P, non-peptidergic P2X3, and myelinated NF-200 nerve fibers in epidermis and dermis of rats with neuropathic pain. Exp Neurol. 2013; 241:13–24

[8] Kambiz S, Baas M, Duraku LS, et al. Innervation mapping of the hind paw of the rat using Evans Blue extravasation, Optical Surface Mapping and CASAM. J Neurosci Methods. 2014; 229:15–27

[9] Kambiz S, Duraku LS, Baas M, et al. Long-term follow-up of peptidergic and nonpeptidergic reinnervation of the epidermis following sciatic nerve reconstruction in rats. J Neurosurg. 2015; 123(1):254–269

[10] Rayner M, Brown H, Wilcox M, Phillips J, Quick T. Quantifying regeneration in patients following peripheral nerve injury Journal of Plastic. Reconstructive & Aesthetic Surgery. 2019; 73(2):201–208

[11] Lee EY, Karjalainen TV, Sebastin SJ, Lim AY. The value of the tender muscle sign in detecting motor recovery after peripheral nerve reconstruction. J Hand Surg Am. 2015; 40(3):433–437

[12] Sokol DK, Wilson J. What is a surgical complication? World J Surg. 2008; 32(6):942–944

[13] Dindo D, Demartines N, Clavien PA. Classification of surgical complications: a new proposal with evaluation in a cohort of 6336 patients and results of a survey. Ann Surg. 2004; 240(2):205–213

[14] Sink EL, Leunig M, Zaltz I, Gilbert JC, Clohisy J, Academic Network for Conservational Hip Outcomes Research Group. Reliability of a complication classification system for orthopaedic surgery. Clin Orthop Relat Res. 2012; 470(8):2220–2226

[15] Davis G, Curtin CM. Management of pain in complex nerve injuries. Hand Clin. 2016; 32(2):257–262

[16] Taylor KS, Anastakis DJ, Davis KD. Chronic pain and sensorimotor deficits following peripheral nerve injury. Pain. 2010; 151(3):582–591

[17] Ciaramitaro P, Mondelli M, Logullo F, et al. Italian Network for Traumatic Neuropathies. Traumatic peripheral nerve injuries: epidemiological findings, neuropathic pain and quality of life in 158 patients. J Peripher Nerv Syst. 2010; 15(2):120–127

[18] Sunderland IR, Brenner MJ, Singham J, Rickman SR, Hunter DA, Mackinnon SE. Effect of tension on nerve regeneration in rat sciatic nerve transection model. Ann Plast Surg. 2004; 53(4):382–387

[19] Starkweather RJ, Neviaser RJ, Adams JP, Parsons DB. The effect of devascularization on the regeneration of lacerated peripheral nerves: an experimental study. J Hand Surg Am. 1978; 3(2):163–167

[20] Nath RK, Kwon B, Mackinnon SE, Jensen JN, Reznik S, Boutros S. Antibody to transforming growth factor beta reduces collagen production in injured peripheral nerve. Plast Reconstr Surg. 1998; 102(4):1100–1106, discussion 1107–1108

[21] Atkins S, Smith KG, Loescher AR, et al. Scarring impedes regeneration at sites of peripheral nerve repair. Neuroreport. 2006; 17(12):1245–1249

[22] Parthiban S, Foster MA, Beale S, Power D. Interim analysis of recruitment data for a randomized control trial of digital nerve repair. J Musculoskelet Surg Res. 2019; 3(1):86–89

[23] Neubrech F, Heider S, Harhaus L, Bickert B, Kneser U, Kremer T. Chitosan nerve tube for primary repair of traumatic sensory nerve lesions of the hand without a gap: study protocol for a randomized controlled trial. Trials. 2016; 17(1):48

[24] Zhu X, Wei H, Zhu H. Nerve wrap after end-to-end and tension-free neurorrhaphy attenuates neuropathic pain: A prospective study based on cohorts of digit replantation. Sci Rep. 2018; 8(1):620

[25] Jordaan PW, Uhiara O, Power D. Management of the scarred nerve using porcine submucosa extracellular matrix nerve wraps. Journal of Musculoskeletal Surgery and Research. 2019; 3(1):128–133

[26] Watson J, Gonzalez M, Romero A, Kerns J. Neuromas of the hand and upper extremity. J Hand Surg Am. 2010; 35(3):499–510

[27] Arnold DMJ, Wilkens SC, Coert JH, Chen NC, Ducic I, Eberlin KR. Diagnostic criteria for symptomatic neuroma. Ann Plast Surg. 2019; 82 (4):420–427

[28] van der Avoort DJ, Hovius SE, Selles RW, van Neck JW, Coert JH. The incidence of symptomatic neuroma in amputation and neurorrhaphy patients. J Plast Reconstr Aesthet Surg. 2013; 66(10):1330–1334

[29] Dunlop RLE, Wormald JCR, Jain A. Outcome of surgical repair of adult digital nerve injury: a systematic review. BMJ Open. 2019; 9(3): e025443

[30] Smits ES, Selles RW, Huygen FJ, Duraku LS, Hovius SE, Walbeehm ET. Disordered conditioned pain modulation system in patients with posttraumatic cold intolerance. J Plast Reconstr Aesthet Surg. 2014; 67(1):68–73

[31] Safa B, Buncke G. Autograft Substitutes. Hand Clin. 2016; 32(2):127–140

[32] Dumanian GA, Potter BK, Mioton LM, et al. Targeted muscle reinnervation treats neuroma and phantom pain in major limb amputees: a randomized clinical trial. Ann Surg. 2019; 270(2):238–246

[33] Kozusko S, Kaminsky A, Boyd L, Konofaos P. Sensory neurotization of muscle: past, present and future considerations. J Plast Surg Hand Surg. 2018; 4:1–6

[34] Lundborg G, Rosén B. The two-point discrimination test: time for a re-appraisal? J Hand Surg [Br]. 2004; 29(5):418–422

[35] Dellon AL, Mackinnon SE, Crosby PM. Reliability of two-point discrimination measurements. J Hand Surg Am. 1987; 12(5 Pt 1):693–696

[36] Wilder-Smith OH. Chronic pain and surgery: a review of new insights from sensory testing. J Pain Palliat Care Pharmacother. 2011; 25 (2):146–159

[37] Holmes W, Young JZ. Nerve regeneration after immediate and delayed suture. J Anat. 1942; 77(Pt 1):63–96, 10

[38] Fu SY, Gordon T. Contributing factors to poor functional recovery after delayed nerve repair: prolonged axotomy. J Neurosci. 1995; 15 (5 Pt 2):3876–3885

[39] Fu SY, Gordon T. Contributing factors to poor functional recovery after delayed nerve repair: prolonged denervation. J Neurosci. 1995; 15(5 Pt 2):3886–3895

[40] Barbour J, Yee A, Kahn LC, Mackinnon SE. Supercharged end-to-side anterior interosseous to ulnar motor nerve transfer for intrinsic musculature reinnervation. J Hand Surg Am. 2012; 37(10):2150–2159

[41] Johnston RB, Zachary L, Dellon AL, Mackinnon SE, Gottlieb L. The effect of a distal site of compression on neural regeneration. J Reconstr Microsurg. 1993; 9(4):271–274, discussion 274–275

[42] Żyluk A, Puchalski P, Szlosser Z. Development of carpal tunnel syndrome after repair of the median nerve in the distal forearm. J Hand Surg Eur Vol. 2018; 43(3):332–333

[43] Schoeller T, Otto A, Wechselberger G, Pommer B, Papp C. Distal nerve entrapment following nerve repair. Br J Plast Surg. 1998; 51(3):227–229, discussion 230

[44] Wilson TJ, Kleiber GM, Nunley RM, Mackinnon SE, Spinner RJ. Distal peroneal nerve decompression after sciatic nerve injury secondary to total hip arthroplasty. J Neurosurg. 2018; 130(1):179–183

[45] Holzgrefe RE, Wagner ER, Singer AD, Daly CA. Imaging of the peripheral nerve: concepts and future direction of magnetic resonance neurography and ultrasound. J Hand Surg Am. 2019; 44(12):1066–1079

[46] Leckenby JI, Furrer C, Haug L, Juon Personeni B, Vögelin E. A retrospective case series reporting the outcomes of advance nerve allografts in the treatment of peripheral nerve injuries. Plast Reconstr Surg. 2020; 145(2):368e–381e

[47] Bertelli JA, Soldado F, Rodrígues-Baeza A, Ghizoni MF. Transfer of the motor branch of the abductor digiti quinti for thenar muscle reinnervation in high median nerve injuries. J Hand Surg Am. 2018; 43(1):8–15

[48] Brown JM, Mackinnon SE. Nerve transfers in the forearm and hand. Hand Clin. 2008; 24(4):319–340, v

[49] Soldado F, Bertelli JA, Ghizoni MF. High median nerve injury: motor and sensory nerve transfers to restore function. Hand Clin. 2016; 32 (2):209–217

[50] Loewenstein SN, Adkinson JM. Tendon transfers for peripheral nerve palsies. Clin Plast Surg. 2019; 46(3):307–315

[51] Barrett JE, Farooq H, Merrell GA. Reliability of focal identification of motor fascicles of the ulnar nerve proximal to the wrist: an anatomical study. J Hand Surg Eur Vol. 2020; 45(3):237–241

[52] Revol M, Servant JM. Paralysis of the intrinsic muscles of the hand. Chir Main. 2008; 27(1):1–11

[53] Hentz VR. Tendon transfers after peripheral nerve injuries: my preferred techniques. J Hand Surg Eur Vol. 2019; 44(8):775–784

[54] Brown JM, Yee A, Mackinnon SE. Distal median to ulnar nerve transfers to restore ulnar motor and sensory function within the hand: technical nuances. Neurosurgery. 2009; 65(5):966–977, discussion 977–978

[55] Bertelli JA, Soldado F, Rodrígues-Baeza A, Ghizoni MF. Transferring the motor branch of the opponens pollicis to the terminal division of the deep branch of the ulnar nerve for pinch reconstruction. J Hand Surg Am. 2019; 44(1):9–17

[56] Mackinnon SE, Roque B, Tung TH. Median to radial nerve transfer for treatment of radial nerve palsy. Case report. J Neurosurg. 2007; 107 (3):666–671

[57] Bertelli JA. Nerve versus tendon transfer for radial nerve paralysis reconstruction. J Hand Surg Am. 2020; 45(5):418–426

2

6 Management of Complications of Nerve Decompression Surgery

6.1 Part A: Complications of Carpal Tunnel Release

Daniel J. Nagle

Abstract

Carpal tunnel syndrome is the most common nerve compression in the upper extremity. Carpal tunnel release surgery provides patients with predictably good outcomes; however, complications do occur infrequently. This chapter will review the diagnosis, treatment, and outcomes of intraoperative and postoperative complications associated with carpal tunnel release.

Keywords: carpal tunnel surgery, carpal tunnel release, complications

6.1.1 Introduction

Carpal tunnel syndrome is the most common nerve compression in the upper extremity. The prevalence of carpal tunnel syndrome in the United States general population has been estimated to be 3.72%,[1] and in 2006 approximately 577,000 carpal tunnel releases were performed.[2] Carpal tunnel release surgery provides patients with predictably good outcomes; however, complications do occur infrequently. This chapter will review the diagnosis, treatment, and outcomes of intraoperative and postoperative complications associated with carpal tunnel release.

6.1.2 Intraoperative Complications

Nerve Injury

Nerve injury can be the most devastating of all the intraoperative complications that can occur during a carpal tunnel release. The median nerve trunk, the palmer cutaneous branch and motor branch of the median nerve, the ulnar nerve, and the digital nerves are all at risk. Benson et al[3] report that a Medline review of the medical literature from 1966 through 2001 for reports of structural damage to nerves, arteries, or tendons during carpal tunnel release revealed an incidence of transient neurapraxias of 1.45% in endoscopic carpal tunnel release (ECTR) cases and 0.25% of open carpal tunnel release (OCTR) cases. Major nerve injuries (median or ulnar nerve) were reported in 0.13% of ECTRs and 0.10% of OCTRs. A review of 54 publications by Boeckstyns and Sorensen[4] found the frequency of irreversible nerve damage to be 0.3% for ECTRs and 0.2% for OCTRs.

Ruijs et al[5] and others have demonstrated that the shorter the time from nerve injury to repair, the better the outcome. Also, there is abundant evidence that primary repair of nerve injuries produces superior results when compared to delayed repair using nerve grafts or conduits. Immediate repair allows the surgeon to more accurately identify the fascicular pattern of the nerve and thus aid in the preservation of the correct fascicular orientation during the repair. It is therefore critical that the diagnosis of an intraoperative nerve injury be made at the time of the incident in order to afford the patient the best chance of a good outcome. Ideally, any nerve laceration that occurs during a carpal tunnel release would be identified at the time of the surgery and repaired using standard microsurgical techniques. A delay in the diagnosis renders the repair more complex due to the retraction of the nerve ends, the need for extensive neurolysis, and the need for nerve grafts to bridge the inevitable nerve gap. Given what is stated above, if during surgery there is any doubt whatsoever that there may have been a nerve injury, the surgeon should explore the area to rule out any injury.

The communicating branch of Berrettini carries sensory fibers between the median and ulnar common digital nerves. This communicating branch is present in up to 94% of patients,[6] and can run very close to the distal edge of the transverse carpal ligament (TCL), placing it at risk during carpal tunnel release. Injury of the communicating branch of Berrettini can lead to decreased digital sensation usually in the long and ring fingers[7] as well as an annoying neuroma in the palm. As with any nerve injury, early repair of a lacerated communicating branch of Berrettini offers the best chance of a good recovery.

Vascular Injury

Vascular injuries are very rarely encountered during carpal tunnel release. Benson et al[3] reported the incidence of injuries to the superficial palmar arch to be 0.02% in ECTRs and 0.00% in OCTRs. Zhang et al[8] report one hematoma among 1144 mini-OCTRs. The vascular supply to the hand is assured by both the radial and ulnar arteries and their anastomoses in the superficial and deep palmar arches.[9] This anatomy is protective of the blood supply to the hand in case of a laceration of the superficial palmar arch. The treatment of an injury to the superficial palmar arch is a function of the arterial anatomy of the patient's hand. In most cases, simple ligation of the lacerated artery is reasonable. However, in the rare situation in which the laceration leads to vascular compromise of a portion of the hand, primary microsurgical repair of the superficial palmer arch would be indicated.

As many hand surgeons perform carpal tunnel surgery under tourniquet control and do not release the tourniquet until the postoperative compressive dressing is applied, the possibility of an undiagnosed arterial injury exists. Such an injury could lead to a postoperative hematoma which could compress the median nerve and cause significant scarring within the carpal tunnel. Early detection and evacuation of the hematoma is the treatment of choice. However, even after appropriate treatment, Kaltenborn et al[10] report that patients who suffered from bleeding complications after carpal tunnel release had significantly worse functional results.

Tendon Injuries

The flexor tendons are in harm's way during a carpal tunnel release. Fortunately, flexor tendon injuries are quite rare. Benson et al[3] reported an incidence of flexor tendon injury in 0.008% of ECTRs and 0.00% of OCTRs. Just as with nerve injuries, a flexor tendon injury should, in general, be identified as quickly as possible and repaired. The surgeon has some latitude however, in regard to the need for tendon repair. If, for example, the superficial flexor (FDS) is lacerated and the flexor digitorum profundus (FDP) to that finger is intact, one could, given that fingers can function quite well without the FDS, opt to not repair the lacerated flexor tendon, thus sparing the patient the rigors and complications associated with a flexor tendon repair. Clearly, clinical judgment is required in every case. Flexor tendon repair in the face of a carpal tunnel release presents unique challenges. The loss of the flexor retinaculum precludes placing the wrist in flexion during the postoperative rehabilitation since placing the wrist in flexion would lead to bowstringing of the flexor tendons and median nerve and compromise the surgical outcome. To overcome this, the flexor retinaculum can be reconstructed at the time of the flexor tendon repair using a rotation flap of the residual flexor retinaculum or with a palmaris longus tendon graft.[11,12] Of course, reconstruction carries with it the possibility of persistence or recurrence of the carpal tunnel syndrome.

6.1.3 Postoperative Complications

Persistent Symptoms

Unidentified Nerve Injury

Postoperative paresthesias can pose a vexing diagnostic dilemma. Are the paresthesias due to the severity of the presenting carpal tunnel syndrome? Was there an injury to one of the nerves? If there was a nerve injury, was it simply a neurapraxia or was there a laceration? Was the carpal tunnel release incomplete? Given the fact that the outcome of a nerve repair is directly related to the delay between the injury and repair, it is critical to differentiate between these various causes of sensory or motor dys-

function in the immediate postoperative period. Assuming that the surgeon did not identify any nerve injury at the time of wound closure, the first opportunity to make the postoperative diagnosis of a nerve injury would be in the recovery area. Unless faced with a significant deterioration of the nerve function compared to preoperative testing (in which case, serious considerations would have to be given to immediate exploration of the surgical wound), most surgeons would attribute the abnormal postop exam to the effects of residual anesthesia or neurapraxia, and assume the nerve function will improve by the first postoperative visit. A lack of improvement at the first postoperative visit should trigger some concern that an occult nerve injury has occurred. Clinical signs are, however, not always reliable. Median nerve neurapraxia can lead to significant motor and sensory impairment that can completely resolve. The severity of the carpal tunnel syndrome can render the postoperative diagnosis of a nerve injury difficult. A patient presenting with preoperative decreased sensation and weakness of the abductor pollicis brevis is unlikely to miraculously have resolution of those symptoms at the first office visit. If the surgeon is certain the surgery was well performed and can explain the altered nerve status (advanced carpal tunnel syndrome, neurapraxia), he/she might elect to follow the patient expectantly. Otherwise, advanced imaging including high-resolution ultrasound,[13] magnetic resonance imaging (MRI), and/or MR neurogram should be performed as soon as possible to rule out nerve laceration. The ultrasound of the median nerve will typically continue to demonstrate findings consistent with median nerve compression[14] in addition to any laceration.[15] A lacerated nerve should be repaired as soon as possible to avoid nerve retraction and the need for nerve grafting.

Undetected nerve injury can lead to chronic hand pain, motor and sensory dysfunction, as well as complex regional pain syndrome (CRPS). The symptoms associated with partial injuries to the median nerve and its branches are often dismissed as stemming from a neurapraxia. However, nerve dysfunction and pain that does not improve with time should alert the surgeon to the possibility of an underlying healing nerve laceration. The diagnostic steps listed above including ultrasound and MR imaging should be pursued to clearly identify and characterize the nerve injury. Nerve studies can also be performed if the injury occurred more than 30 days earlier. The delayed treatment of a completely or partially lacerated nerve will typically require neurolysis and nerve grafting.

The diagnosis of postoperative neurapraxia is one of exclusion. Only if the surgeon is confident no intraoperative nerve laceration occurred can a "wait-and-see" posture be adopted. If there is any question regarding the presence of a nerve injury, advanced imaging should be pursued as discussed above. If, however, a neurapraxia is the correct diagnosis, one can be relatively confident that with the passage of time the patient will improve. However, there are a few caveats. Clearly a neurapraxia of a median nerve in a patient with an advanced carpal tunnel syndrome will recover more slowly than a neurapraxia in a patient with a mild carpal tunnel syndrome. Advanced age and diabetes can negatively impact the recovery after any nerve injury including neurapraxia. Recovery after a severe neurapraxia can require months and even years.

The discussion of injuries to the palmer cutaneous branch of the median nerve was not undertaken earlier in this chapter as it is typically not identified until well into the postoperative period. Patients who suffer this injury complain of numbness in the proximal thenar eminence. They also complain of shooting pain at the volar wrist. The clinical exam can include decreased sensation in the distribution of the nerve and also a Tinel's sign over the resultant neuroma. Injuries to this nerve are relatively rare and are associated with incisions that are placed radial to the palmaris longus near the flexor carpi radialis at the wrist flexion crease. The diagnosis is typically based on the clinical examination, though occasionally high-resolution ultrasound can demonstrate the neuroma.[16] A diagnostic local anesthetic block performed proximal to the area of the suspected neuroma can be helpful. The treatment of this problem is surgical. The neuroma of the palmar cutaneous nerve must be identified, and the palmar cutaneous branch followed back to its origin off the median nerve. The neuroma is then buried in soft tissue or bone depending upon the surgeon's preference. While repair of the palmar cutaneous branch of the median can be performed, due to the typical delay in diagnosis and the distal nature of the nerve injury in the region of its arborization, primary repair is rarely possible.

Incomplete Release

Incomplete release of the TCL can occur with both OCTR and ECTR. The possibility of an incomplete release should be considered when confronted with a patient who has undergone a carpal tunnel release whose symptoms worsen or do not improve after what is thought to be a successful carpal tunnel release. It is rare that a patient who has undergone a successful carpal tunnel release does not notice some improvement in their symptoms within the first couple of days or weeks of surgery. Of course, if the patient presents with a very advanced carpal tunnel syndrome the improvement will be more nuanced and may take longer. A patient that undergoes a carpal tunnel release and is no better or worse after the surgery, assuming there has been no nerve injury (see above), must be considered to have residual compression of the median nerve in spite of what appeared to be an adequate release of the TCL. In this situation, it is reasonable to follow the patient's progress over a few weeks. If, however, the patient shows no improvement, an ultrasound and possibly an MRI of the carpal tunnel, distal

forearm, and palm should be carried out in order to rule out residual compression of the median nerve. While one could perform postoperative nerve studies to confirm the presence of continued or worsened nerve compression, the fact that even after a successful nerve decompression the nerve studies do not improve for several months makes the interpretation of early postoperative nerve studies difficult. X-rays of the wrist should be used to rule out any undiagnosed advanced arthrosis (scapholunate advanced collapse deformity [SLAC] and scaphoid non-union advance collapse deformity [SNAC]), gout, or pseudogout, all of which can produce abundant synovitis which can erode through the volar wrist capsule and cause continued median nerve compression. Should the above-mentioned diagnostic tests fail to clearly identify a site of residual compression, a diagnostic steroid injection can be helpful. If the patient's symptoms temporarily improve after injection, exploration of the carpal tunnel should be undertaken. If the patient experiences absolutely no improvement after the steroid injection, another source of the patient's symptoms should be considered (e.g., cervical radiculopathy, brachial plexopathy, thoracic outlet syndrome, pronator syndrome, diffuse peripheral neuropathy, multiple sclerosis, Waldenstrom's macroglobulinemia[17]).

The exploration of the median nerve for any sign of residual compression should start in the distal forearm taking care to open the distal forearm fascia. The nerve should be dissected through the carpal tunnel all the way into the palm visualizing the median nerve and all its branches. Postoperative splinting with the wrist in mild extension should be used to avoid the development of bowstringing of the flexor tendons and median nerve.[18]

Occasionally, the median nerve will be severely scarred and simple decompression will not be sufficient and more complex treatment may be required. Such treatment can include wrapping the nerve with a vein graft,[19] the use of local rotation flaps such as a hypothenar fat pad flap,[20] and local muscle flaps utilizing the abductor digiti minimi,[21] the pronator quadratus,[22] or the palmaris brevis.[23] Synovial flaps have been used as well.[24] Pedicled flaps such as the reverse radial forearm adipofascial flap,[25] and even free omental transfer[26] have been used with some success.

Typically, the identification and decompression of the residual median nerve compression leads to good recovery. Stang et al[27] reported that 84% of patients who underwent surgery for incomplete release of the carpal tunnel were satisfied with the outcome of the surgery. However, 78% of patients complained of persistent neurological symptoms.

Flexor Tendon Complications

Postoperative complications related to the flexor tendons are rare. There are two major complications that can be encountered. One is the subluxation of the ulnar flexor tendons over the hook of the hamate. The other is bow-stringing of the flexor tendons.

Subluxation of the flexors over the hook of the hamate may be the consequence of the TCL incision being carried out through or very close to its bony attachment on the hook of the hamate without leaving a remnant of the ulnar edge of the TCL to inhibit flexor tendon subluxation. Symptoms consist of a popping sensation along the volar aspect of the wrist when the wrist is flexed and ulnarly deviated while the patient makes a fist. If this is noticed early in the postoperative period, splinting the wrist in extension for several weeks can be curative. Should nonoperative treatment not succeed, excision of the hook of the hamate should be considered.[28]

Bowstringing can occur after an extended carpal tunnel release in which the distal forearm fascia and TCL are completely released combined with mobilization of the median nerve out of its bed. The palmar displacement of the flexor tendons pushes the median nerve out of the carpal tunnel into the subcutaneous tissue. The subcutaneous position of the median nerve renders it susceptible to trauma. Even light pressure applied to the displaced median nerve will cause paresthesias and pain. Just as with subluxation of the flexor tendons over the hook of the hamate, if the bowstringing is noted early during the postoperative period, splinting with the wrist in extension can be helpful. However, if this conservative approach does not solve the problem, reconstruction of the TCL can be performed using either residual TCL or a free palmaris longus graft.[11,12]

Rarely, postoperative scarring of the flexor tendons can lead to "triggering" of the enlarged scarred tendons as they pass beneath the distal edge of brachial fascia. This entity should not be confused with the slightly more common "trigger wrist" which is associated with pathology affecting the flexor tendons in patients with an intact TCL, the treatment of which includes carpal tunnel release.[29] The treatment of a post-carpal tunnel release "trigger" wrist consists of the surgical release of the distal aspect of the antebrachial fascia as well as release of the neo-TCL that will have formed after the prior carpal tunnel release. Postoperative splinting should be used to prevent bowstringing of the flexor tendons and median nerve.

Trigger fingers are often noticed after carpal tunnel release but are not, strictly speaking, a complication of carpal tunnel release surgery. King et al[30] reported the incidence of trigger finger in 1185 patients during the first 6 months after carpal tunnel release to be 6.6% on the operated side as opposed to 3.5% in the unoperated contralateral hand. The thumb was the most frequently involved digit. The incidence of triggering in the index, long, ring, and small fingers was similar in the operated and nonoperated hands. Lin et al[31] noted the increased incidence of trigger finger after carpal tunnel release primarily during the first 6 postoperative months. The treat-

ment for a trigger finger is well established and includes steroid injections and, if needed, release of the A1 pulley.

Infection

The likelihood of developing an infection after a carpal tunnel release has been reported to be as low as 0.32%.[32] Werner et al[32] noted several independent positive risk factors for infection following an open carpal release, including younger age, male sex, obesity, tobacco use, alcohol use, diabetes, inflammatory arthritis, peripheral vascular disease, chronic liver disease, chronic kidney disease, chronic lung disease, and depression. Werner et al in another study[33] noted an increase in surgical site infection after OCTR in patients with poorly controlled diabetes and a perioperative (within 3 months of surgery) HbA1c of greater than 8 mg/dL. While multiple studies[34,35] suggest that prophylactic antibiotics are of no benefit when used for procedures such as carpal tunnel release, some authors have suggested prophylactic antibiotics should be considered when performing a carpal tunnel release in diabetic patients.[36]

The surgeon must be ever vigilant regarding patient complaints of increasing pain and erythema at the surgical site. Even a simple stitch abscess can rapidly devolve into a deep infection. Early treatment including stitch removal and antibiotics will often lead to the resolution of a superficial infection. In the unfortunate case in which a deep infection develops, the treatment includes incision and drainage and appropriate IV antibiotic therapy. Unfortunately, in such situations the patient is likely to develop extensive scarring of the flexor tendons and median nerve that could possibly require tenolysis, neurolysis, and vascularized soft tissue coverage.

Pillar Pain

"Pillar" pain is characterized by discomfort over the "pillars" of the hand centered over the hook of the hamate and the unciform process of the trapezium. Pillar pain is typically not noted immediately after surgery but becomes apparent as the patient applies pressure to the palm while pushing off to rise from a chair or when doing a pushup. Larsen et al[37] noted that 73% of 90 patients undergoing standard OCTR, mini-OCTR, and ECTR (30 patients in each group) developed pillar pain. The operative technique had no impact on the incidence of pillar pain. The etiology of pillar pain has been thought to possibly be related to changes in the carpal anatomy though the exact etiology is still unknown.[38] The patient presenting pillar pain should be counseled to avoid aggravating activities though this can delay the return to work. The use of the antioxidant alpha-lipoic acid (ALA) for 40 days has been reported to reduce pillar pain in a small cohort of patients.[39] Extracorporeal shock wave therapy has also been shown in a small controlled study by Haghighat et al[40] to be beneficial in the treatment of pillar pain. Fortunately, pillar pain almost always resolves spontaneously during the first few postoperative months and reassuring the patient of this fact is typically the only treatment needed.

Pisiform Pain

Occasionally, patients develop discomfort at the pisotriquetral joint after carpal tunnel release. Patients who develop this problem will complain of discomfort with direct compression of the pisotriquetral joint. Stahl et al[41] have opined this is related to latent pisotriquetral arthritis that is unmasked as a result of a change in the biomechanics of the pisotriquetral articulation noted after carpal tunnel release. The transection of the TCL is thought to lead to a loss of the radial restraint of the pisotriquetral joint, which in turn leads to maltracking of the pisiform and aggravation of the underlying arthrosis. Stahl et al[41] reviewed the charts and X-rays of 700 patients who had undergone either OCTR or ECTR and identified 14 cases of pisotriquetral dysfunction and arthrosis. Both the diagnosis and treatment can include a steroid injection carried out under fluoroscopic control. If the steroid injection does not lead to long-term relief, excision of the pisiform is typically curative.

Scar Tenderness

The incidence of scar tenderness after carpal tunnel release has been reported to be between 19% and 61%.[42,43] ECTR appears to be associated with less scar pain than OCTR.[44] The possibility that scar tenderness after OCTR is related to injury of the terminal branches of the palmar cutaneous branches of the median and ulnar nerves has been suggested. Siegmeth et al[45] performed a prospective randomized study comparing postoperative scar pain in two cohorts of 42 patients each. One cohort underwent an OCTR during which no attempt was made to preserve the superficial nerve branches. The other cohort underwent a similar OCTR during which the superficial nerve branches were meticulously protected. The authors noted no difference in scar pain between the two methods at 6 weeks, 3 months, and 6 months. The treatment of scar tenderness can include postoperative scar massage (once the wound is healed), and the application of silicone padding and steroid cream. The avoidance of heavy hand use during the early healing phase is also beneficial.

Complex Regional Pain Syndrome

Complex regional pain syndrome (CRPS) is encountered in 2 to 8% of patients who have undergone carpal tunnel release regardless of the surgical technique. Post carpal tunnel release, CRPS is more frequently noted in middle aged (40–64 y) women.[46] The hand surgeon must consider CRPS in the differential diagnosis of patients who are noted to have postoperative pain out of proportion to what one would expect. Also, CRPS should be considered in patients who seem to be doing relatively well after surgery but subsequently develop pain and swelling for no apparent reason. The hand surgeon can treat early cases of CRPS with a 2-week course of oral steroids as well as frequent gentle therapy. Should this initial treatment not lead to the resolution of the patient's symptoms, referral to a pain clinic for more aggressive treatment should be considered.

Prolonged Neurological Symptoms

Elderly patients who present with very advanced carpal tunnel syndrome can occasionally develop postoperative nerve pain that seems to be associated with the gradual recovery of median nerve function. This is a relatively rare phenomenon. The treatment of this can include the use of gabapentin as well as duloxetine, though the mainstay of treatment is constant reassurance that the symptoms will resolve. Serial light touch localization and two-point discrimination testing and nerve studies can provide the patient with "objective" encouraging evidence of nerve improvement. Unfortunately, the recovery can be very slow and require a year or two.

6.2 Part B: Complications and Failure of Cubital Tunnel Surgery

Godard C.W. de Ruiter

Abstract

In cubital tunnel surgery, various procedures are available to the surgeon to choose from, ranging from simple decompression to different techniques of ulnar nerve transposition. In this chapter, an overview of the different complications for the various procedures is provided. In addition, technical issues associated with these procedures are discussed, as well as possible reasons for failure (persistence or recurrence of symptoms) and different options for revision surgery. Finally, treatment recommendations are presented for the management of the different complications and practical tips are provided for the detection and surgical treatment of potential anatomical variations.

Keywords: ulnar nerve, neuropathy, elbow, decompression, transposition, subcutaneous, submuscular, neuroma

6.2.1 Introduction

Cubital tunnel syndrome (CuTS), also known as ulnar neuropathy at the elbow (UNE), is the second most common neuropathy after carpal tunnel syndrome. The severity of symptoms can be classified as mild, moderate, or severe, according to the classification introduced by Dellon.[47] Conservation treatment, consisting of pain medication, the elimination or reduction of the frequency of external compression on the nerve and sometimes a night splint, often is the first treatment especially in mild cases. Surgery is offered to the patient in case conservative treatment fails or in case the patient presents with moderate-to-severe symptoms.[47]

6.2.2 Surgery for Ulnar Neuropathy: Different Procedures and Potential Complications

There are various surgical procedures available to the surgeon and patient to choose from, ranging from simple and endoscopic decompression to different techniques of ulnar nerve transposition (subcutaneous, submuscular, and intramuscular).[48] These procedures all have different pros and cons. In the Cochrane review from 2016 no difference in outcome was found for the various procedures (clinical improvement averaged around 70%), but a higher chance for complications following transposition, especially the risk on superficial and deep wound infection.[48] Simple decompression, therefore, nowadays is the first surgical treatment of choice, but in some cases (e.g., in case of luxation or severe neurologic deficit) the surgeon can decide, together with the patient, to directly transpose the ulnar nerve in addition to the decompression. Below, the different surgical treatments for CuTS are discussed and specifically the complications associated with these procedures and potential reasons for failure. In the second part of this chapter (6.2.3) options for revision surgery are discussed. Finally, in the last part (6.2.4) recommendations are provided to prevent and manage com-

plications, and practical tips for the detection and surgical treatment of anatomical variations.

Complications after Decompression of the Ulnar Nerve

The most standard procedure in CuTS is simple decompression of the ulnar nerve. A slightly curved incision is made between the medial epicondyle and the olecranon (▶ Fig. 6.1) to identify the nerve. Subsequently, potential compression sites are inspected (most often Osborne's ligament or the aponeurosis of the flexor carpi ulnaris [FCU] muscle). The most frequent side effect of this procedure, which is often probably not even reported as complication, is numbness around the elbow due to injury to the posterior branches of the medial antebrachial cutaneous nerve (MABCN). This might be caused by traction, which most likely will recover slowly in time, but in severe cases (complete transection) sometimes a neuroma might develop which can be quite debilitating to the patient (▶ Fig. 6.2). The risk for the development of a MABCN neuroma after simple decompression is not exactly known, but in a study by Mackinnon and Novak in 73 out of 100 cases that underwent revision cubital tunnel surgery, a neuroma of the MABCN was found.[49] Management of MABCN neuroma will be discussed in the final part of this chapter (6.2.4), but it is important to realize that, even in the absence of a neuroma, pain/numbness around the elbow can substantially reduce patient satisfaction with the outcome, despite the relief of tingling sensation in the hand, and therefore care should be taken during the exposure of the ulnar nerve to prevent MABCN injury.

Other complications that have been reported after simple decompression are hematoma/seroma, direct injury to the ulnar nerve or branches to the FCU muscle and CRPS.[51,52] In addition, the ulnar nerve may have been inadequately released, either at the usual compression

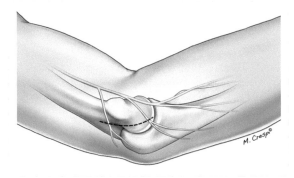

Fig. 6.1 Anatomical drawing illustrating the course of the medial antebrachial cutaneous nerve (MABCN) that divides into a posterior (PB) and anterior branch (AB). Most commonly the posterior branch crosses the usual site of incision (*dashed black line*) 2 cm distally to the medial epicondyle (ME), but in about 23% of the cases crossing branches are also found proximal to or at the level of the ME (*as in this drawing*).[50]

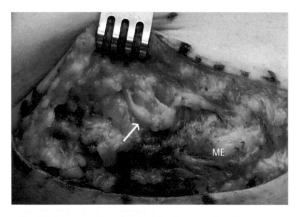

Fig. 6.2 Intraoperative photograph of a case of medial antebrachial cutaneous nerve (MABCN) neuroma (*arrow*) after previous subcutaneous transposition. ME, medial epicondyle.

sites (▸ Fig. 6.1) or due to unusual causes/anatomical variations such as an arcade of Struthers proximal to the cubital tunnel,[53] an epitrochleoanconeus muscle and prominent medial head of triceps (see Chapter 6.2.4 for practical tips on detection and surgical treatment).[54,55] Finally, decompression might lead to ulnar nerve (sub)luxation, which sometimes leads to persistence of symptoms requiring revision surgery (subcutaneous, submuscular, or intramuscular transposition).

An alternative to simple decompression is endoscopically assisted decompression of the ulnar nerve in a proximal and distal direction after in situ release of the ulnar nerve at the cubital tunnel. In a randomized controlled trial, the endoscopic procedure has been shown to indeed significantly increase the length of the ulnar nerve that can be decompressed (using the same 3-cm incision, as for the open procedure it increased from 9 to 16 cm), but significantly more postoperative hematomas occurred in the endoscopic group and there was no significant difference in short- and long-term outcome.[56]

Subcutaneous Transposition of the Ulnar Nerve at the Elbow

The risks for the development of the complications mentioned above are significantly higher after subcutaneous transposition than after simple decompression as shown in the Cochrane review from 2016[48] and recent meta-analysis (with odds ratio of 0.449 and 0.469 for fixed and random effect models, respectively),[52] whereas in most studies there is no difference in outcome. Transposition of the ulnar, therefore, frequently is not performed as primary procedure. Exception is if there is preoperative (sub)luxation of the ulnar nerve, although in the randomized trial by Bartels et al, subgroup analysis for the presence of (sub)luxation showed no difference in outcome for simple decompression and subcutaneous transposition.[57]

In addition to the previously mentioned complications for simple decompression, subcutaneous transposition also has other potential complications, including devascularization of the ulnar nerve,[58] kinking proximal or distal to the cubital tunnel, residual compression at the intermuscular septum, and/or "scarring" around the nerve in the subcutaneous plane[59] (▸ Fig. 6.3 and ▸ Fig. 6.4), which (except for the latter) are mostly technical issues.

Kinking of the ulnar nerve may occur proximally to the transposition due to an unrecognized arcade of Struthers,[53] an insufficiently incised brachial fascia,[60] and distally due to a remnant of the FCU aponeurosis.[59] Another rare complication is secondary compression due to failure to recognize dislocation/snapping of the medial part of the triceps during elbow flexion[61] (see Chapter 6.2.4). Finally, recurrent dislocation of the ulnar nerve may occur, especially when the skin is sutured to the medial epicondyle using a single subcutaneous suture. The formation of a fasciodermal sling, using the technique described by Eaton et al,[62] may prevent this recurrence of dislocation.

Submuscular Transposition of the Ulnar Nerve at the Elbow

Submuscular transposition of the ulnar nerve is an alternative to the subcutaneous transposition mentioned above. There are different techniques of submuscular transposition, including the Learmonth[63] and Z-lengthening technique.[64] Compared to the subcutaneous transposition, the advantages of submuscular transposition is that nerve lies protected under a well-vascularized

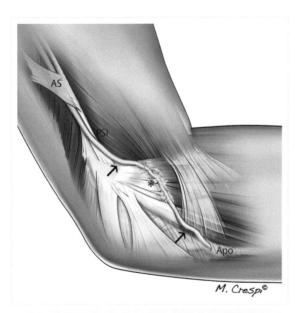

Fig. 6.3 Anatomical drawing showing the course of the ulnar nerve after subcutaneous transposition with potential kinking sites (proximal and distal to the transposition, *arrows*), secondary compression sites (at the arcade of Struthers (AS), the proximal septum intermuscular (PSI), and the aponeurosis (Apo) of the flexor carpi ulnaris (FCU), and the formation of scar tissue in the subcutaneous plane around the ulnar nerve (*).

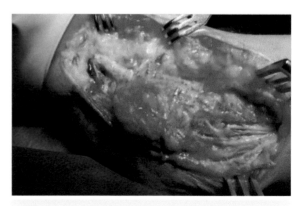

Fig. 6.4 Intraoperative picture showing extensive scarring around the ulnar nerve after subcutaneous transposition.

muscle, while after subcutaneous transposition the ulnar nerves lies more superficial, making it more vulnerable to trauma and hypersensitivity.[65] General complications are similar to the ones mentioned for simple decompression, and technical issues are similar to the ones mentioned for subcutaneous transposition (potential kinking of the ulnar nerve and/or compression at the intermuscular septum). In addition, submuscular transposition may be complicated by secondary compression under the muscle. The Z-lengthening technique has been shown in cadavers to reduce the intraneural pressure compared with, for example, the Learmonth technique[66] and may reduce the chance for secondary compression. Another technical issue specific for submuscular transposition is secondary compression by the distal intermuscular septum (DIS) in the forearm (▶ Fig. 6.5). Finally, patients postoperatively may experience muscular pain in the region of the reattached/sutured flexor pronator muscle, and in case the arm has been immobilized postoperatively, an extension contracture of the elbow may develop (see Chapter 6.2.4). Postoperative hematoma/seroma can develop after submuscular transposition due to transection of a well-vascularized muscle.

Intramuscular Transposition of the Ulnar Nerve at the Elbow

Some surgeons favor intramuscular over submuscular transposition, because the ulnar nerve is placed in a bed

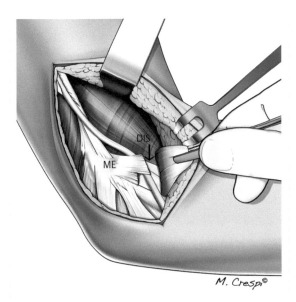

Fig. 6.5 Anatomical drawing of potential compression after submuscular transposition due to an underlying distal inter-muscular septum (DIS; *black arrow*). The ulnar nerve in this drawing has been transposed after Z-wise incision of the flexorpronator mass and the muscle is retracted with forceps to illustrate the relation of the ulnar nerve to this DIS.

of muscular fibers instead of directly on the elbow joint capsule.[67] Important in this technique is to identify the longitudinal septa inside the flexor pronator mass (at least three).[67] No other complications than the ones mentioned above have been reported for this technique.

Minimal Medial Epicondylectomy

Finally, other surgeons (mostly orthopedic) prefer the minimal medial epicondylectomy over transposition, because in their view it reduces the risk for ulnar nerve devascularization compared with transposition, and the same time prevents tethering of the ulnar nerve behind the medial epicondyle, which might persist after simple decompression.[68] A major disadvantage is that about one-third of the patients postoperatively complain of tenderness at the osteotomy site.[68] In addition, there is the risk of iatrogenic injury to the anterior band of the medial collateral ligament, which might lead to instability of the elbow. Other reported side effects are loss of pinch and grip strength to the weakness of the flexor pronator muscle and anterior subluxation of the ulnar nerve.

6.2.3 Persistence or Recurrence of CuTS despite Previous Surgery
Follow-Up after Surgery

Persistence of recurrence of symptoms after cubital tunnel surgery occurs in up to 30% of the cases after primary decompression[57,69]; some of which will require revision surgery. When considering reoperation for CuTS, it is important to realize that recovery of nerve function takes time (sometimes up to a year).[57] It is also important to discuss this preoperatively with the patient, because patients otherwise may have different expectations. When informing about residual symptoms, the impact of paresthesias/pain in digit IV/V should be distinguished from potential pain at elbow. Finally, the surgeon should be aware of a potential double crush injury (such as cervical radiculopathy or thoracic outlet syndrome). EMG or ultrasound (US) can best be repeated if symptoms persist for more than 3 to 6 months after the first surgery, depending on the severity of pain symptoms (recovery of nerve function often takes longer). In case the results show improved ulnar nerve conduction and/or decreased cross-sectional surface area of the ulnar nerve it is best to wait for further recovery to occur, but if no improvement is observed on EMG and/or US, a secondary procedure should be considered in case of persistent paresthesias. In case of persistent muscle weakness, it is best to wait for 1 year. Persistence of numbness (without pain) is not a good indication for revision surgery.

Recently, a "supercharge" technique (end-to-side transfer of the anterior interosseous to the motor component of the ulnar nerve in addition to ulnar nerve decompression/transposition) has been reported to improve the results of motor recovery, but this technique should be reserved for severe cases of ulnar neuropathy (with signs of denervation on EMG)[70] and results are still preliminary; prospective cohort studies and RCTs with standardized outcome measures are necessary to determine the beneficial effect of this additional technique.[71]

Finally, luxation of the ulnar nerve following decompression is not an indication for revision surgery unless the patient is still bothered by tingling sensations in digit IV and V.

Revision Surgery for CuTS

The procedures that are most frequently performed in revision surgery, subcutaneous and submuscular transposition,[69,72] have already been discussed above. Currently, there are no randomized trials that have compared the effectiveness of both procedures. Results of one prospective and several retrospective studies are difficult to compare, because different patients have been included (sometimes multiple revision surgeries) and often different outcome measures have been used to evaluate results.[72] Overall, the chance for improvement after revision surgery is high (85%), although there also is a small chance for worsening of preoperative symptoms (2.4%).[72] When deciding on the type of procedure, it is best to discuss the different advantages and disadvantages of the procedures with the patient. Certain patient-related factors may be reasons to prefer subcutaneous over submuscular transposition (for example, in musicians, weight-lifters, patients that have had previous elbow trauma with heterotopic ossifications, and the use of anticoagulants that cannot be discontinued preoperatively).

6.2.4 Prevention and Management of Complications; Tips and Tricks

Most important factor that reduces the chance for complications in cubital tunnel surgery is knowledge of the anatomy and potential anatomic variations. First, during exposure of the ulnar nerve the posterior branch of the MABCN should be identified and spared (▶ Fig. 6.1). If it is transected accidentally, the proximal end of the branch can best be dissected further up and transected again so the proximal end falls back into the subcutaneous tissue of the upper arm, away from the surgical site, where there is a higher chance for the neuroma to become symptomatic, probably because there it is embedded in scar tissue.

Patients that present with a neuroma of the MABCN often are reoperated. During the surgery, the neuroma is resected and the proximal end is again transected higher up (as described above). Sometimes, the freshly cut nerve end is covered with autologous fat or the end is implanted into adjacent muscle tissue.[73] The use of artificial nerve grafts to cap the nerve end and prevent reformation of the neuroma is currently being investigated.

Kinking of the ulnar nerve after transposition can be prevented by sufficient release of the brachial fascia in the upper arm and a potential arcade of Struthers that can be found up to 5 to 7 cm proximal to the medial epicondyle.[53] Also, in the forearm the aponeuroses of the FCU should be sufficiently opened to prevent distal kinking. Sometimes it is also necessary to separately dissect out the first motor branches to the FCU, because these might restrict ulnar transposition, and if not mobilized sufficiently, may also lead to tethering of the ulnar nerve.

Secondary compression should be prevented by V-shaped incision of the intermuscular septum proximal to the medial epicondyle[67] and the distal septa in the forearm during intra- and submuscular transposition.[67,74] The proximal intermuscular septum should be cauterized/ligated before incision, because there are a variable number of large-caliber vessels running through the base of this septum and bipolar coagulation after transection will cause them to retract, but still bleed.[67]

Careful hemostasis anyway is important in cubital tunnel surgery, especially after transposition, because it increases the subcutaneous area that is exposed and hematoma in this area may increase the chance for postoperative fibrosis. Therefore, compression bandage can best be applied after the surgery, especially when a tourniquet has been used to operate under blood void. The latter is not standard practice in cubital tunnel surgery, because it can be quite painful when performed under local anesthesia, but especially for transposition of the ulnar nerve it improves the visibility and therefore probably reduces the risk for MABCN injury. The bandage is removed after 2 days and the patient is instructed to frequently flex and extend the elbow to promote nerve gliding, and to prevent the formation of adhesions and contractures. After submuscular transposition the patient is instructed to additionally wear an elbow brace for 3 weeks and after that not to lift heavy objects for an additional 3 weeks. Sometimes patients, after this 6-week period, may experience muscle soreness at the site of transection of the flexor pronator mass, but this frequently resolves with physical therapy.

In addition to the technical issues mentioned above, various anatomical variations may complicate CuTS, including the presence of an epitrochleoanconeus muscle and a snapping medial part of the triceps muscle.

The epitrochleoanconeus muscle was found by Gervasio et al in 3.2% of their patients that underwent CuTS surgery, and in all cases[5] it was associated with a prominent head of the triceps muscle that covered the ulnar nerve proximally to the cubital tunnel,[54] which makes it difficult to identify the ulnar nerve during cubital tunnel surgery. Therefore, it is helpful to know before the start of the surgery if this anatomical variation is present, because the ulnar nerve can then first best be exposed distal to the cubital tunnel and followed in a proximal direction. Another reason why it is helpful to know if an epitrochleoanconeus muscle is present before the surgery is that the procedure can best be performed under general anesthesia, because removal of the epitrochleoanconeus muscle (myectomy) and part of the triceps muscle is often too painful to perform under local anesthesia.[54,55] An alternative is to just transect the muscle (myotomy), but this may lead to persistence of CuTS due to residual compression of the ulnar nerve by the hypertrophic epitrochleoanconeus muscle.[55] Further there is no need to transpose the nerve, because the pathophysiologic mechanism is not stretch injury, but compression. This may explain why surgical results are often favorable.[54,55]

Another anatomical variation that is sometimes encountered during CuTS is a snapping medial part of the triceps muscle. It often coexists with ulnar nerve luxation and therefore is frequently misdiagnosed as an isolated ulnar nerve dislocation. Failure to recognize a snapping triceps may lead to persistence of CuTS despite an otherwise successful ulnar nerve transposition.[61] Both epitrochleoanconeus muscle and snapping triceps can be detected preoperatively with ultrasound.

6.2.5 Conclusions

Different potential complications and technical issues should be considered when performing surgery for CuTS. Understanding anatomy and potential anatomical variations is thereby important. Secondary surgery in case of failure can be quite successful, but it is important to set the right indication and discuss the different pros and cons of the various options that are available with the patient.

References

[1] Papanicolaou GD, McCabe SJ, Firrell J. The prevalence and characteristics of nerve compression symptoms in the general population. J Hand Surg Am. 2001; 26(3):460–466

[2] Fajardo M, Kim SH, Szabo RM. Incidence of carpal tunnel release: trends and implications within the United States ambulatory care setting. J Hand Surg Am. 2012; 37(8):1599–1605

[3] Benson LS, Bare AA, Nagle DJ, Harder VS, Williams CS, Visotsky JL. Complications of endoscopic and open carpal tunnel release. Arthroscopy. 2006; 22(9):919–924, 924.e1–924.e2. Review

[4] Boeckstyns ME, Sørensen AI. Does endoscopic carpal tunnel release have a higher rate of complications than open carpal tunnel release? An analysis of published series. J Hand Surg [Br]. 1999; 24(1):9–15

[5] Ruijs AC, Jaquet JB, Kalmijn S, Giele H, Hovius SE. Median and ulnar nerve injuries: a meta-analysis of predictors of motor and sensory recovery after modern microsurgical nerve repair. Plast Reconstr Surg. 2005; 116(2):484–494, discussion 495–496

[6] Kaur N, Singla RK, Kullar JS. Cadaveric Study of Berretini communications in North Indian population. J Clin Diagn Res. 2016; 10(6):AC07–AC09

[7] Ferrari GP, Gilbert A. The superficial anastomosis on the palm of the hand between the ulnar and median nerves. J Hand Surg [Br]. 1991; 16(5):511–514

[8] Zhang D, Blazar P, Earp BE. Rates of complications and secondary surgeries of mini-open carpal tunnel release. Hand (N Y). 2019; 14(4):471–476

[9] Coleman SS, Anson BJ. Arterial patterns in the hand based upon a study of 650 specimens. Surg Gynecol Obstet. 1961; 113:409–424

[10] Kaltenborn A, Frey-Wille S, Hoffmann S, et al. The risk of complications after carpal tunnel release in patients taking acetylsalicylic acid as platelet inhibition: a Multicenter Propensity Score-Matched Study. Plast Reconstr Surg. 2020; 145(2):360e–367e

[11] Hunter JM. Reconstruction of the transverse carpal ligament to restore median nerve gliding. The rationale of a new technique for revision of recurrent median nerve neuropathy. Hand Clin. 1996; 12(2):365–378

[12] Whitaker I, Cairns S, Josty I. The palmaris longus tendon weave: a novel method of reconstructing the transverse carpal ligament. Plast Reconstr Surg. 2008; 122(6):227e–228e

[13] Holzgrefe RE, Wagner ER, Singer AD, Daly CA. Imaging of the peripheral nerve: concepts and future direction of magnetic resonance neurography and ultrasound. J Hand Surg Am. 2019; 44(12):1066–1079

[14] Steinkohl F, Gruber L, Gruber H, et al. Memory effect of the median nerve: can ultrasound reliably depict carpal tunnel release success? Röfo Fortschr Geb Röntgenstr Nuklearmed. 2017; 189(1):57–62

[15] Brown JM, Yablon CM, Morag Y, Brandon CJ, Jacobson JA. Use of the peripheral nerves of the upper extremity: a landmark approach. Radiographics. 2016; 36(2):452–463

[16] Zanette G, Tamburin P. The diagnostic value of nerve ultrasound in an atypical palmar cutaneous nerve lesion.

[17] Briani C, Visentin A, Campagnolo M, et al. Peripheral nervous system involvement in lymphomas. J Peripher Nerv Syst. 2019; 24(1):5–18

[18] Cook AC, Szabo RM, Birkholz SW, King EF. Early mobilization following carpal tunnel release. A prospective randomized study. J Hand Surg [Br]. 1995; 20(2):228–230

[19] Varitimidis SE, Riano F, Vardakas DG, Sotereanos DG. Recurrent compressive neuropathy of the median nerve at the wrist: treatment with autogenous saphenous vein wrapping. J Hand Surg [Br]. 2000; 25(3):271–275

[20] Plancher KD, Idler RS, Lourie GM, Strickland JW. Recalcitrant carpal tunnel. The hypothenar fat pad flap. Hand Clin. 1996; 12(2):337–349

[21] Milward TM, Stott WG, Kleinert HE. The abductor digiti minimi muscle flap. Hand. 1977; 9(1):82–85

[22] Dellon AL, Mackinnon SE. The pronator quadratus muscle flap. J Hand Surg Am. 1984; 9(3):423–427

[23] Rose EH, Norris MS, Kowalski TA, Lucas A, Flegler EJ. Palmaris brevis turnover flap as an adjunct to internal neurolysis of the chronically scarred median nerve in recurrent carpal tunnel syndrome. J Hand Surg Am. 1991; 16(2):191–201

[24] Wulle C. Treatment of recurrence of the carpal tunnel syndrome. Ann Chir Main. 1987; 6(3):203–209

[25] Luchetti R, Riccio M, Papini Zorli I, Fairplay T. Protective coverage of the median nerve using fascial, fasciocutaneous or island flaps. Handchir Mikrochir Plast Chir. 2006; 38(5):317–330

[26] Harii K. Clinical application of free omental flap transfer. Clin Plast Surg. 1978; 5(2):273–281

[27] Stang F, Stütz N, Lanz U, van Schoonhoven J, Prommersberger KJ. Results after revision surgery for carpal tunnel release. Handchir Mikrochir Plast Chir. 2008; 40(5):289–293

[28] Itsubo T, Uchiyama S, Takahara K, Nakagawa H, Kamimura M, Miyasaka T. Snapping wrist after surgery for carpal tunnel syndrome and trigger digit: a case report. J Hand Surg Am. 2004; 29(3):384–386

[29] Park IJ, Lee YM, Kim HM, et al. Multiple etiologies of trigger wrist. J Plast Reconstr Aesthet Surg. 2016; 69(3):335–340

[30] King BA, Stern PJ, Kiefhaber TR. The incidence of trigger finger or de Quervain's tendinitis after carpal tunnel release. J Hand Surg Eur Vol. 2013; 38(1):82–83

[31] Lin F-Y, Manrique OJ, Lin CL, Cheng HT. Incidence of trigger digits following carpal tunnel release: a nationwide, population-based retrospective cohort study. Medicine (Baltimore). 2017; 96(27):e7355

[32] Werner BC, Teran VA, Deal DN. Patient-related risk factors for infection following open carpal tunnel release: an analysis of over 450,000 Medicare patients. J Hand Surg Am. 2018; 43(3):214–219

[33] Werner BC, Teran VA, Cancienne J, Deal DN. The Association of Perioperative Glycemic Control with postoperative surgical site infection following open carpal tunnel release in patients with diabetes. Hand (N Y). 2019; 14(3):324–328

[34] Li K, Sambare TD, Jiang SY, Shearer EJ, Douglass NP, Kamal RN. Effectiveness of preoperative antibiotics in preventing surgical site infection after common soft tissue procedures of the hand. Clin Orthop Relat Res. 2018; 476(4):664–673

[35] Harness NG, Inacio MC, Pfeil FF, Paxton LW. Rate of infection after carpal tunnel release surgery and effect of antibiotic prophylaxis. J Hand Surg Am. 2010; 35(2):189–196

[36] Ko JS, Zwiebel S, Wilson B, Becker DB. Perioperative antibiotic use in diabetic patients: a retrospective review of 670 surgeries. J Plast Reconstr Aesthet Surg. 2017; 70(11):1629–1634

[37] Larsen MB, Sørensen AI, Crone KL, Weis T, Boeckstyns MEH. Carpal tunnel release: a randomized comparison of three surgical methods. Journal Hand Surg (E). 2013; 38E(6):646–650

[38] Brooks JJ, Schiller JR, Allen SD, Akelman E. Biomechanical and anatomical consequences of carpal tunnel release. Clin Biomech (Bristol, Avon). 2003; 18(8):685–693

[39] Boriani F, Granchi D, Roatti G, Merlini L, Sabattini T, Baldini N. Alpha-lipoic acid after median nerve decompression at the carpal tunnel: a randomized controlled trial. J Hand Surg Am. 2017; 42(4):236–242

[40] Haghighat S, Zarezadeh A, Khosrawi S, Oreizi A. Extracorporeal shockwave therapy in pillar pain after carpal tunnel release: a prospective randomized controlled trial. Adv Biomed Res. 2019; 8:31

[41] Stahl S, Stahl S, Calif E. Latent pisotriquetral arthrosis unmasked following carpal tunnel release. Orthopedics. 2010; 33(9):673

[42] Kluge W, Simpson RG, Nicol AC. Late complications after open carpal tunnel decompression. J Hand Surg [Br]. 1996; 21(2):205–207

[43] Brown RA, Gelberman RH, Seiler JG, III, et al. Carpal tunnel release. A prospective, randomized assessment of open and endoscopic methods. J Bone Joint Surg Am. 1993; 75(9):1265–1275

[44] Shin EK. Endoscopic versus open carpal tunnel release. Curr Rev Musculoskelet Med. 2019; 12(4):509–514

[45] Siegmeth AW, Hopkinson-Woolley JA. Standard open decompression in carpal tunnel syndrome compared with a modified open technique preserving the superficial skin nerves: a prospective randomized study. J Hand Surg Am. 2006; 31(9):1483–1489

[46] Mertz K, Trunzter J, Wu E, Barnes J, Eppler SL, Kamal RN. National trends in the diagnosis of CRPS after open and endoscopic carpal tunnel release. J Wrist Surg. 2019; 8(3):209–214

[47] Dellon AL. Review of treatment results for ulnar nerve entrapment at the elbow. J Hand Surg Am. 1989; 14(4):688–700

[48] Caliandro P, La Torre G, Padua R, Giannini F, Padua L. Treatment for ulnar neuropathy at the elbow. Cochrane Database Syst Rev. 2016; 11:CD006839

[49] Mackinnon SE, Novak CB. Operative findings in reoperation of patients with cubital tunnel syndrome. Hand (N Y). 2007; 2(3):137–143

[50] Benedikt S, Parvizi D, Feigl G, Koch H. Anatomy of the medial antebrachial cutaneous nerve and its significance in ulnar nerve surgery: an anatomical study. J Plast Reconstr Aesthet Surg. 2017; 70(11):1582–1588

[51] Zhang D, Earp BE, Blazar P. Rates of complications and secondary surgeries after in situ cubital tunnel release compared with ulnar nerve transposition: a retrospective review. J Hand Surg Am. 2017; 42(4):294.e1–294.e5

[52] Said J, Van Nest D, Foltz C, Ilyas AM. Ulnar nerve in situ decompression versus transposition for idiopathic cubital tunnel syndrome: an updated meta-analysis. J Hand Microsurg. 2019; 11(1):18–27

[53] Spinner M, Kaplan EB. The relationship of the ulnar nerve to the medial intermuscular septum in the arm and its clinical significance. Hand. 1976; 8(3):239–242

[54] Gervasio O, Zaccone C. Surgical approach to ulnar nerve compression at the elbow caused by the epitrochleoanconeus muscle and a prominent medial head of the triceps. Neurosurgery. 2008; 62(3) Suppl 1:186–192, discussion 192–193

[55] de Ruiter GCW, van Duinen SG. Complete removal of the epitrochleoanconeus muscles in patients with cubital tunnel syndrome: results from a small prospective case series. World Neurosurg. 2017; 104:142–147

[56] Schmidt S, Kleist Welch-Guerra W, Matthes M, Baldauf J, Schminke U, Schroeder HW. Endoscopic vs open decompression of the ulnar nerve in cubital tunnel syndrome: a prospective randomized double-blind study. Neurosurgery. 2015; 77(6):960–970, discussion 970–971

[57] Bartels RH, Verhagen WI, van der Wilt GJ, Meulstee J, van Rossum LG, Grotenhuis JA. Prospective randomized controlled study comparing simple decompression versus anterior subcutaneous transposition for idiopathic neuropathy of the ulnar nerve at the elbow: Part 1. Neurosurgery. 2005; 56(3):522–530, discussion 522–530

[58] Messina A, Messina JC. Transposition of the ulnar nerve and its vascular bundle for the entrapment syndrome at the elbow. J Hand Surg [Br]. 1995; 20(5):638–648

[59] Rogers MR, Bergfield TG, Aulicino PL. The failed ulnar nerve transposition. Etiology and treatment. Clin Orthop Relat Res. 1991 (269):193–200

[60] Dellon AL. Musculotendinous variations about the medial humeral epicondyle. J Hand Surg [Br]. 1986; 11(2):175–181

[61] Spinner RJ, O'Driscoll SW, Jupiter JB, Goldner RD. Unrecognized dislocation of the medial portion of the triceps: another cause of failed ulnar nerve transposition. J Neurosurg. 2000; 92(1):52–57

[62] Eaton RG, Crowe JF, Parkes JC, III. Anterior transposition of the ulnar nerve using a non-compressing fasciodermal sling. J Bone Joint Surg Am. 1980; 62(5):820–825

[63] Learmonth JR. A technique for transplanting the ulnar nerve. Surg Gynecol Obstet. 1942; 75:792–793

[64] Dellon AL, Coert JH. Results of the musculofascial lengthening technique for submuscular transposition of the ulnar nerve at the elbow. J Bone Joint Surg Am. 2003; 85(7):1314–1320

[65] Gervasio O, Gambardella G, Zaccone C, Branca D. Simple decompression versus anterior submuscular transposition of the ulnar nerve in severe cubital tunnel syndrome: a prospective randomized study. Neurosurgery. 2005; 56(1):108–117, discussion 117

[66] Dellon AL, Chang E, Coert JH, Campbell KR. Intraneural ulnar nerve pressure changes related to operative techniques for cubital tunnel decompression. J Hand Surg Am. 1994; 19(6):923–930

[67] Henry M. Modified intramuscular transposition of the ulnar nerve. J Hand Surg Am. 2006; 31(9):1535–1542

[68] Göbel F, Musgrave DS, Vardakas DG, Vogt MT, Sotereanos DG. Minimal medial epicondylectomy and decompression for cubital tunnel syndrome. Clin Orthop Relat Res. 2001(393):228–236

[69] Wever N, de Ruiter GCW, Coert JH. Submuscular transposition with musculofascial lengthening for persistent or recurrent cubital tunnel syndrome in 34 patients. J Hand Surg Eur Vol. 2018; 43(3):310–315

[70] Power HA, Kahn LC, Patterson MM, Yee A, Moore AM, Mackinnon SE. Refining indications for the supercharge end-to-side anterior interosseous to ulnar motor nerve transfer in cubital tunnel syndrome. Plast Reconstr Surg. 2020; 145(1):106e–116e

[71] Dengler J, Dolen U, Patterson JMM, et al. Supercharge end-to-side anterior interosseous-to-ulnar motor nerve transfer restores intrinsic function in cubital tunnel syndrome. Plast Reconstr Surg. 2020; 146(4):808–818

[72] Natroshvili T, Walbeehm ET, van Alfen N, Bartels RHMA. Results of reoperation for failed ulnar nerve surgery at the elbow: a systematic review and meta-analysis. J Neurosurg. 2018; 130(3):686–701

[73] Dellon AL, Mackinnon SE. Treatment of the painful neuroma by neuroma resection and muscle implantation. Plast Reconstr Surg. 1986; 77(3):427–438

[74] Felder JM, III, Mackinnon SE, Patterson MM. The 7 structures distal to the elbow that are critical to successful anterior transposition of the ulnar nerve. Hand (N Y). 2019; 14(6):776–781

Section 3

Bone Surgery: Fracture

7 Management of Finger Fracture Complications

Mick Kreulen

Abstract

Finger stiffness and pain, resulting in permanent impairment, and salvage procedures are the ultimate sequelae of finger fractures in dire straits. All due to a myriad of possible complications that may occur after trauma to the sophisticated and vulnerable anatomical harmony in the hand. The injury itself and all subsequent events, treatment as well as complications, will add to the risk of the dreaded permanent loss of finger function. It is simply because a lot more tissues than bone are involved in a fracture and its treatment. A finger fracture should therefore be regarded as a treacherous soft tissue injury around a small broken bone. In that way, the path of fracture treatment is paved in the service of soft tissue healing and restoring the biomechanical equilibrium of multiple tissues in close proximity.

A book chapter does not allow for a full appreciation of all possible finger fracture complications and their treatment. Especially the prevention, early diagnosis, and treatment of osteomyelitis and infection deserve separate attention. The aim here is to advocate a systematic approach to all complications appreciating all involved tissues in phalangeal and metacarpal fractures in order to avoid the pitfalls of doing more harm than good. Three complications are discussed to illustrate this; nonunions, malunions, and, of course, the ultimate foe, finger stiffness.

Keywords: finger stiffness, malunion, nonunion, tendon adhesions, capsular contracture, ligament contracture, splint therapy, stepwise release surgery, osteotomy, bone reconstruction

7.1 Finger Stiffness

Joint stiffness is indeed the most common and notorious complication of a phalangeal fracture and can easily lead to a permanent functional impairment. The initial trauma, prolonged immobilization, surgery, but also overzealous therapy, all have a strong tendency to result in joint stiffness. Subsequent complications of whatever nature will increase this risk. Contractures in any position and stiffness in any direction is possible in all metacarpophalangeal (MCP) and interphalangeal (IP) joints. However, to maximize joint space in the swollen, injured hand, the MCP joints will tend to stiffen in extension and the IP joints in flexion.[1,2,3] Joints do not have to be involved in the trauma to become stiff. The tendency toward stiffness expands to joints of uninjured fingers.[4] Preventative measures should involve the entire hand, regardless of the injury.

The first causative agent in this tendency is edema from the inflammatory cascade. Edema itself is not a complication. The accumulation of edema is a natural response in the inflammation phase of any event within the layers of motion around tendons, ligaments, capsular structures, synovial spaces, and it acutely impairs joint motion. Edema control is one of the very first measures to take after a finger fracture. When edema continues or exacerbation occurs from interventions or early complications during the overlap with the fibroblastic phase of wound healing, the distended synovial spaces will transform with fibroblast proliferation. Adhesions and ligament shortening will effectively occur, promoted by collagen cross-linking.[1,2] Eventually, the changes become fixed and joint contractures will develop. As with infection and osteomyelitis, prevention is paramount:

- Edema control from the very start including elevation and compressive dressings.
- Infection prevention in open fractures and invasive procedures.
- Fracture treatment that allows for early PIP and MCP motion. This is actually a prerequisite for all surgical or nonsurgical treatment. From this perspective, stability of the fracture outweighs (but not eliminates) the discussion whether the position of the fracture is acceptable. An anatomical position of a fracture is only acceptable if it is stable enough to allow for stiffness prevention measures.
- In case of surgery, choose the least invasive fixation technique that is stable enough to allow for early protected motion. This is not automatically a plea for percutaneous K-wires as the best choice. If it fits the requirements, fine. But, all available techniques should be considered every time. Open reduction with screws, cerclage wires, or plates could very well be this "least invasive procedure."
- Gentle tissue handling at all times. This also includes nonsurgical interventions.
- Immobilize as short as possible in the proper joint positions and provide removable splints for intermittent rest and protected motion during inflammatory healing phases.
- Unambiguously clear patient instructions. Prevent excessive active therapy during inflammatory healing phases.

The path of treatment for a finger fracture can either set the stage for an excellent outcome or provide a recipe for disaster.[2] Of course, the cascade toward stiffness cannot always be prevented. In high-energy traumas with serious soft tissue injury or in cases with fulminant complications like progressive osteomyelitis, the focus will divert to reducing the inevitable impairment. Proper alignment and functional joint positioning are secured to allow for residual dexterity or subsequent salvage procedures. Special consideration is needed for the presence of a complex regional pain syndrome (CRPS).[5,6] The treatment of CRPS is beyond the scope of this chapter, but the presence of painful dystrophic symptoms will definitely postpone or at least change the path of treatment as outlined here. CRPS will be discussed in Chapter 25.

7.1.1 Evaluation of the Stiff Finger

Joint stiffness after a finger fracture needs a systematic evaluation of all contributing factors. The pitfall here is the tendency of the patient, the doctor, and the hand therapist to first and only focus on the fracture and to treat the X-ray, rather than the patient. "If hand function does not return to normal, even after hand therapy, it must be because the fracture has not healed properly in an anatomic position and/or because any hardware is still in place that wasn't there when everything was still okay." And subsequently assume that a correction osteotomy or simple removal of hardware will automatically restore hand function to normal or expect this from a hand therapist. Of course, this might be true in a range of cases. But, to disregard complex finger biomechanics is to invite failure in a well-meant surgical attempt. A systematic and stepwise diagnostic approach is warranted and documented for each different type of tissue.[1,4,6] Although it seems recommendable to avoid tunnel vision and start with physical examination before radiologic examination, it is better to be aware of hardware problems, a delayed or nonunion before manipulating the finger. The following six consecutive steps are the author's preference to investigate a stiff finger as well as the adjacent uninjured fingers:

1. Needless to say, but often forgotten, is to first determine whether a preexisting stiffness was present before the injury. Any history of trauma, Dupuytren's disease, musculoskeletal or neurologic disorders, rheumatoid disorders, gout or degenerative arthritis is first recorded. Of course, the nature of the trauma combined with the treatment path so far will be the first direction indicator for the causes of stiffness.

2. Next is an X-ray examination in three directions. A posteroanterior, a lateral, and an oblique view to assess delayed or nonunion, the presence and position of implants, osteomyelitis, callus formation, degenerative arthritis, joint incongruity, and any other malunion or exostoses. These may all disturb the biomechanical equilibrium of the musculoskeletal system, add to stiffness, and cause pain and/or a structural motion blockage. A CT-scan can help in mapping joint surface incongruity as will be discussed in the paragraph on malunions.

3. Inspection and observation of the entire hand can be very informative. The aspect of the hand can show signs of infection, residual edema, scars, dystrophic symptoms, and the deformity at rest. Finger motion is observed during the attempts of different functional grips. Some deformities concomitant to stiffness and pointing to contributing factors will only become apparent in motion. For example, the "loss" of a knuckle or scissoring of fingers during flexion, and a swan neck deformity or finger deviation during extension. Paradoxical DIP-extension as the patient pulls the FDP tendon at end-range flexion may indicate the contribution of lumbrical tightness which, in isolation, can only be found by observation. However, limited joint flexion, interosseous muscle tightness, or adherence of the flexor tendons within zones 1 or 2 can prevent demonstration of lumbrical muscle tightness.

4. Palpation and manipulation of the finger for residual edema, skin turgor, scar contractures, subcutaneous fibrosis, hardware prominence, flexor bowstringing, etc. Painful neuromas, hypersensitive skin, and disturbed soft tissue vascularization are also detected by touch and could also contribute in the cascade toward stiffness and/or will at least affect any treatment regime. The location of the fracture and adjacent joints are palpated and tested for clinical instability or rigidity. If joints are very stiff or fixed in a contracture, distinction between musculotendinous, ligamentous, and capsular contributions is not possible on physical examination and might probably be all involved.[5] In such cases, the next step is impossible to perform and can be skipped.

5. Still holding the hand, joint motion is tested relative to the position of adjacent joints. Is the limitation of joint movement fixed, or does it vary with the position of other joints? First, the intrinsic tightness test where PIP joint flexion is affected by the position of the MCP joint. A decreased passive PIP flexion with the MCP joint held in extension as compared to the MCP held in flexion and to uninjured fingers indicates involvement of the intrinsic muscles. As said, this test might be impossible to perform in the presence of structural ligamentous contractures, adhesions, malunions, or pain. If applicable, it should be documented that intrinsic muscle tightness is not excluded yet and be examined at a later stage. Intrinsic muscle involvement is too often overlooked. Second, the Oblique Retinacular Ligament (ORL) tightness test is performed (Landsmeer test). If passive extension of the PIP joint brings the DIP joint in full and stiff extension and when DIP flexion is only possible with the PIP joint in flexion, this is suggestive for ORL tightness. A contracture that might develop in pseudoboutonniere deformities, for example after dorsal angular malunions of the proximal phalanx. The third relative motion test is for extrinsic tightness, when IP-joint flexion decreases with MCP

3

and wrist flexion, suggestive for extrinsic extensor muscle contracture.[1,3,5] Likewise, extrinsic flexor muscle contracture is suspected when IP-joint extension decreases with MCP and wrist extension.

6. Measurement of passive versus active range of motion of all finger joints of the affected hand. Extrinsic extensor- or flexor tendon adhesions are most likely the predominant contributors if passive motion exceeds active motion.[1,3,6] However, a discrepancy in passive and active extension could as well be caused by tendon disruption,[6] a shortening malunion or angulation in the sagittal plane found in step 2. Again, joints can be completely stiff with an equally limited passive and active motion in any position of the adjacent joints.

In all cases, a systematic examination and documentation will always provide necessary information for any treatment plan, also in the presence of an obvious and predominant malunion, nonunion or in the presence of a completely fixed joint that does not respond to any provocative testing. Additional radiologic examination might help. The development of sophisticated ultrasound probes and high-resolution 3T-MRI with dedicated coils are capable of an increasingly meticulous scrutiny of the injured tissues but also require increased understanding of the radiologist on local anatomy and pathofysiology.[7] In general, it is best to proceed with a nonsurgical treatment protocol based on the findings of examination. Besides a high chance of improvement, it serves a diagnostic purpose because different elements of stiffness are revealed only as others are resolved.[1] Treatment of the stiff finger is also a stepwise process with repeated examination after every improvement.

7.1.2 Treatment of the Stiff Finger

Nonoperative Therapy

As a general rule, nonoperative therapy precedes surgical intervention.[1,3] It serves more purposes than just the attempt to resolve finger stiffness. As stated above, it might have a diagnostic value. For example: the extent of a rotation malunion and its effect on functional grips will only become apparent when finger flexion increases, any intrinsic tightness will only become apparent when capsular contractures resolve, and the distinction between capsular tightness and tendon adhesions can only be made when passive motion increases. Furthermore, a hand therapist will invest in patient education, shared decision making and setting realistic functional goals tailored to the patient's needs. The educated patient is a strong ally[2] and a clear motivation is paramount to embark on a journey stretching over many months of rehabilitation and possible surgical interventions.[5]

The basis of nonoperative therapy to resolve finger stiffness is to put a low-load prolonged stress on the contracted soft tissues in order to gain plastic deformation in the desired direction.[1,3] Both static and dynamic splinting regimes have proven to be quite successful in resolving fingers stiffness.[2,4,5,6] Proper splinting is adjusted to the desired direction of plastic deformation, the support of any instability, the amount of allowed protected motion, the control of edema, and the relaxation needed to relieve inflammatory signs. A skilled hand therapist will be able to compose the right splinting regime for each individual stiff finger:

• Serial casting.
• Static-progressive splinting.
• Dynamic splinting.
• Relative motion splinting.

Serial casting and static-progressive splinting are gaining preference as the first choice. Plastic deformation of the contracted tissues appears to be best achieved by a stress-relaxation method and, especially in serial casting (▶ Fig. 7.1a), this method is less prone to overzealous exercising and the dreaded exacerbation of inflammation. Inflammatory signs will need a regime that allows for periods of relaxation. Both in static-progressive splinting and serial casting the joint is held at a constant position without continuous pull. The amount of force required to maintain that position decreases with time, as the tissue stretches by plastic deformation, until an equilibrium is reached and the cast can be adjusted or replaced.[1,2] A static-progressive splinting regime (▶ Fig. 7.1b) also works according to the stress-relaxation method but in contrast to serial casting, the splint can be made adjustable and removable to allow for motion exercises.[4,5]

Dynamic splinting with some kind of continuous traction device (▶ Fig. 7.1c) is preferred in later and persistent stages of stiffness, after the inflammatory cascade has subsided and when motion exercises are necessary to preserve residual gliding qualities of soft tissues. The greatest risk of a dynamic regime is to put too much force on the tissues.[3,4] Overzealous redression and forceful exercise by either a hastily patient or an inexperienced therapist will do more harm than good. On the other hand, a properly adjusted continuous traction device and well-educated exercises may offer a beneficial regime for both gliding surfaces and tissue contractures. Plastic deformation of the contracted tissues in dynamic splinting is achieved by creep. Creep is the deformation of tissues while placed under constant traction-stress for an extended period of time.[2]

A well-known but not often applied splinting technique for PIP or even DIP joint stiffness is the relative motion splint (▶ Fig. 7.1d). The technique is widely accepted to aid in the recovery of tendon repair and boutonniere deformities. It allows immediate active motion relative to adjacent fingers with tendons from a shared muscle.[8] The same splint might also enforce active PIP extension or flexion by restricting the MCP joint. In other words, the force for extension or flexion is diverted to the PIP joint

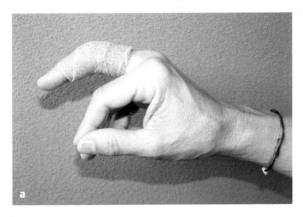
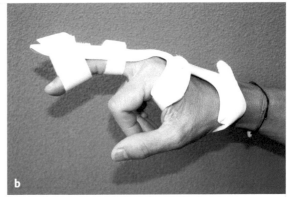
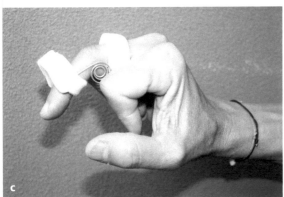
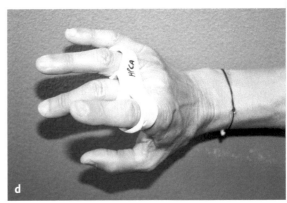

Fig. 7.1 Examples of the four different splinting principles for a proximal interphalangeal (PIP) flexion contracture of the middle finger. (I acknowledge the input of the hand therapists of the Amsterdam Hand & Wrist Centre, HPCA, for these photographs.) **(a)** An example of serial casting. **(b)** An example of a static-progressive splint. **(c)** A dynamic traction device. **(d)** A relative motion splint to enforce active PIP extension.

because it cannot be taken up by the hypermobile MCP joint.[9] This might be of beneficial aid to active motion exercises. Especially intrinsic tightness, muscle contractures, or tendon adhesions can be directly addressed with the relative motion method. In summary, seven principles of nonoperative therapy can be distracted from this paragraph:

1. Patient education.
2. Edema control.
3. Assessment of inflammatory signs.
4. Proper splinting regime.
5. Active and passive motion exercises of all fingers.
6. Measuring progress and repeated examination of the contributing factors to residual stiffness.
7. Supporting the patient to resume daily activities and return to work.

Surgical Treatment of the Stiff Finger

Nonoperative therapy should continue as long as there is improvement, even if it is only a slight or slow progress.[3] The treatment regime is only reconsidered if an objective plateau has been reached and several weeks or even months pass with no further resolution of stiffness.[1,2,5,6]

Surgery is not an alternative to nonoperative therapy or vice versa. Both treatments should facilitate each other to achieve the optimal result. At some point, surgery might be needed for nonoperative therapy to proceed and vice versa. For example, a malunion might need to be corrected first before therapy can be resumed, or therapy is needed first to resolve capsular stiffness before surgical tenolysis or tendon reconstruction can be successful. Again, a stepwise and systematic approach is warranted. This paragraph will focus on this approach rather than outlining details of surgical techniques. As said, the first step is to repeat full examination of the stiff finger and to make an inventory of contributing factors to the persistent stiffness. Next is to determine the timing and sequence of interventions. In the ideal timing for surgery:

- The inflammatory phase has subsided.
- There is no longer fluctuating edema.
- Therapy has reached a plateau in positive progress.
- Scars are fully matured.

Any divergence from this ideal timing needs appreciation of the risk of associated complications weighed against the need for earlier surgery. Of course, complications like the presence of active infections, paronychia, panaritium, osteomyelitis, or purulent arthritis will immediately bypass any timing criterium for surgery in a stiff finger. These need acute treatment. But also, failed, insufficient, prominent, or broken hardware are examples that might need earlier surgery. Painful neuromas or foreign bodies can seriously impede therapy and also warrant earlier surgery. In those cases, a single and least invasive procedure is chosen that fully resolves the problem at hand. Any further elective procedures on the inventory list should wait until the timing criteria above are met.

As a rule of thumb, one surgical session should only combine multiple procedures that can be performed through a single approach (dorsal, volar, or lateral) and that do not require conflicting postoperative therapy. Combining multiple approaches in one surgical session should be avoided.[2] The risk of creating more complications and disappointing results increases exponentially with the extent of surgery.[4] Moreover, it is false to assume that the same result can be achieved in a reduced rehabilitation time when all contributing factors are surgically treated in one session. Stepwise and well-timed multiple surgical sessions are aimed to facilitate nonoperative therapy in a continued resolving of stiffness that might even reduce the need for further surgery.[6] On the other hand, all procedures that *can* be combined in one session through the same approach *should* be combined. Intraoperative stepwise surgery in one session is possible with a wide awake patient under local anesthesia. It enables to determine the progress from each procedure and the need to proceed with subsequent procedures in the same session.[2,3,5,6] From this perspective, surgical procedures that might be necessary can be grouped into three categories of possible combinations:

1. Bone and skin reconstruction. Primary surgical attention should be directed toward problems with skin and bone. Malunions, nonunions, exostoses, or malposition of implants are addressed in the first surgical step.[6] The paragraphs on malunion and nonunion will elaborate on this. Also, bone reconstruction needs a well-vascularized soft tissue coverage. Scar contractures and soft tissue coverage of questionable quality are preferably reconstructed at the same time. Bone reconstruction should not be combined with extensive release procedures beyond the approach for the skin and bone procedure or with tendon reconstructions. The goal here is to achieve functional and stable anatomy of the joints, phalanges, and/or metacarpals with well-vascularized soft tissue coverage to allow for optimal resumption of nonoperative therapy.

2. Release procedures and hardware removal. When nonoperative therapy is no longer able to further improve stiffness and bone and skin have healed properly, the focus will be on persistent capsular and ligament contractures, muscle contractures, and tendon adhesions. Ideally, a single approach is selected for a stepwise

release of all adhesions and contracted structures under local anesthesia. For example, the preferred midlateral approach dorsal to the neurovascular bundle might allow for dorsal and palmar exposure of all structures that need release in a PIP flexion contracture.[3,5,6] However, the concomitant need for flexor tendon tenolysis or a pulley reconstruction will prefer a palmar approach.[5] Previous surgery, hardware location, or a full extensorhood release may prefer a dorsal approach. Multiple approaches should not be combined in one session and the need for extensive release procedures on both the dorsal and palmar aspect of the digit will require a staged surgical treatment.[2,6] Regardless of the approach and techniques, less than full range of motion should be anticipated following multiple necessary surgical release procedures.[3] When a two-staged release in this category is planned, the ratio to first address either the dorsal or palmar side depends on the functional desire of the patient and the position and extent of the contractures. In general, it is preferred to first improve lost flexion of the MCP and PIP joints.[2] Any hardware on the dorsal or lateral aspect is removed. From proximal to distal and only if needed, a stepwise consecutive release of zone 5 and 6 extensor tendon and sagittal band adhesions, the dorsal capsule of the MCP joint, the entire extensorhood and the intrinsics, the dorsal capsule of the PIP joint, the oblique retinacular ligament, further distal extensor tenolysis, or even Fowler's tenotomy are all combined at this stage.[2,5,6] The goal here is to at least restore passive MCP, PIP, and DIP flexion and facilitate active extension to the point of maximal passive extension. In a later stage, palmar release procedures will address residual PIP and DIP flexion contractures.[2] A palmar Bruner's or midlateral approach under local anesthesia is used to consecutively release zone 1 and 2 flexor tendon adhesions, the transverse retinacular ligament, the accessory collateral and checkrein ligaments, and, if still needed, a resection of the proximal volar plate. Although release procedures are preferably not combined with reconstructions, an exception is made for a pulley reconstruction. A skilled therapist will be able to protect a reconstructed pulley while exercising tendon excursion. Successful release procedures are aimed to achieve both passive extension and flexion to the level of functional desire. Postoperative therapy is started immediately after surgery and will focus on edema control, maintaining the gained passive motion and exercising active flexion and extension. In the majority of cases, no further surgery will be necessary. Silastic rods are implanted in this step in the exceptional case that needs a staged flexor tendon reconstruction.

3. A final and last category is reserved for tendon reconstructions. Tendon reconstructions or transpositions require optimal results of all previous steps: bone and

joint stability, a well-vascularized gliding soft tissue environment, and a full passive motion in the desired functional range. Either flexor digitorum profundus reconstruction or extensor tendon reconstruction at the level of the PIP joint is most common at this stage.

When multiple surgical steps are necessary, it is important to start the next step only if the timing criteria have been met again. Needless to repeat, the entire treatment is a long process that requires a close threefold collaboration of hand surgeon, hand therapist, and patient. After each step, whether it is surgical or nonsurgical, gained results are shared as a team and new goals are set for the next step. A motivated and diligent team with realistic goals will be able to achieve the maximal functional result in the challenge to overcome a stiff finger. However, at any point in this trajectory an acceptance and coping with residual stiffness should also be considered and weighed against a realistic improvement from continued treatment. The next two paragraphs will illustrate that also salvage procedures should be considered in seriously injured fingers. Against wishful judgment, an arthrodesis or even amputation can be the best option in severe cases.

7.2 Malunion

A malunion is generally defined as an incomplete bone union or union in a faulty position. Its definition does not include a minimum degree of incompleteness or faulty position. It also does not include any relationship to functional impairment or long-term degenerative risks. As clinical hand surgeons, we have a natural tendency to use the term "malunion" as a diagnosis instead of a symptom. It is not a diagnosis. It is an objective finding that might have a cause-and-effect relationship with a functional deficit. There are three additional pitfalls in looking at malunions of phalangeal and metacarpal fractures:

1. A malunion is commonly described in a single plane. Similar to fracture dislocations as an angulation-, translocation-, shortening-, or rotational deformity. Each referring to a dislocation in only one plane. Most often in the sagittal (volar versus dorsal) or coronal (lateral) planes. While in reality, it should always be considered as a three-dimensional deformity in multiple planes. We tend to use its most prominent deformity in its most obvious plane for characterization of the malunion. For example, "a rotational deformity" or "a dorsal angulation malunion." It should be noticed that a rotational deformity probably also has a component of shortening and angulation, and a dorsal angulation malunion will also angulate in the coronal plane and could have a component of rotation and translocation. When planning a reconstructive procedure, all planes of malunion and their contribution to the functional deficit should be recognized.

2. It is difficult to get a reliable measure of the actual extent of the malunion on standard radiographs. Again, it should be remembered that we are looking at a two-dimensional representation of a three-dimensional problem. The slightest difference in view will affect the angle of the dislocation, the amount of shortening, the widening of the gap. Keep this in mind when you compare your measurements to reference values in the literature. It is important to realize that measurements on standard radiographs are mere indications of the degree of malunion in only one plane, and also as only one part of the analysis of the patient's complaints and functional deficit. A 3D CT-scan will help in cases where a reliable measurement of the malunion in multiple planes is needed.

3. It can be difficult to predict functional deficit from a malunion. Is the malunion the main (and only) accountable source of the functional deficit? And to what extent? We are often provided with maximum acceptable degrees of angulation, maximum millimeters of shortening, or a maximum percentage of joint surface involvement. Our stock of knowledge includes well-supported data from biomechanical and anatomical research or widely accepted expert opinions. From this base, it is tempting to jump to a fast conclusion putting a cause-and-effect relationship between an objective malunion and an objective functional deficit. And subsequently, to expect that surgical correction of only that malunion should be able to correct the functional deficit in full. This pitfall carries the risk of inviting failure to your procedure. Even if we are confident in our measurements and the deformity is significant, we should be aware that the malunion is not necessarily the only causative agent of the functional deficit of the affected ray. There are always exceptions to this rule. For example, it is safe to fully attribute finger scissoring to an objective isolated rotational deformity in the presence of a painless full range of motion. In the paragraph on finger stiffness, the quality and integrity of all soft tissues in the zone of injury are addressed as important possible contributors to complaints and functional deficits after phalangeal and metacarpal fractures.

7.2.1 Treatment of Malunions

Surgical correction of a malunion is indicated when a realistic expectation of satisfactory relief of symptoms outweighs the investment of a surgical procedure, the risk of new complications and the time needed for healing and rehabilitation. It can be only the first step in resolving finger stiffness as explained in the previous paragraph. From this perspective, the surgical plan should be aimed at a functional gain tailored to the needs of each specific patient. On the other hand, not all malunions cause a disabling functional deficit. A slight malunion might only present as an apparent loss of a knuckle, a minimal change in alignment of the finger, a minimal rotation of the nail, or only a slight loss in range of motion. All without the loss of functional ability. Intact functional grips of the hand might feel unusual to the patient without actual impairment. The patient's desire for surgical correction of a minor malunion is sometimes only based on frustration about a nonanatomical healing of the fracture and a changed appearance of the hand as compared to the other hand, without any functional deficit. It should be discussed whether the combination of a correction osteotomy with (secondary) multiple release procedures to gain those last 20 degrees of motion is realistic and worth the risk of new complications. On the other hand, the aesthetically displeasing loss of the knuckle in a volar angulation malunion of the fifth metacarpal neck with maybe a slight loss of finger extension might not pose any functional limit to hand function, but still worthwhile to consider surgical correction in a well-informed and motivated patient. Of course, these considerations should have been taken into account in the acute stage of fracture treatment when a certain degree of dislocation was accepted to heal in malunion, especially in metacarpal neck fractures.

The first step before making a surgical treatment plan is to resolve any concurrent joint stiffness as much as possible by an optimal nonoperative therapy regime as outlined above. Ideally, edema and inflammation should have subsided, soft tissues should be healed, and any fibrotic scarring matured. As with the stiff finger, the hand therapist plays a valuable role in this process and helps to determine the functional goals tailored to the patient's needs. The surgical malunion correction plan should include the following:
- Infection prevention.
- The approach, site, and type of correction osteotomy.
- The possible need of a cancellous or structural bone graft.
- The choice of implant.
- Adjunct soft tissue procedures.
- Postoperative rehabilitation regime.

Metacarpal Malunions

The most common malunions of metacarpal neck fractures are volar angulated due to the pull of the intrinsic muscles. The angle that can be tolerated increases toward the fifth ray. As said, exact tolerable angles can be treacherous to use, vary considerably, and do not address the needs and desire of the patient. That said, the reported tolerable angles range from 10 degrees in the index and middle finger[10,11] increasing to a tolerable angle in the little finger beyond the commonly assumed 30 degrees[12] up to a maximum of 70 degrees.[13] Take into account that angulation is often combined with a less prominent rotation deformity and shortening. In general, correction

osteotomy is best performed at (or very close to) the site of the old fracture where normal anatomy can be restored and multiple planes of malunion can be corrected. A closing wedge osteotomy is easier than an opening wedge osteotomy but shortens the metacarpal further. An opening wedge osteotomy is preferred in cases with a surgical goal to correct an extension lag combined with a significant loss of power. A stable fixation (plate & screws) will be needed to allow for early mobilization.[14]

The second common metacarpal malunion is a dominant rotational deformity after oblique or spiraled metacarpal shaft fractures. Because of its distance to the finger-tip crossing three joints, only a slight metacarpal rotation error can result in disabling scissoring of the fingers during functional grips. The immobilization period of metacarpal fractures has shortened considerably in the last decades and early finger movement is encouraged. This has resulted in the possibility of an early detection of a developing rotation malunion. Because full osseous union will not be complete in the first months, it might still be possible to open the original plane of the fracture and restore normal anatomy. This is an additional argument for planning the osteotomy at the site of the malunion. Alternative classic sites of osteotomy are described proximal to the malunion at the metacarpal base as a transverse or step-cut osteotomy. These can be considered in cases with a full osseous union, without other planes of malunion to correct, without adhesions to release and with a limited need of derotation or in cases where the malunion site has questionable bone stock or soft tissue coverage. However, a clinically significant rotational deformity is typically a malunion to correct early at the site of the deformity, either opening the original plane or with a derotational osteotomy and a stable fixation to allow for early mobilization.

Phalangeal Malunions

Treatment of phalangeal malunions is far more challenging. The proximal phalanx is encapsulated in the ingenious intrinsic and extrinsic assembly of tendons with a high tendency for malunion in unstable fractures, tendon adhesions, and the development of PIP and DIP contractures. Typical dorsal angulation of fractures in the base of the proximal phalanx can be insidious to assess on standard radiographs. The proximal fragment of base and shaft fractures is flexed by intrinsic muscle force while the dorsal fragment is extended. The dorsal surface of the phalanx shortens relative to the length of the extensor apparatus, creating a biomechanical dysbalance and a pseudoboutonnière deformity. If left untreated, a staged and stepwise approach is necessary as outlined in the paragraph on the stiff finger. In general, a closing wedge osteotomy and a lateral plate at the site of the original fracture is preferred.[10] This might be challenging due to its proximity to the PIP or MCP joint, the close relation to the extensor assembly and the desire to fit a stable fixation. Some divergence from the old fracture site might be necessary to avoid further complications. Dorsal plating is second best and should be avoided in the distal half of the proximal phalanx, closer to the PIP joint. It interferes with the extensor assembly and a later plate removal and tenolysis should be anticipated. However, the proximal phalanx base close to the MCP joint in the middle and ring finger will often require dorsal plating or alternatively, a crossed K-wire fixation. Opening wedge osteotomy with a bone graft also carries the risk of new adhesions and contractures with a high chance of subsequent tenolysis and/or capsulolysis.[15] These are reserved for the need to correct significant phalangeal shortening or malunions in the coronal plane.

The relation of the middle phalanx to the extensor assembly does allow for small dorsal plating at its base or small well-fitted lateral plating at its shaft or distal half. But, crossed K-wire fixation with good bone contact that allows for early mobilization is generally preferred in the middle phalanx.

Intra-articular Malunions

In addition to malalignment in multiple planes and all aforementioned issues to consider, an intra-articular incongruity and chondral injury may further complicate the malunion with pain, arthritis, and the risk of progressive degeneration. A developing intra-articular malunion is therefore best corrected early. Ideally, the old fracture line is opened to restore normal anatomy. However, this should only be performed in the presence of large fragments. The risk of creating multiple small fragments with questionable viability without the possibility of a stable fixation should be avoided to prevent nonunion, osteonecrosis or fixation failures. Therefore, the first step is to evaluate the size and course of the original fragments and the quality of the joint surfaces. A 3D CT scan is often necessary for proper assessment. Combined with patient characteristics and functional desire the following four options are considered:

1. Early osteotomy within the first months when osseous union is not yet complete. This creates the advantage of restoring normal anatomy but is only reliable in the presence of one or two large viable fragments. The case in ▶ Fig. 7.2 is a 16-year-old female, 10 weeks after trauma. The fracture site of the large fragment could be opened and intra-articular anatomy restored.
2. Advancement osteotomy[16] is a smart technique that enables to focus on joint congruity and malunion correction but ignores the old fracture lines. Osseous union should be complete because osteotomy is planned at the site of the original fracture, but not in the fracture itself. It is described for malunited condylar fractures but can also be applied in other intra-articular malunions. Preferably, one new large

fragment is created at the site of the old fracture and advanced to correct the malunion and restore the joint surface (▶ Fig. 7.3). Some challenging creativity is sometimes needed to plan the osteotomy keeping three goals in mind: (1) restoring joint congruity, (2) restoring phalangeal alignment in all planes, and (3) creating one or two new large viable fragments that allow for stable screw fixation.
3. Accept the articular incongruity and instead perform an extra-articular osteotomy to correct the angular and/or rotational deformity produced by the malunion.[10,14] Although this technique might feel suboptimal, it eliminates the risk of further intra-articular complications and restores proper alignment for the residual range of motion. This is especially suitable for patients with malaligned fingers without pain, with an acceptable range of motion and with multiple small intra-articular malunited fractures in the more forgiving MCP and DIP joints.
4. While beyond the scope of this chapter, reconstruction or salvage should always be on the list of options.[3] For example, the experience with a Hemi-Hamate arthroplasty for a partially destroyed volar base of the middle phalanx has optimized this technique to yield a reliable option for these intra-articular malunions. Smaller defects might be salvaged by a volar plate advancement arthroplasty. Larger chondral defects in stiff, painful joints might not benefit from osteotomies or reconstruction and are best treated with arthrodesis or a prosthetic arthroplasty. Typically, in painful and destructed DIP-joints, thumb and index PIP finger joints, an arthrodesis is the first choice, and in all other MCP and PIP joints a prosthetic arthroplasty is the first choice. This depends, of course, on the complaints and functional desire of the patient.

7.3 Nonunion

Nonunion of uncomplicated phalangeal or metacarpal fractures is rare. Almost all cases are atrophic nonunions secondary to vascular compromise or infection. Reconstruction to achieve osseous union in such atrophic nonunions can be quite challenging and disappointing. The sequelae of poorly vascularized bone and its surroundings, osteomyelitis, and/or soft tissue infections yield an environment with little potential of bone-regeneration. Especially crush injuries and complex injuries where fractures are combined with extensive soft tissue damage or even bone loss fall in that category. Furthermore, phalanges tend to have a lot of difficulty to bridge a bone defect. It is, therefore, of essential importance to ensure measures for the prevention of infection and to prevent any unnecessary vascular compromise by iatrogenic soft tissue or bone damage. Here, we encounter the challenge to balance between (1) the need for a stable fracture fixation

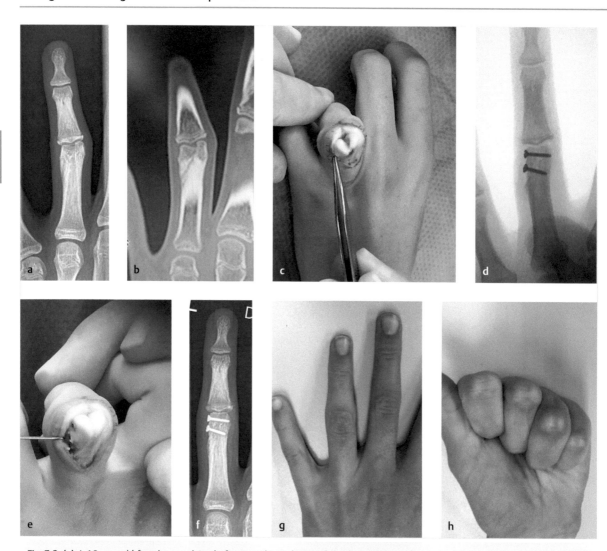

Fig. 7.2 **(a)** A 16-year-old female complained of pain and angulation of the fourth finger after nonsurgical treatment of an accepted dislocation in an intra-articular proximal interphalangeal (PIP) fracture in her left nondominant hand. **(b)** Computed tomography (CT) scan image of the finger shows a malunion of a proximally dislocated monocondylar fracture with an intra-articular step-off and angulation in the PIP joint. **(c)** The intraoperative view, 10 weeks after trauma, still reveals an intra-articular gap and a rotation of the proximally displaced ulnar condyle. The original fracture-site could be used for osteotomy. **(d)** Advancement and derotation of the large viable fragment and screw fixation. **(e)** Original intra-articular anatomy is restored. **(f)** Complete union and malunion correction is achieved. **(g)** Postoperative active extension of the finger. **(h)** Postoperative active flexion of the finger.

that allows for early unloaded functional exercise of the fingers and (2) the need to be as less invasive and to be as gentle to all tissues as possible to reach that goal. Excessive surgical exposure, denuding the fractured bone, and the heat from high-speed drilling in open procedures as well as from high-speed (repeated) K-wire drilling in percutaneous fixation, will all comprise tissue viability and bone regeneration potential at the fracture site. From this perspective, we can identify cases of phalangeal or metacarpal fractures where the possibility of a nonunion should be anticipated:

1. Cases with a high level of suspicion for avascular necrosis of the fracture-site due to:

- Extensive soft tissue injury, crush injuries, explosion (fireworks), and shotgun injuries.
- Iatrogenic surgical soft tissue or bone damage.
2. Cases with postoperative or posttraumatic wound infection and/or osteomyelitis.
3. Cases with traumatic bone loss with a defect exceeding 3 mm.
4. Cases with fractures in large enchondromas or pathological fractures.

The anticipation of the possibility of a nonunion in high-risk cases requires active countermeasures:
1. Proper infection prevention measures.

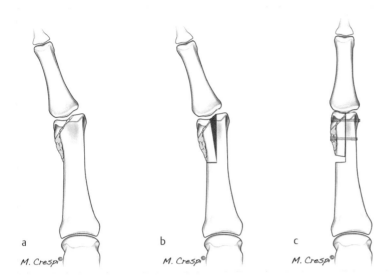

Fig. 7.3 **(a)** Intra-articular malunion in the proximal interphalangeal (PIP) joint of a small dislocated condylar fragment and a coronal angulation deformity. **(b)** Proximal transverse osteotomy to create a large viable fragment including the original fragment and a three-dimensional closing wedge osteotomy to advance, derotate, and angulate the large fragment to reconstruct functional anatomy. **(c)** Stable screw fixation of the large fragment to allow for early mobilization.

a

b

c

2. A stable fracture fixation that can remain in situ for an extended period, using gentle surgical tissue handling with the least invasive technique needed for such fixation.
3. Primary bone reconstruction and, if necessary, soft tissue reconstruction in cases with a significantly devascularized zone of injury or tissue loss.
4. Active monitoring, early recognition, and aggressive treatment at the onset of an infection.

7.3.1 Treatment of Nonunions

Do all nonunions need surgery? Clinical stability and functional recovery can be complete while radiolucent lines are still visible on radiographs. Even in the presence of an objective long-term nonunion, it remains obvious that it's not the radiograph that might require treatment, but the patient. The "diagnosis nonunion" harbors an intention to treat and should therefore include associated functionally relevant symptoms as pain, instability, and/or stiffness. As such, the nonunion is labelled symptomatic and a reconstructive procedure can be considered.

Although uncommon, cases of hypertrophic nonunion are relatively easy to treat, as they need a more stable fixation with proper bone contact. Open reduction and internal plate and screw fixation will provide this, combined with a (cancellous) bone graft if this is necessary to achieve proper bone contact. Symptomatic atrophic nonunions should not be simply refixated but will always need a bone reconstruction. As a general rule, five technical principles need to be addressed in planning the reconstruction of an atrophic phalangeal or metacarpal nonunion:

1. Infection prevention.
2. Resection of all atrophic and nonviable bone.
3. Autologous, cancellous, or structural bone graft to bridge the bone defect.

4. A strong, stable fixation of the reconstruction by plating.
5. Viable soft tissue coverage of the reconstruction.

Nonunions of the distal phalanx are somewhat more common. Pain or instability of the finger-tip and nail deformities can be present and the reason for a reconstruction. In hypertrophic nonunions and without the need to address concomitant nail deformities, a closed percutaneous compression screw can provide sufficient stability to achieve final union. Open reconstruction is needed in cases with a displaced or atrophic nonunion needing a graft. Both need an open debridement and reduction of the nonunion.[17] In cases with nail deformities, the exposure is best performed through the nail bed, allowing for matrix repair and realignment of the nail bed on the reconstructed phalanx. Alternatively, a lateral incision can be used. A cancellous or structural graft can be harvested from the distal radius or the olecranon.[18] Fixation should provide a strong and durable stability and small compression screws or even cerclage wires are preferred over K-wires, although good results have been reported.[18]

It should also be anticipated that the result of a reconstruction of any nonunion can be unsuccessful. Patient characteristics, a strong motivation to succeed combined with realistic expectations should be in accordance with the treatment plan. It may require a long period of healing and rehabilitation. Salvage procedures should also be considered and discussed with the patient. Arthrodesis or arthroplasty should be considered in cases of intra-articular nonunions with pain, severe stiffness, questionable soft tissue quality, and/or signs of (degenerative) cartilage damage. At least, it should be discussed with the patient before a reconstructive venture with a long period of hand therapy is started. It could all still end in an arthrodesis. Amputation should be considered in cases with severe soft tissue injury, extensive fibrosis, stiffness, permanent sensory loss, and/or pain. Especially, when combined with significant bone loss that would require a reconstruction with poor soft tissue coverage. A successful bone reconstruction in a stiff finger with bad sensation or even pain should be considered a failure. A hesitation toward amputation is natural for patients and surgeons. But, a well-advised amputation can relieve hopeless symptoms in a short rehabilitation period, facilitating (or even restoring) the functional ability of the adjacent fingers.

7.4 Take-Home Message

A finger fracture is a treacherous soft tissue injury around a small broken bone. The first pitfall in complications after finger fractures is to focus on the bone, while all surrounding soft tissues collaborating in a delicate equilibrium should be considered to be involved. A myriad of complications create a complex challenge that requires a systematic and stepwise approach in both repeated examination and treatment. A thorough understanding of the intricate anatomy, biomechanics, and pathophysiology is needed to avoid the many pitfalls of doing more harm than good. Nonoperative therapy and a well-tailored splinting regime might obviate surgical treatment and should always come first. Moreover, in the process of slowly resolving stiffness, the distinction between multiple causative agents might become apparent. Elective surgery is considered when the inflammatory cascade has subsided, fibrotic tissue has matured, and nonoperative therapy has failed or reached an objective plateau. Three-dimensional malunions and nonunions harbor pitfalls in their assessment and treatment, and should never be regarded as separate from their soft tissue envelope. This might necessitate carefully planned staged surgical procedures alternated with long periods of therapy. A well-informed and motivated patient is a strong ally for the hand surgeon and hand therapist working in a close relationship. Realistic goals of the treatment plan are tailored to the needs and desire of the individual patient. However, despite a successful treatment and team effort, it should be anticipated that complications in finger fractures might result in a permanent impairment. Acceptance of suboptimal results and salvage procedures like arthrodesis and even amputation are always on the list to consider, albeit only by a team of hand surgeon and hand therapist specialized in complications after finger fractures and their treatment.

References

[1] Shin AY, Amadio PC. The stiff finger. In: Wolfe SW, et al. Green's operative hand surgery. Philadelphia: Elsevier Churchill Livingstone; 2017
[2] Kaplan FTD. The stiff finger. Hand Clin. 2010; 26(2):191–204
[3] Tuffaha SH, Lee WPA. Treatment of proximal interphalangeal joint contracture. Hand Clin. 2018; 34(2):229–235
[4] Yang G, McGlinn EP, Chung KC. Management of the stiff finger: evidence and outcomes. Clin Plast Surg. 2014; 41(3):501–512
[5] Catalano LW, III, Barron OA, Glickel SZ, Minhas SV. Etiology, evaluation, and management options for the stiff digit. J Am Acad Orthop Surg. 2019; 27(15):e676–e684
[6] Wang ED, Rahgozar P. The pathogenesis and treatment of the stiff finger. Clin Plast Surg. 2019; 46(3):339–345
[7] Petchprapa CN, Vaswani D. MRI of the fingers: an update. AJR Am J Roentgenol. 2019; 213(3):534–548
[8] Hirth MJ, Howell JW, O'Brien L. Relative motion orthoses in the management of various hand conditions: a scoping review. J Hand Ther. 2016; 29(4):405–432
[9] Colditz JC. Active redirection instead of passive motion for joint stiffness. IFSSH Ezine. 2014; 4(4):41–44
[10] Gajendran VK, Gajendran VK, Malone KJ. Management of complications with hand fractures. Hand Clin. 2015; 31(2):165–177
[11] Balaram AK, Bednar MS. Complications after the fractures of metacarpal and phalanges. Hand Clin. 2010; 26(2):169–177
[12] Sletten IN, Hellund JC, Olsen B, Clementsen S, Kvernmo HD, Nordsletten L. Conservative treatment has comparable outcome with bouquet pinning of little finger metacarpal neck fractures: a multicentre randomized controlled study of 85 patients. J Hand Surg Eur Vol. 2015; 40(1):76–83
[13] Strub B, Schindele S, Sonderegger J, Sproedt J, von Campe A, Gruenert JG. Intramedullary splinting or conservative treatment for displaced fractures of the little finger metacarpal neck? A prospective study. J Hand Surg Eur Vol. 2010; 35(9):725–729
[14] Ring D. Malunion and nonunion of the metacarpals and phalanges. Instr Course Lect. 2006; 55:121–128
[15] Büchler U, Gupta A, Ruf S. Corrective osteotomy for post-traumatic malunion of the phalanges in the hand. J Hand Surg [Br]. 1996; 21 (1):33–42
[16] Teoh LC, Yong FC, Chong KC. Condylar advancement osteotomy for correcting condylar malunion of the finger. J Hand Surg [Br]. 2002; 27(1):31–35
[17] Chim H, Teoh LC, Yong FC. Open reduction and interfragmentary screw fixation for symptomatic nonunion of distal phalangeal fractures. J Hand Surg Eur Vol. 2008; 33(1):71–76
[18] Ozçelik IB, Kabakas F, Mersa B, Purisa H, Sezer I, Ertürer E. Treatment of nonunions of the distal phalanx with olecranon bone graft. J Hand Surg Eur Vol. 2009; 34(5):638–642

8 Management of Complications in Carpal Fractures (Malunion, Nonunion)

Florian M.D. Lampert, Ayla Hohenstein, and Max Haerle

Abstract

Fractures of the carpal bones differ substantially in incidence. Apart from the scaphoid, they can frequently be treated conservatively with good results. Relevant concomitant soft tissue injuries are rare. Although scaphoid fracture is the most common fracture of the carpal bones, its treatment is still burdened with various unresolved difficulties and risks in the course of treatment. An overview of the most common complications is given in this chapter, with specific emphasis on scaphoid nonunion. Different treatment options are discussed, along with their indications and limitations, and a treatment algorithm is suggested.

Keywords: carpal fracture, scaphoid fracture, malunion, nonunion, humpback deformity, bone graft, osteosynthesis

8.1 Introduction

Fracture of the carpal bones can occur as a principle in any carpal bone. The frequency with which they occur is illustrated in ▶ Fig. 8.1. Besides the scaphoid, the triquetrum is most affected, but rarely presents a source of complication. Most times in carpal bones, conservative treatment is sufficient and complications are rare. This is true for most fractures besides the scaphoid, unless they occur in a feature of massive trauma of the wrist, which is difficult to be analyzed in a statically reproducible way. Uncommon fractures of the wrist, which may be a recurrent source of complications, are the fractures of the hook of the hamate and the pisiform fractures.

In the treatment of scaphoid fractures, many pitfalls lurk along the path during the whole course from the initial injury to the—at best—restitutio ad integrum. In particular, a delayed or absent bony union occurs in approximately 10% of all fractures.[1] Risk factors for scaphoid nonunion are: location of fracture (proximal third), fracture displacement, carpal instability, time to treatment, heavy labor, and smoking.[2,3] The long-term consequence of an untreated scaphoid nonunion could be severe osteoarthritis and pain in the vast majority of cases (75–100%) after 10 years,[4,5] which occurs in the typical pattern of a scaphoid nonunion advanced collapse (SNAC-Wrist).[5]

A number of frequent main problems in the treatment of scaphoid fractures can be identified[6]:

- The patient trivializes the injury and does not turn to a doctor.
- The doctor does not initiate adequate imaging diagnostics.
- The fracture is not detected in imaging diagnostics.
- The grade of dislocation or instability of a detected fracture is not adequately assessed.
- Despite a correct diagnosis, no adequate therapy is initiated.
- Despite an adequate indication, therapy is not carried out correctly.
- Despite state-of-the-art diagnostics and therapy, the fracture does not heal due to anatomical peculiarities of the scaphoid or secondary factors.

8.2 Uncommon Carpal Fractures

Hook of hamate and pisiform fractures are by far less frequent than fractures of the scaphoid. Fractures of the hamate and pisiform occur as isolated injuries, in many cases on direct impact of a club or bat in athletes or tool handles or grips in workers. Both fracture types have in common a considerable risk of being missed on clinical examination and standard plain radiographs with the consequence of the development of complications. Most common are painful nonunions, as well as irritation or injury to the deep or superficial branch of the ulnar nerve from either direct impact or pressure from hematoma or edema. Furthermore, hook of hamate fractures can lead to flexor digitorum profundus (FDP) tendinopathy or even rupture. Both fracture types usually present with tenderness over the hypothenar eminence. On clinical

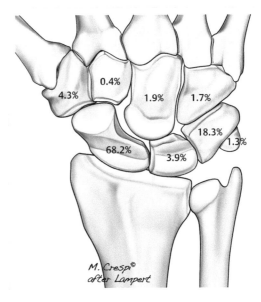

Fig. 8.1 Relative incidence of carpal bone fractures.

suspicion, a radiograph with carpal tunnel or special pisiform projection should be acquired; in case of doubt, a computed tomography reliably visualizes the fracture.

In the absence of dislocation, these fractures are commonly treated conservatively; in cases of dislocated fractures, minimally invasive placement of cannulated screws can be considered. In cases of nonunion after unsuccessful conservative treatment or for undiagnosed as well as comminuted fractures, excision of the respective bone commonly leads to good results without relevant functional impairments.[7,8]

8.3 Scaphoid Fractures

8.3.1 (Patho-)Physiology of Fracture Healing in the Scaphoid

Approximately 80% of the scaphoid is covered with cartilage; therefore, secondary (i.e., periosteal) bone healing with formation of callus does not take place in a significant manner. Being the major mechanical link between the proximal and the distal row of carpal bones, the scaphoid is exposed to severe shearing and bending forces especially on its distal part, thus creating repeated interfragmentary motion in case of a fracture, with a tendency to collapse into a dorsally angulated "humpback deformity."

The major blood supply to the scaphoid is from the radial artery, whose branches enter the nonarticular portion of the scaphoid at the dorsal ridge at the level of the waist or distal part and supply the proximal 70 to 80% of the bone. The volar scaphoid branches from the radial artery and its superficial palmar branch supply the distal 20 to 30% of the scaphoid. Both the volar and the dorsal branches reach the scaphoid on more distal level; therefore, the vascularity of the proximal pole predominantly depends on retrograde intraosseous blood flow, which poses a high risk for avascular necrosis.[9]

Taking this into account, it becomes evident that the factors' stability and blood supply are alternately dependent on each other. Neither will a sufficient neovascularization be likely to cross an unstable fracture site, nor will poorly vascularized bone fragments be likely to unite. Although both factors are crucial for successful fracture treatment, in the clinical setting, direct bone contact and rigid stability are absolute conditions but there is no evidence for the principle "the more—the better" concerning the compression forces of different devices.[10,11] Too much compressive strain might rather impair intraosseous blood flow and increase the risk for hardware complications.

8.3.2 Complications in Fracture Healing

Unavoidable Complications

Due to its particular geometry, the local biomechanical strain, and its tenuous vascular pattern, fractures of the scaphoid are prone to complications during any kind of therapy. Even in state-of-the-art operative treatment with correct placement of implant, nonunion may occur in up to 10% of scaphoids.[1] Conservative treatment of nondisplaced scaphoid fractures is accompanied with similar nonunion rates as the operative therapy, but the latter have a faster return to work and less time spent in a cast, traded in for the risks of the operative procedure.[12] Considering the location, proximal pole fractures are more likely to develop complications.[3] Primary fracture dislocation > 1 mm is another major risk factor for complications.

Sources of Complications

Failed Primary Nonsurgical Treatment

Although there is a trend toward a more aggressive indication for an operative therapy using minimally invasive screw fixation of *un*displaced scaphoid fractures classified A1/A2 according to Herbert/Krimmer, operative therapy is still not proven to yield superior long-term results in comparison to conservative treatment. Nevertheless, it enables an earlier return to activity (work/sport) in the predominantly young and active population suffering from scaphoid fractures.[12] If immobilization is started duly, conservative therapy provides an equivalent end result.[13] Immobilization is carried out in a short arm cast in slight wrist extension, usually with inclusion of the first carpometacarpal joint, although there is no evidence, that this is necessary. Immobilization of the elbow, however, is generally considered obsolete, since it does neither provide superior immobilization nor higher union rates, but is associated with the risk of permanent restrictions of elbow motion. Fractures of the tuberculum (A1) usually heal within 4 weeks, fractures of the waist (A2) within 6 to 8 weeks. Nevertheless, even with correct indication and execution of the conservative therapy, nonunions still occur in 5 to 12% of cases.[1]

Malreduction of Fractures

A condition sine qua non for success of the operative treatment of a scaphoid fracture is an anatomical reposition. It is generally accepted that computed tomography is the modality of choice for staging of scaphoid fractures and thus for initiation of an adequate therapy.[14] During the operation, however, the usual imaging modality is fluoroscopy, which has improved the results substantially; nevertheless, it suffers from the limited information content of any two-dimensional imaging technique and a relatively poor spatial resolution. Failure to recognize and address displacement or associated carpal lesions can be a predisposition for pseudarthrosis, axial (e.g., "humpback"), or rotational deviations.

Malpositioning of Implants

Proper intraosseous placement of the screw is crucial for successful treatment of scaphoid fractures. For maximal

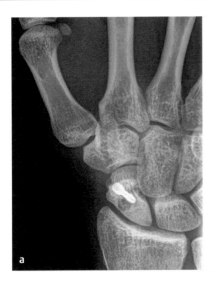 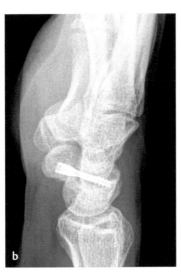

Fig. 8.2 (a, b) Malpositioning of headless screw.

biomechanical stability, and thus increase in the likelihood of bone union, screws should be placed in the central axis of the scaphoid in scaphoid waist fractures. In cases of small proximal pole fragments or oblique fractures, screw placement perpendicular to the fracture line may be necessary and also provides sufficient stability. The dorsal approach is more prone to technical errors and associated with the risk of impairing blood supply to the scaphoid[9] and affecting the cartilage as well as the scapholunate ligament. Choosing the maximal possible screw length does not seem to provide superior stability. Due to its curvature in two planes, screw placement is technically demanding and misplacements still occur even in experienced hands despite the routine use of fluoroscopic control (▶ Fig. 8.2). To overcome this problem, intraoperative 3D-imaging and even robot-assisted screw placement have been suggested in pilot studies.

Failure of Bone Healing

As stated above, osteosynthesis in the scaphoid has to create equilibrium between the competing demands of providing rigid stability to the fracture without compromising the precarious intraosseous blood supply. Therefore, both mechanically insufficient and overaggressive placements of implants are inappropriate. Yet, exact definition of complication rates according to single implants is difficult to impossible.

8.3.3 Surgical Interventions for Complication in the Healing Process

Malunion

The first goal of the treatment in scaphoid fractures is to achieve bone union. However, it has been shown that malunions of the scaphoid, namely the so-called "humpback deformity," result in pain and restriction in the range of motion and are prone to the development of posttrau-

matic osteoarthritis. The option of a correction osteotomy should therefore be taken into consideration in cases of malunion. Nevertheless, correction osteotomy is a complex invasive procedure, and its results are not necessarily superior to conservative therapy; therefore, the benefits and risks have to be discussed thoroughly with the patient. In asymptomatic cases, restraint is called in most instances. Technically, in cases of torsion or a lateral offset, osteotomy is performed in the former fracture site, followed by open reposition under fluoroscopic control and (re-)osteosynthesis, usually using a volar approach. In the most common deformity, the "humpback," the Linscheid maneuver is often helpful for reposition and correction of the dorsal intercalated segment instability (DISI) deformity, which will then result in a wedge-shaped palmar defect due to the initial bone resorption. In these cases, a bone graft in size and shape of the defect is compulsory, with the usual harvesting site being the iliac crest. Osteosynthesis is performed with cannulated screws, plates, or K-wires in most instances. Options for salvage procedures are dorsal cheilectomy, radial styloidectomy, or other methods, which can also be applied in cases of SNAC-wrist, such as four-corner fusion, proximal-row carpectomy, or d-enervation of the wrist.[15]

Nonunion

A much more frequent complication is the formation of a nonunion subsequent to a scaphoid fracture. By definition, a delayed union is considered a pseudarthrosis after 6 months. In the scaphoid, however, the above-mentioned biomechanical and vascular peculiarities often cause an irreversible nonunion as recently as 8 weeks after trauma (▶ Fig. 8.3). The underlying principle of the multitude of reconstructive options is the transformation of the pseudoarthrotic zone into an "acute-injury" setting, which is then attended with appropriate immobilization and solid blood supply. Depending on the time

3

3

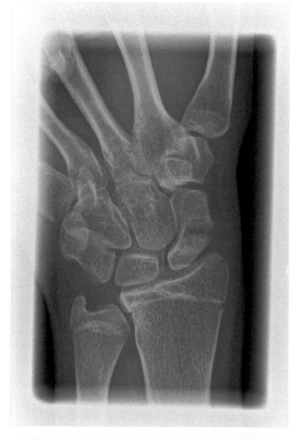

Fig. 8.3 Scaphoid nonunion following an unrecognized fracture.

elapsed since the primary injury, its location, and the extent of the nonunion interface as well as eventual deformities, different operative approaches will apply. Slade and Dodds[16] introduced a classification scheme as a guide for decision-making in treatment (▶ Table 8.1).

Resection

In selected cases with no or minimal displacement and without extensive sclerosis or bone resorption at the nonunion site (Grade I-III), a percutaneous approach without debridement of the bone may be justified. Traditionally, even for nondisplaced scaphoid nonunions, full debridement of the nonunion is recommended before bone grafting and fixation. If the gap width exceeds 1 to 2 mm, the likeliness of bridging without bone grafting is minimal; therefore, thorough debridement is mandatory. The most common approach is the limitation of the resection of the actual nonunion zone until vital bone is exposed (punctuate bleeding on tourniquet release, "paprika sign"). Cysts within the fragments are debrided using small curettes. In the Matti-Russe technique, an egg-shell-shaped cavity is created, allowing the placement of 1–2 iliac corticocancellous bone struts within both fractured fragments. The choice of a palmar or dorsal approach depends on the

location of the nonunion and the surgeon's preferences. If no relevant deformity is present, resection can be carried out arthroscopically. In doing so, impairment of the local vascular and ligamentous structures can be preserved to a large extent.[17] In cases of early stages of degenerative alterations of the radial styloid (SNAC I), a radial styloidectomy can be performed in the same session.

Bone Grafting

Bone grafts can be classified as either avascular or vascularized, with a further subdivision according to their structure (cancellous, corticocancellous, osteocartilaginous), origin (radius, iliac crest, rib, femur, allogenic...), or type of vascularization (palmar or dorsally pedicled, free).

For the choice of bone graft, the location, shape, size, and vascularity have to be taken into consideration, as well as the hitherto course and the possible presence of deformities. Typical indications for avascular bone grafting are nonunions with sufficient perfusion of the fragments, in particular the proximal pole. In case of doubt, this should be assessed by magnetic resonance imaging (MRI). If no relevant defect or deformity is present and the grafted bone is primarily employed for its osteogenic potential, autologous cancellous bone is usually sufficient, and typical harvesting sites are the distal radius or the iliac crest. The least invasive way of bone insertion is the arthroscopic approach. Following arthroscopic identification and thorough debridement of the fibrous tissue and sclerotic bone, eventual minor deformities can be reduced by closed means and a guidewire for a cannulated compression screw is inserted. Subsequently, the unstructured bone graft (harvested from the distal radius or the iliac crest via a mini open approach or using a biopsy cannula) is introduced into the defect and compacted tightly, followed by insertion of an adequate screw or K-wires to provide stability and compression.[17] For scaphoid nonunions with greater bone loss and/or significant deformities, however, the arthroscopic approach may not provide adequate correction and bone stock. In these cases, the treatment of choice is open debridement and grafting of (cortico-)cancellous bone. The dimensions of the graft are determined by the shape of the defect after debridement and reduction, in which the latter can substantially increase the actual defect size. Typically, a generously dimensioned triangular or trapezoid-shaped wedge of bone is placed between the debrided ends of the nonunion site using a palmar open approach (▶ Fig. 8.4). Nonunions of the proximal pole, however, are not easily accessible in this manner and do not lead to a typical humpback deformity; in such cases, a dorsal approach is often preferred.

8.3.4 Types of Bone Grafts
Avascular Bone Grafts

The typical harvesting sites for avascular bone grafts are the iliac crest (▶ Fig. 8.5) and the distal radius. The

Table 8.1 Classification system for scaphoid nonunions

Grade	Category	Characteristics of Scaphoid Nonunions
I	Delayed presentation	Scaphoid fractures with delayed presentation (4–8 weeks).
II	Fibrous nonunion	Intact cartilaginous envelope, minimal fracture line at nonunion interface, no cyst or sclerosis.
III	Minimal sclerosis	Bone resorption at nonunion interface < 1 mm with minimal sclerosis.
IV	Cyst formation and sclerosis	Bone resorption at nonunion interface < 5 mm, cyst formation, and maintained scaphoid alignment.
V	Cyst formation and sclerosis	Bone resorption at nonunion interface > 5 mm and < 10 mm, cyst formation, and maintained scaphoid alignment.
VI	Pseudarthrosis	Separate bone fracture fragments with profound bone resorption at nonunion interface. Gross fragment motion and deformity is often present.
Subtypes	Category	Associated Characteristics
a	Proximal pole nonunion	The proximal pole has a tenuous blood supply and a mechanical disadvantage that places it at greater risk of delayed or failed union
b	Avascular necrosis	Scaphoid nonunion with avascular necrosis confirmed by MRI or intraoperative lack of punctate bleeding. The fracture must heal and revitalize.
c	Ligamentous injury	Injury suggested by static and dynamic imaging of the carpal bones or arthroscopic, direct observation.
d	Deformity	Scaphoid deformity must be corrected. This requires a bicortical structural bone graft and rigid fixation.

Source: Used with permission from Slade JF 3rd, Dodds SD. Minimally invasive management of scaphoid nonunions. Clin Orthop Relat Res. 2006; 445: 108–119.
Abbreviation: MRI, magnetic resonance imaging.

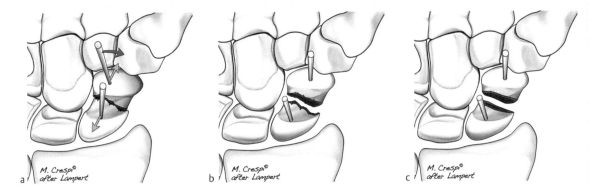

Fig. 8.4 (a–c) Reposition using the Linscheid maneuver.

former allows the retrieval of large bone volumes with up to three cortical surfaces with donor site morbidity that is generally considered relatively benign; nevertheless, complications such as hematoma, pain, injuries of the lateral femoral cutaneous nerve, and even fractures occur in approx. 20% of the patients. The distal radius lends itself for harvesting smaller volumes of unstructured cancellous bone, but with the advantage of avoiding a second operation site and general anesthesia. Usually, a curette or a biopsy punch is used; the latter can also be utilized for arthroscopic bone grafting.

Allogenic bone grafts are appealing, because they avoid any donor site morbidity, and microbiological and immunological concerns are largely negligible in certified GMP products. Otherwise, representing solely avital scaffolds, this graft lacks the osteogenic potential that is urgently required in this setting.

3

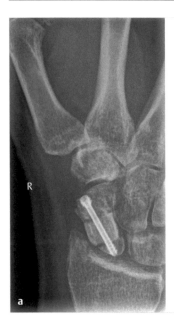
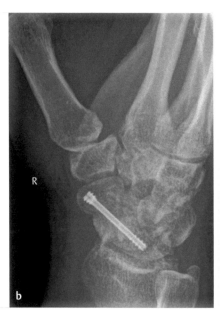

Fig. 8.5 (a, b) Scaphoid reconstruction with iliac crest bone graft.

Vascularized Bone Grafts (VBGs)

Due to the precarious vascularity of the scaphoid, in particular its proximal pole,[9] ample revascularization techniques have been suggested for cases of impaired blood supply or avascular necrosis. Numerous authors suggest that vascularized bone grafting may be beneficial in cases of avascular necrosis[2,18] due to the transfer and preservation of vital osteocytes. Nevertheless, indications and choice of grafts are frequent areas of debate. Also, in the non-VBGs, rigid fixation of VBGs is mandatory employing the above-mentioned techniques. Only few studies directly compared the outcomes of different treatment options for scaphoid nonunions; data for superiority of one technique is sparse. Nevertheless, with regard to VBGs, several studies were able to show favorable results, especially in technically demanding cases such as severe deformity or proximal pole necrosis.[18] This supports the assumption that the insertion of vascularized bone tissue is beneficial for the process of bone union by providing a graft with not only osteoconductive but also osteogenic properties. One exemplary recent study reports on union rates of 71% using a nonvascularized iliac crest bone graft compared to 79% with a radial bone graft pedicled on the 1,2-intercompartmental supraretinacular artery and 89% using a medial femoral condyle vascularized free graft, whereas there was no statistical significance. Reoperation rates for persistent nonunion and salvage procedures were 23%, 12%, 16%, again not being statistically significant.[18]

Pedicled Vascularized Bone Grafts

Pedicled VBGs have been described based on the 1,2 or 2,3 intercompartmental supraretinacular artery (ICSRA), the palmar carpal artery, or the first dorsal metacarpal artery. Grafts from the dorsal distal radius, such as the 1,2

ICSRA or 2,3 ICSRA, are largely used as inlay grafts rather than structural wedge grafts, since dorsally pedicled grafts are restricted in restoring scaphoid anatomy due to the risk of torsion or tension on the pedicle. For this reason, dorsally pedicled grafts may not be the first choice in cases of humpback deformity or carpal collapse. Volarly based pedicled grafts have proven to be capable to restore scaphoid geometry and carpal alignment[19]; nevertheless, they may not be the first choice for extensive bone defects, or eventually have to be combined with grafting of cancellous avascular bone, which may be harvested through the same distal radius approach (▸ Fig. 8.6).

Free Vascularized Bone Grafts

In certain cases, pedicled VBGs are not expedient. This may be the case, if the intended vascular pedicle has been compromised in previous surgeries such as radius fractures or release of the first extensor compartment. A complete avascular necrosis of the proximal pole with fragmentation or large volume bone defects can also not be sufficiently addressed using pedicled VBGs. In such situations, the use of free VBGs may be suitable. The first graft of this type was the deep circumflex iliac artery bone flap. Although high union rates have been reported, this flap is accompanied with considerable donor site morbidity. It has declined in importance since the free VBG from the medial femoral condyle was introduced, which offers a number of advantages: pedicled on a branch of the descending geniculate artery, this osteocartilaginous flap from the convex surface of the medial femoral trochlea can be harvested relatively uncomplicated; due to the cartilage cover and the similarity of its shape with the proximal pole of the scaphoid, it is suitable for its replacement.[20] The use of the flap without its cartilag-

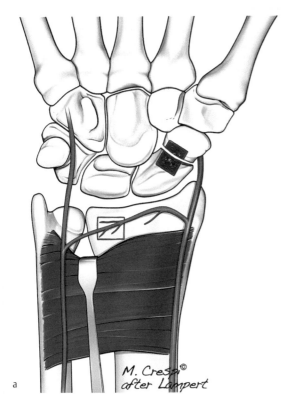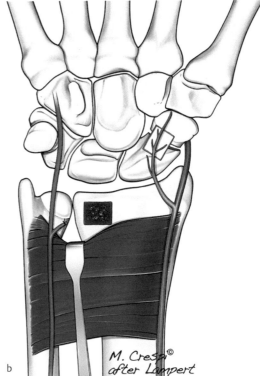

Fig. 8.6 (a, b) Scaphoid reconstruction with volar pedicled graft.

inous portion for sole bone replacement is possible as well. Usually, the arterial anastomosis is performed end-to-side to the radial artery, or end-to-end to its palmar branch. Especially in cases of failed previous reconstructive surgery, this flap can be an option to avoid salvage procedures such as partial wrist fusion or proximal row carpectomy, especially in younger and high-demand patients.

8.3.5 Other Options for Proximal Pole Replacement

Free Medial Femoral Condyle

The free medial femoral condyle VBG (see above) is one solution among various others, which have been proposed for the challenge of scaphoid proximal pole replacement. A generally accepted gold standard does not yet exist.

Hamate Autograft

Introduced in 2016, the ipsilateral proximal hamate autograft is a relatively new and auspicious option for proximal pole replacement. Long-term results, however, are still pending.[21] In this technique, the proximal pole of the ipsilateral hamate is harvested as an osteochondral graft

in the size of the defect to be replaced, together with the adhering portions of the volar capitohamate ligament. Hence, replacement of the proximal pole with reconstruction of the scapholunate ligament is possible using the same operative approach without the morbidity of a second donor site. Further studies are needed for a profound judgment of the appropriateness of this technique.

Rib Autograft

Osteochondral grafts have also been described for proximal pole replacement. They are harvested at the level of the osteochondral junction; descriptions vary in the harvesting site between the fourth and the eighth rib. Fixation is usually carried out with K-wires, because the chondral portion of the graft does not offer sufficient hold for a compression screw and tends to split during insertion. Although these procedures do not really replace "like with like," and are burdened with an unfavorable donor site, good results have been reported.[22]

Synthetic Spacers

Silicone spacers still have some merit in degenerative joint replacement in the hand. In scaphoid proximal pole replacement, however, unfavorable results (i.e., lytic bone lesions, silicone synovitis, and high explantation rates) have led to their abandoning. A spacer, which gained a certain degree of popularity, is the pyrocarbon Adaptive Proximal Scaphoid Implant (APSI). This ovoid-shaped device has the advantage of a relatively easy and little invasive implantation procedure, which can also be carried out arthroscopically assisted. Despite a considerable complication rate, the long-term results are fairly satisfactory, but not superior to the usual salvage procedures. The natural progress of SLAC-wrist development could not be halted.[23]

8.3.6 Treatment Algorithm for Scaphoid Nonunion

The algorithm in ▶ Fig. 8.7 reflects the approach in the authors' institution and may serve as a decision-making aid.

8.4 Osteosynthesis Devices

The importance of rigid bone fixation has repeatedly been stated above. During the past decades, headless intramedullary compression screws have gradually gained benchmark status for the majority of applications in the scaphoid, even the more, since most of the current devices are not only cannulated, but also self-drilling and self-tapping and therefore comfortable in handling. Relevant differences in outcome among different screw manufacturers, however, cannot be derived from the current literature.[10] If a screw cannot be securely placed in the bone satisfyingly, K-wires still pose a reasonable alternative, although they provide less compression and bending stiffness in comparison to screws[11] and are associated with lower union rates in wedge grafting compared to screw fixation (77% vs. 94% union).[2] If neither of these options appears to be expedient, i.e., in cases of large pal-

mar defects or previous surgeries with placement of screws, palmar angular stable plate fixation is an option, which is considered a valuable complement of their surgical armamentarium for selected cases by many surgeons.[24] Disadvantages of this technique are the risk of erosion of the radial cartilage and the need of hardware removal after consolidation. Using compression staples in the scaphoid is also an option, which is not widespread, but reported on with good results (▶ Fig. 8.8).

8.5 The Role of Arthroscopic Techniques

The main drawbacks of open techniques on the scaphoid are their risk of further compromising the already critical local vascularity, as well as detachment of the surrounding capsular and ligamentous stabilizing structures. Along with the continuous evolution of arthroscopic techniques in the wrist, the treatment of fractures and nonunions of the scaphoid has gained new features to circumvent these problems. This technique demand significant experience with arthroscopic procedures. In acute fractures, arthroscopically assisted percutaneous fixation allows reduction under direct visualization as well as the assessment of possible concomitant injuries.

In cases of scaphoid nonunions, an appraisal of the stability of the nonunion site can be carried out arthroscopically; if no instability is detectable even on testing with a hook probe and no deformity is present, the indication for a reconstruction might be reconsidered. If the indication for reconstruction is confirmed after diagnostic evaluation of the complete wrist, both ends of the nonunion are thoroughly debrided with a burr until vital cancellous bone is reached. If existent, a deformity can now be corrected using the so-called Linscheid maneuver, and a guidewire is placed centrally in the long axis of the

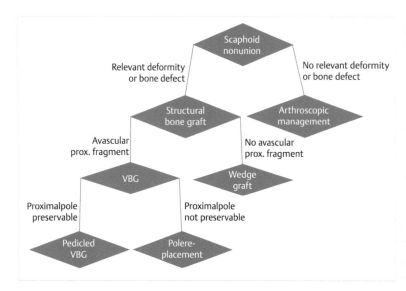

Fig. 8.7 Treatment algorithm for scaphoid nonunion.

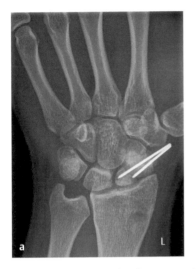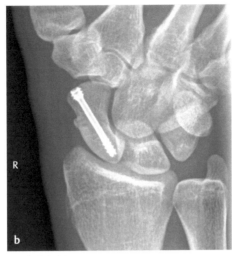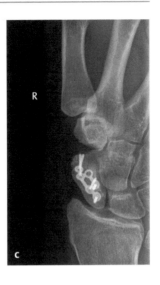

Fig. 8.8 (a–c) K-Wires, headless intramedullary screw, plate.

bone. Now, the cancellous bone graft from the distal radius or the iliac crest is introduced through the midcarpal joint and impacted in the defect, followed by the placement of a percutaneous screw. In selected cases, this technique can provide high union rates, along with minimal invasiveness and the possibility to treat concomitant injuries.[17,25]

8.6 Take-Home Messages

- Fractures of the hook of the hamate and pisiform have good potential for conservative therapy. Excision of the fractured segment show little complications in case of nonunions.
- Scaphoid fractures are technically demanding injuries, complications are not uncommon.
- Being the most relevant complication, nonunion most frequently occurs due to suboptimal conditions for fixation or vascular supply.
- Consequently, mechanical stability and vascularity are two major factors to be considered in planning revision surgery.
- VBGs have a firmly established role in the treatment of scaphoid nonunion.
- Arthroscopic techniques can demonstrate their benefits of reducing invasiveness and treating accompanying lesions.

References

[1] Kawamura K, Chung KC. Treatment of scaphoid fractures and nonunions. J Hand Surg Am. 2008; 33(6):988–997

[2] Merrell GA, Wolfe SW, Slade JF, III. Treatment of scaphoid nonunions: quantitative meta-analysis of the literature. J Hand Surg Am. 2002; 27(4):685–691

[3] Shah J, Jones WA. Factors affecting the outcome in 50 cases of scaphoid nonunion treated with Herbert screw fixation. J Hand Surg [Br]. 1998; 23(5):680–685

[4] Ruby LK, Stinson J, Belsky MR. The natural history of scaphoid nonunion. A review of fifty-five cases. J Bone Joint Surg Am. 1985; 67(3):428–432

[5] Vender MI, Watson HK, Wiener BD, Black DM. Degenerative change in symptomatic scaphoid nonunion. J Hand Surg Am. 1987; 12(4):514–519

[6] AWMF. Leitlinie Skaphoidfraktur. 2015 Nr. 012–016 Contract No.: AWMF

[7] Pulos N, Kakar S. Hand and wrist injuries: common problems and solutions. Clin Sports Med. 2018; 37(2):217–243

[8] Schädel-Höpfner M, Prommersberger KJ, Eisenschenk A, Windolf J. Treatment of carpal fractures. Recommendations of the Hand Surgery Group of the German Trauma Society. Unfallchirurg. 2010; 113(9):741–754, quiz 755– Behandlung von Handwurzelfrakturen. Empfehlungen der Sektion Handchirurgie der Deutschen Gesellschaft fur Unfallchirurgie

[9] Gelberman RH, Menon J. The vascularity of the scaphoid bone. J Hand Surg Am. 1980; 5(5):508–513

[10] Fowler JR, Ilyas AM. Headless compression screw fixation of scaphoid fractures. Hand Clin. 2010; 26(3):351–361, vi. Epub 2010/07/31

[11] Panchal A, Kubiak EN, Keshner M, Fulkerson E, Paksima N. Comparison of fixation methods for scaphoid nonunions: a biomechanical model. Bull NYU Hosp Jt Dis. 2007; 65(4):271–275

[12] Grewal R, King GJ. An evidence-based approach to the management of acute scaphoid fractures. J Hand Surg Am. 2009; 34(4):732–734

[13] Ibrahim T, Qureshi A, Sutton AJ, Dias JJ. Surgical versus nonsurgical treatment of acute minimally displaced and undisplaced scaphoid waist fractures: pairwise and network meta-analyses of randomized controlled trials. J Hand Surg Am. 2011; 36(11):1759–1768.e1

[14] Krimmer H, Schmitt R, Herbert T. Scaphoid fractures: diagnosis, classification and therapy. Unfallchirurg. 2000; 103(10):812–819– Kahnbeinfrakturen–Diagnostik, Klassifikation und Therapie

[15] Boe CC, Amadio PC, Kakar S. The management of the healed scaphoid malunion: what to do? Hand Clin. 2019; 35(3):373–379

[16] Slade JF, III, Dodds SD. Minimally invasive management of scaphoid nonunions. Clin Orthop Relat Res. 2006; 445(445):108–119

[17] Wong WC, Ho PC. Arthroscopic management of scaphoid nonunion. Hand Clin. 2019; 35(3):295–313

[18] Aibinder WR, Wagner ER, Bishop AT, Shin AY. Bone grafting for scaphoid nonunions: is free vascularized bone grafting superior for scaphoid nonunion? Hand (N Y). 2019; 14(2):217–222

[19] Mathoulin C, Haerle M. Vascularized bone graft from the palmar carpal artery for treatment of scaphoid nonunion. J Hand Surg [Br]. 1998; 23(3):318–323

[20] Bürger HK, Windhofer C, Gaggl AJ, Higgins JP. Vascularized medial femoral trochlea osteocartilaginous flap reconstruction of proximal pole scaphoid nonunions. J Hand Surg Am. 2013; 38(4):690–700

[21] Elhassan B, Noureldin M, Kakar S. Proximal scaphoid pole reconstruction utilizing ipsilateral proximal hamate autograft. Hand (N Y). 2016; 11(4):495–499

[22] Sandow MJ. Costo-osteochondral grafts in the wrist. Tech Hand Up Extrem Surg. 2001; 5(3):165–172

[23] Poumellec MA, Camuzard O, Pequignot JP, Dreant N. Adaptive proximal scaphoid implant: indications and long-term results. J Wrist Surg. 2019; 8(4):344–350

[24] Quadlbauer S, Pezzei C, Jurkowitsch J, et al. Palmar angular stable plate fixation of nonunions and comminuted fractures of the scaphoid. Oper Orthop Traumatol. 2019; 31(5):433–446—Palmare winkelstabile Verplattung von Pseudarthrosen und Trummerfrakturen des Kahnbeins

[25] Lee YK, Choi KW, Woo SH, Ho PC, Lee M. The clinical result of arthroscopic bone grafting and percutaneous K-wires fixation for management of scaphoid nonunions. Medicine (Baltimore). 2018; 97(13): e9987

3

9 Management of Complications of Scaphoid Fracture Fixation

Geert Alexander Buijze, Anne Eva J. Bulstra, and Pak Cheong Ho

Abstract

Scaphoid fractures are notorious for their troublesome healing. Operative scaphoid fracture fixation is reportedly a safe procedure with predictable high rates of union and a low complication rate. However, some series have highlighted complication rates of up to 30% and pertaining mostly to hardware issues and (recalcitrant) nonunion.

This chapter offers guidelines for prevention and management of the most frequent complications after surgical treatment of scaphoid fractures: hardware issues, (recalcitrant) nonunion and malunion.

Hardware problems can be prevented by using slightly shorter screws than traditionally recommended and checking both length and central screw placement with four to five standard intraoperative fluoroscopy views. Nonunion with or without avascular necrosis (AVN) can be successfully treated by nonvascularized, vascularized, or arthroscopic-assisted bone grafting (ABG) procedures with comparable good outcomes. Humpback deformity and dorsal intercalated segment instability (DISI) can be corrected with either anterior corticocancellous wedge grafting or external maneuvers combined with temporary K-wire fixation and cancellous bone grafting. Malunion after operative fixation seems preventable by meticulous surgical technique. Treatment combines a correction osteotomy to the exact same principles as nonunion surgery.

Recalcitrant nonunions may still be treated by revision repair using vascularized grafts or ABG, although salvage procedures may be preferable in certain cases. Concomitant degenerative arthritis—leading to so-called scaphoid nonunion advanced collapse (SNAC)—as well as poor healing potential will direct treatment options toward salvage procedures. Common salvage for SNAC stage 1 is distal pole resection whereas for SNAC stages 2 and 3, proximal row carpectomy and four corner fusion are most common. Long-term outcomes of the various procedures are comparably satisfactory.

Keywords: scaphoid fracture, scaphoid nonunion, treatment, screw fixation, complications

9.1 Introduction

There is no progress without failure. Complications after operative treatment of scaphoid fractures due to a technical imperfection, an unfavorable indication, incautious rehabilitation, or plainly by misfortune occur to every surgeon in up to a 30% of cases.[1] Hardware problems, delayed union, and (recalcitrant) nonunion and malunion are the main complications seen after operative fixation.

This chapter aims to guide the prevention and management of the most frequent complications after surgical treatment of scaphoid fractures and nonunions.

9.2 Hardware Complications

Although under-reported or under-emphasized with highly variably cited rates in the literature, problems related to hardware are likely the most common complication of scaphoid fracture fixation. These include erroneous screw placement protruding in the scaphotrapezial or radiocarpal joint, screw breakage, intraoperative equipment breakage (involving K-wire and/or screw), and K-wire migration. Migration and loosening of any hardware material should alert the surgeon's suspicion of delayed union.

In one of the scarce papers highlighting complications, Bushnell et al reported a 29% complication rate using the dorsal antegrade percutaneous cannulated screw technique of nondisplaced scaphoid waist fractures.[1] They had 21% (5/24) major complications including three cases involving hardware problems, one nonunion, and one fracture of the proximal pole; and 8% (2/24) minor complications including intraoperative equipment breakage of a K-wire and screw, respectively. Three cases involved problems with the screws, necessitating an additional operation. One patient's postoperative computed tomography (CT) scan showed errant screw placement with dorsal malpositioning and inadequate capture of the distal fragment. Healing occurred after hardware removal and revision retrograde percutaneous screw fixation. A second patient's screw was too long distally and caused symptomatic irritation at the scaphotrapezial joint. A third patient had a delayed union that allowed the screw to settle and became symptomatic. The latter two patients had their symptoms resolved with removal of the screws. Another patient had insidious pain several months after consolidation with radiographic evidence of proximal pole fracture around the head of the screw. The idiopathic etiology could be related to devascularization as well as creating fragility of the proximal pole after drilling and advancing a relatively large screw head through the proximal pole. Similarly, we here report a case of proximal third nonunion following retrograde screw fixation with avascular fragmentation of the proximal pole around the tip of the screw.

The authors give a plausible explanation for the highly variable reported rate of complications including the fact that certain authors do not label hardware removal to be one. In addition, the short-term nature of most series will miss long-term complications such as arthritis of the scaphotrapezial joint related to screw prominence.

Long-term osteoarthritic changes at the scaphotrapezial joint have been related to attrition from prominence of the screw. Dias et al reported this problem in four of eight patients with scaphotrapezial joint space narrowing at a mean follow-up of 93 months after screw fixation.[2] At 12-year follow-up, Saeden et al reported an incidence of scaphotrapezial osteoarthritis of 61% (14/23) following fixation, and only 25% (4/16) after nonoperative treatment and suggested this difference resulted from possible injury to the scaphotrapezial joint surface during surgery.[3] In a meta-analysis comparing operative versus conservative treatment for nondisplaced scaphoid waist fractures, these two studies were pooled for risk of osteoarthritis. It developed in 40% of patients after surgery as compared with 10% of patients after cast immobilization, a nearly significant difference (p = 0.05).[4]

As described in these studies, radiographic scaphotrapezial joint narrowing is seldom symptomatic. In case of several millimeter screw protrusion with attritional degeneration, it is advisable to remove the screw and eventual associated trapezial osteophyte. Otherwise treatment can be conservative most of the time. Advanced symptomatic scaphotrapezial arthritis may require either a 3-mm distal scaphoid pole resection or proximal pole trapezoidotrapezial resection by open or arthroscopic means. In case of associated DISI, pyrocarbon implants or interposition grafts can be added to maintain height of the "radial carpal column" which seems to limit further progression and, in some cases, even correct DISI.

To err on the safe side with screw lengths and avoid prominence, authors have recommended subtracting 6 mm instead of 4 mm from the measured length and to confirm it using a parallel-guidewire technique.[1] Arguments in favor were recently strengthened in a biomechanical model of 18 scaphoids undergoing an osteotomy simulating an oblique proximal fracture.[5] Screws of three lengths (10, 18, and 24 mm) were randomly assigned for fixation and scaphoids cyclically loaded to failure. The 10-mm screw proved inferior but there was no significant difference in ultimate load between the 18- and 24-mm screw. The authors advocate that as the fracture site is closer to the 18-mm screw midpoint, the distal threads are engaged closer to the fracture.

In a retrospective study of medical records of 43 professional American football players who underwent scaphoid fracture fixation, there were hardware complications in as much as 15% of patients.[6] Problems related to hardware included screw loosening, hardware breakage, and erosion on the neighboring carpal bones due to prominent hardware. Hence, even though cannulated compression screw fixation is routinely stable and may allow for direct functional range of motion, there is a clear role for careful rehabilitation to be adapted on case-to-case basis. It seems prudent to err on the safe side and protect active patients against overenthusiastic quick return to heavy labor and contact sports. In doubt, the authors recommend obtaining a CT scan to determine early signs of (trouble with) healing to adapt rehabilitation accordingly.

9.2.1 Tips and Tricks

- Subtracting 6 mm (instead of 2–4 mm) of the measured screw length avoids protrusion trouble while still providing adequate stability. Screw lengths longer than 22 to 24 mm are rarely required.
- Be mindful that screw measurement for percutaneous fixation is different from open fixation. For open screw fixation, we may use the measuring gauge as the end can easily press directly onto the bone surface. For percutaneous fixation, as typically the wound is small, using the measuring device can be notoriously inaccurate due to the soft tissue intervening. Therefore, the recommended measuring method should be using a K-wire of same length to mark the length. Second, when measuring the length, one method is to stop the guide pin drilling just before the pin exits from the cortex, i.e., when it is still within the bone. If one measures the pin length when the pin just exits the bone surface, one may need to subtract 2 mm extra. Thus, the screw length measurement depends on how one measures the length and the reference point.
- The four or five standard fluoroscopy views as recommended by the authors will help identify protruding screws (▶ Fig. 9.1). To judge screw length and protrusion, its perpendicular views are most useful: the semipronated oblique view and the posteroanterior (PA) view in ulnar deviation. When the wrist is ulnarly deviated, it extends/erects the scaphoid and thus gives the appearance of "lengthening the screw." Another useful view is the "bean" view, i.e., semisupinated. Because of the dorsal convexity of the scaphoid, the most common mistake is to pass the guide pin too dorsally and hence exiting the dorsal cortex too early. However, from the conventional PA or anteroposterior (AP) view, even in full ulnar deviation, the premature exit of the pin may not be noticeable because of the overlap with the proximal pole. Hence the bean view is important for one to catch the right trajectory. Classically, it should hit the junction between dorsal 2/3 and volar 1/3, while going parallel to the anterior cortex of the scaphoid. A fifth view in standard PA or AP format can be added to exclude a pronation deformity of the distal fragment and helps evaluate the scapholunate (SL) interval; however, it should be interpreted with caution as screw length may be misleading.
- Be mindful that changing a cannulated compression screw intraoperatively may jeopardize adequate screw purchase and compression. In doubt, a parallel K-wire can be either temporarily left in place or added. Otherwise an additional temporary K-wire or screw connecting the distal scaphoid pole to the capitate can be used.
- Immobilize the wrist without the thumb for as long as "radiographically" necessary. In compliant patients,

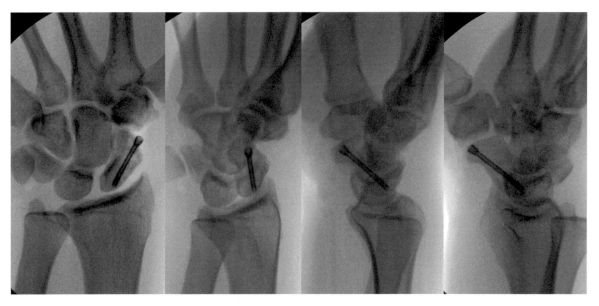

Fig. 9.1 The four intraoperative views of fluoroscopy to realize for every scaphoid screw fixation: anteroposterior (AP) in ulnar deviation, semisupinated oblique "bean" view, lateral view, semipronated oblique view. The AP view in ulnar deviation and semipronated oblique views get the best perpendicular views and show that this 24-mm screw is slightly too proud at the scaphotrapezial joint, which would have been missed on standard AP and lateral views only. A practical open-source smartphone-sized pdf guide can be downloaded at www.pbma.fr/education. © Dr. Buijze 2020.

early active wrist mobilization can be recommended, if the screw fixation is stable. Strengthening and passive mobilization can be commenced when CT scan shows > 50% osseous union and a stable screw fixation. According to biomechanical studies, the strength of the partially united scaphoid augmented with a well-fixed screw approximates that of an intact scaphoid. This is also the time for athletes to resume sport activities.

- Displaced fractures, with or without concomitant perilunate ligament injury, increase the challenge. Under this situation, the most common mistake is the malreduction of the fracture, as reduction based on intraoperative imaging is notoriously unreliable. In specialized centers, it may be recommended to use arthroscopy to assess and facilitate the reduction, particularly at the midcarpal joint. Under direct vision, the two fragments can be controlled with joysticks, or using a probe or freer as equipment to help reducing the gap, step, and rotation problems of the two fragments before passing the guide pin across. Finally, the arthroscope can also be used to assess for any protrusion of the screw from the proximal scaphoid at the radiocarpal joint, if correct screw length is in doubt.

9.3 Scaphoid Nonunion

9.3.1 Risk Factors

Following operative fixation of a scaphoid fracture, 0 to 25% of patients present with nonunion—defined as absent trabecular bridging on CT in the planes of the lon-

gitudinal axis of the scaphoid at 6 months follow-up. Nearly 100% union rates are typically described for non- or minimally displaced scaphoid waist fractures, while fractures of the proximal pole are associated with higher nonunion rates (0–25%). High union rates (98–100%) can also be achieved with screw fixation in displaced fractures,[7] though time to union may be prolonged. Clementson et al described delayed healing (> 14 wk) in 3/17 (18%) patients with a scaphoid fracture, all of which were diagnosed as severely displaced.[8] Smoking and presentation delay have been associated with a higher risk of nonunion among acute fractures managed nonoperatively or established scaphoid nonunions managed operatively. Although there is a paucity of data on factors associated with nonunion following operative management of acute fractures specifically, most patient- and fracture-related risk factors are likely comparable, except those that are corrected operatively such as fracture dislocation and angulation (▶ Table 9.1).

As for surgical technique, no superior fixation method or surgical approach (dorsal vs. volar) has yet been identified with regards to clinical outcomes, union rate, and complications. While multiple fixation methods exist—including single head compression screws as the most common method, K-wires, staples, and plates—comparative studies are scarce. A meta-analysis by Kang et al comparing dorsal and volar percutaneous approaches for screw fixation reported no significant difference in terms of nonunion and other complications (▶ Table 9.1).[9] Importantly, however, a meticulous surgical technique avoiding eccentric screw placement is considered essential

Table 9.1 Risk factors for (recalcitrant) scaphoid nonunion among acute scaphoid fractures and established scaphoid nonunions

	Study design	Patients (studies)	Absolute union rate			RR nonunion	OR nonunion (95% CI)
			Proximal	Waist	Distal		
Fracture location						Proximal versus non-proximal	
Eastley 2013[a]	SR	67 (8)				7.5 (95%CI 4.9–11.5)	
Merrell 2002[*b]	SR	676 (19)	67% p<0.01 (prox vs waist)	85% p<0.05 (waist vs distal)	100% p<0.05 (waist vs distal)	2.2 (prox vs waist)	ND* prox vs distal
Grewal 2013[a]	Retrospective cohort	219 (1)	86% p=underpowered	94% p>0.05 (prox vs waist)	100% p>0.05 (prox vs distal)	2.3 (prox vs waist)	ND* (prox vs distal)
Male gender							Male vs female
Zura 2016[c]	Inception cohort	7149 (1)	-	-	-	-	2.6 (2.1–3.1) p<0.001
Patient age increase by 10 years							Per 10 years increase in age
Zura 2016[c]	Inception cohort	7149 (1)	-	-	-	-	0.80 (0.75–0.80) p<0.001
Smoking			Smoking	No smoking		Smoking versus no smoking	
Dinah & Vickers 2007[b]	Retrospective cohort	34 (1)	40%	82% p<0.01		3.3	
Ditsios 2017[b]	Meta-analysis	256 (5)	56%	93% p<0.01		6.3	
NSAID with opioids							Use versus no use
Zura 2016[c]	Inception cohort	7149 (1)	-	-	-	-	2.6 (2.1–3.2) p<0.001
Opioids only							Use versus no use
Zura 2016[c]	Inception cohort	7149 (1)	-	-	-	-	3.1 (2.6–3.9) p<0.001

(Continued)

Table 9.1 (Continued) Risk factors for (recalcitrant) scaphoid nonunion among acute scaphoid fractures and established scaphoid nonunions

	Study design		Patients (studies)	Absolute union rate		RR nonunion		OR nonunion (95% CI)	
Osteoarthritis								*Osteoarthritis vs no osteoarthritis*	
Zura 2016[c]	Inception cohort		7149 (1)	-		-		2.2 (1.7–2.8) p<0.001	
Osteoporosis								*Osteoporosis vs no osteoporosis*	
Zura 2016[c]	Inception cohort		7149 (1)	-		-		2.5 (1.3–4.6). p<0.005	
Time to surgery				*>12 months*	*<12 months*	*> versus < 12 months*			
Merrel 2002[b]	SR		1046 (28)	80%	90% p<0.01	2.0			
Dorsal or volar approach				*Dorsal approach*	*Volar approach*	*Dorsal versus volar*			
Kang 2016	SR		141 (7)	97%	96%	0.75 p>0.1			

SR: Systematic review; RR: relative risk; OR: odds ratio; CI: confidence interval; u: unknown; prox = proximal pole fracture

[a]Studies reporting union rate among nonoperatively treated acute scaphoid fractures

[b]Studies reporting union rate after operation for established scaphoid nonunions

[c]Study reporting union rates among both operatively and nonoperatively treated acute scaphoid fractures

* ND: relative risk could not be determined due to a 0% nonunion rate in distal fractures.

to reduce surgeon-related preventable complications. Although the most popular approach for percutaneous screw fixation of common waist fractures seems retrograde from volar at the scaphoid tubercle, several authors have argued for more central screw placement, either retrograde transtrapezial or antegrade from dorsal—as is common in proximal pole fractures. Advantages of central screw placement or screw fixation perpendicular to the fracture site remain biomechanical as no series, including the meta-analysis by Kang et al, has found significant differences in clinical outcomes and complications.[9]

Recommendations with regard to postoperative immobilization remain inconsistent. While some allow immediate mobilization, others immobilize for 2 to 4 weeks. Avoiding early strenuous wrist activity including unprotected early return to contact sports is important, as return to athletics is a risk factor, particularly in contact sports.[6] In a retrospective study on professional American football players undergoing scaphoid fracture fixation, there was a 25% nonunion rate and 34% had degenerative changes consistent with scaphoid nonunion advanced collapse (SNAC) stages 2 and 3.[6] No detail was provided on time of return to play and rehabilitation. In contrast Rettig et al reported an acceptable low nonunion rate of 3% with a cautious rehabilitation protocol as follows. Return to play was considered safe after open reduction and internal fixation (ORIF) of a scaphoid waist fracture when range of wrist motion had recovered within 10% of the opposite side in absence of pain.[10] Immobilization averaged 12.5 days and time of return to sports 8 (range, 3–21) weeks. Similarly, use of standard crutches in polytrauma patients[11] should be avoided to reduce the risk of destabilizing operative reduction and risk of subsequent nonunion.

9.3.2 Treatment

Nonunion treatment consists of hardware removal, and surgical take down of the sclerotic nonunion site until bleeding bone, bone grafting, and stable fixation (▶ Fig. 9.2–▶ Fig. 9.12). Percutaneous placed screws are preferably removed under fluoroscopic guidance with the dedicated K-wire and screwdriver. This part can be tedious and time consuming. If primarily treated elsewhere, it is advisable to check the operative report and order the appropriate removal set beforehand.

Take down of the nonunion site is best performed with a high-speed burr, sawblade, and or osteotome. Use of a rongeur can clear a remaining spike. All techniques emphasize the need to resect substantial portions of the scaphoid nonunion site surfaces in order to encourage healing, under the rationale that the sclerotic fracture ends will not support healing. Bleeding bone can be determined by intermittent tourniquet deflation. On the proximal site, absent bone punctate bleeding may confirm AVN of the proximal pole. Despite AVN of the

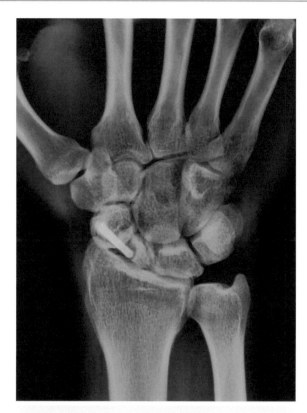

Fig. 9.2 A 38-year-old male with a symptomatic nonunion at the proximal third of the scaphoid, 10 years after screw fixation of an acute scaphoid waist fracture. © Dr. Ho 2020.

proximal pole, both vascularized bone grafting (VBG) and nonvascularized bone grafting (NVBG) can lead to high rate of union (▶ Table 9.2). For ABG, the large series of 20 years' experience of the senior author suggests that in case of AVN, there is still an 81.8% chance of healing through neovascularization from distal and from the ligament of Testut.[12]

Two meta-analyses reported comparable union rates following VBG (84% and 92%) and NVBG (80% and 88%) for established scaphoid nonunions. In the presence of AVN and in case of proximal pole nonunions VBG yielded higher union rates (72% and 97%, respectively) compared to NVBG (62% and 93%).[13,14] With regard to donor site, more complications were reported with the use of iliac crest bone grafts (both VBG and NVBG) (9%) compared to distal radius grafts (1%) while yielding similar union rates (87% and 89%, respectively). Iliac crest grafts are also associated with more pain at the donor site. For all graft types, higher union rates were reported for bone grafting with fixation (88–91%) than for grafting without fixation (79%).[14] Quality of current evidence for the treatment of established nonunions remains limited by high volumes of largely low-level evidence and the inconsistent reporting and use of definitions for AVN, nonunion, and complications. As of yet, no systematic review has identified a

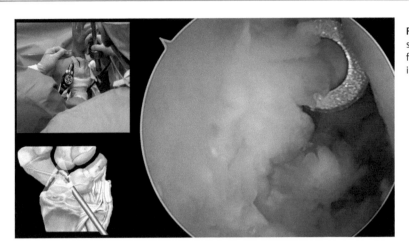

Fig. 9.3 The proximal pole was split in a small volar fragment and a larger dorsal fragment and the screw could be visualized in the nonunion gap. © Dr. Buijze 2020.

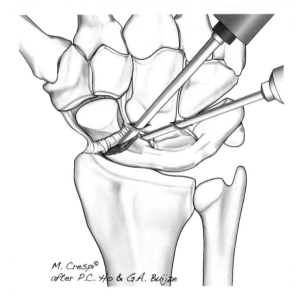

M. Cresp©
after P.C. Ho & G.A. Buijze

Fig. 9.4 Schematic drawing of nonunion take down showing how the sclerotic cap is largely removed until punctate bleeding and/or avascular necrosis of the proximal pole are confirmed upon release of the tourniquet. Leaving fibrotic tissue at the capsular reflection avoids graft spill.

statistically substantiated superior treatment approach for scaphoid nonunion (▸ Table 9.2).

With the increasing popularity of wrist arthroscopy, ABG has recently become a more attractive option for many surgeons. The senior author's outcomes in 124 patients showed an overall union rate of 90.3% (112/124).[12] The average radiological union time was 14 weeks (range, 6–80). Final clinical follow-up showed no pain in 67 patients (54%), whereas in the remaining 57 patients visual analog scale (VAS) pain was on average 1.7 (range, 0–7). ADL performance scores improved from 34.2 to 38.6 ($p < 0.05$) and grip strength from 28.2 to 36.2 kg ($p < 0.05$). Complications included one case of intraoperative screw-

driver breakage, three cases of transient neuropathy, three cases of pin-tract infection, and three cases donor site morbidity at the iliac crest (transient).

Stabilization can be performed by K-wires (with optional temporary scaphocapitate/radiolunate pinning) or volar plate fixation as repeat screw fixation may not provide adequate purchase in the remaining bone. These stabilization methods also reduce the risk of graft extrusion, which is a notorious pitfall in anterior wedge grafting stabilized by a single screw.

Below-elbow cast immobilization with or without thumb immobilization is recommended for 6 up to 12 weeks to diminish risk of K-wire migration (▸ Fig. 9.13). K-wires are removed upon radiographic confirmation of early bony consolidation.

A salvage procedure is considered when union cannot be achieved after one or more attempts or when arthritis becomes established. Salvage options include wrist denervation, radial styloidectomy, excision of the distal pole of the scaphoid, proximal row carpectomy (PRC), scaphoid excision and so-called "four-corner" arthrodesis (4CA; capitate, hamate, triquetrum, and lunate), and total wrist arthrodesis.

In case of scaphoid nonunion with concomitant degeneration of the radial styloid process consistent with stage 1 SNAC wrist, a standard nonunion repair can be associated with a radial styloidectomy. Advantage of performing this procedure arthroscopically includes the improved visualization of the crucial radioscaphoid ligaments and dorsal radiocarpal ligaments that need to be spared. Fluoroscopic control is recommended to prevent under- or over-resection. In chronic scaphoid nonunion or SNAC 1 in patients with unfavorable healing characteristics, in cases with crucial necessity of quick recovery, and in the elderly, a distal pole resection can be preferred. At 15 years follow-up, Malerich et al showed favorable, long-term clinical results and did not result in noteworthy wrist collapse.[15] Midcarpal arthritis, which may develop after the procedure, did not cause appreciable deterioration in patient outcomes. This procedure also did not

3

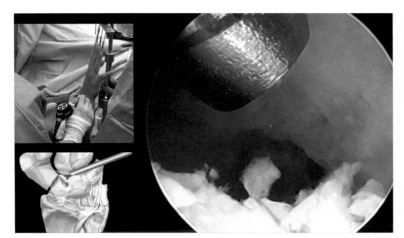

Fig. 9.5 After screw removal, take down of the nonunion site with a 2.0-mm shaver and a 2.9-mm burr, removing the sclerotic bone at the nonunion site until bleeding of the distal fragment, while the proximal pole is avascular. © Dr. Ho & Buijze 2020.

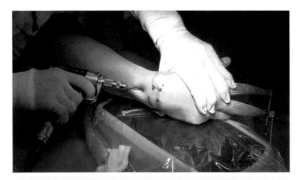

Fig. 9.6 The radiolunate interval is reduced with the Linscheid maneuver. In the presence of an intact scapholunate (SL) ligament, dorsiflexion deformity of the proximal pole of scaphoid is corrected by firstly passive wrist flexion to realign the extended lunate with the radius. © Dr. Ho 2020.

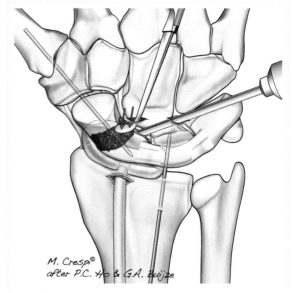

Fig. 9.8 Schematic drawing showing that in case of proximal pole nonunion arthroscopic-assisted bone grafting (ABG), an inflated Foley catheter placed in the radiocarpal joint is required to prevent graft spillage.

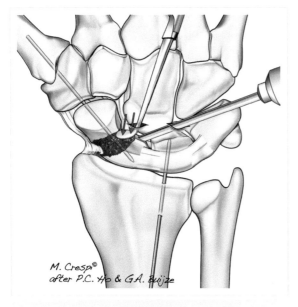

Fig. 9.7 Schematic drawing of arthroscopic-assisted bone grafting (ABG) with abundant stuffing in a waist nonunion through a radial midcarpal portal using downward pressure on an angled spatula.

eliminate the option of using additional, more conventional reconstructive procedures if needed.

In case of further associated degenerative features such as stages 2 and 3 SNAC wrist, palliative procedures can be indicated, including PRC and scaphoidectomy and four corner arthrodesis (4CA, ▶ Table 9.3). 4CA and PRC have proven comparable in terms of pain reduction and patient satisfaction. Although trends of better patient-rated functional outcome following PRC have been described, a meta-analysis by Saltzman et al could not establish a statistically significant difference between PRC and 4CA. 4CA has been associated with greater postoperative grip strength compared to PRC.[16] Importantly, however, the overall complication rate—including nonunion and conversion of fusion—is reported to be higher following 4CA.

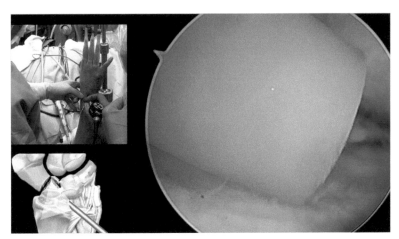

Fig. 9.9 A size 6 Foley catheter is used to block any spillage of the graft. The tip of the catheter is cut off just past the balloon. Then, it is inserted in the radiocarpal joint, either through the 1–2 portal or in this case, through the 3–4 portal. The balloon is inflated with saline solution to fill up the space between the nonunion site and the distal radius. © Dr. Ho & Buijze 2020.

3

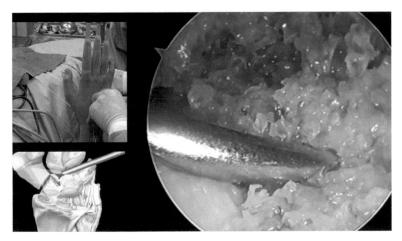

Fig. 9.10 Autogenous cancellous bone graft from the contralateral iliac crest is delivered via the midcarpal radial (MCR) portal using a 4.5-mm cannula and packed tightly and extensively into the nonunion site using an impactor and a spatula. © Dr. Ho & Buijze 2020.

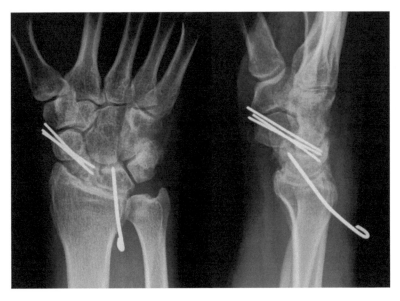

Fig. 9.11 Fixation with two more 1.1-mm K-wires shows good final scaphoid alignment with optimal graft filling and no extrusion to the radiocarpal joint. © Dr. Ho 2020.

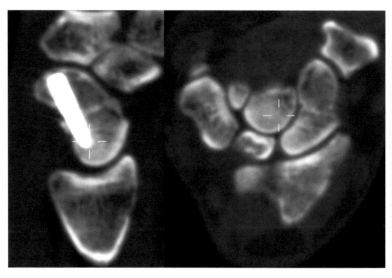

Fig. 9.12 Example of a screw that has been placed too anterior, preventable when using the semisupinated "bean view." When computed tomography (CT) is reconstructed along the longitudinal axis, it shows slight flexion of the distal fragment in the sagittal plane, and ulnar deviation with pronation of the distal fragment in the coronal plane. The lateral intrascaphoid angle (LISA) and/or height to length ratio (HLR) are slightly increased. © Dr. Buijze 2020.

Table 9.2 Union rates and complications following various types of bone grafting for the treatment of established scaphoid nonunions

	Study design	No. of pts (studies) F/U	Overall union rate		Union rate in the presence of AVN or proximal pole fracture		Comments
Vascularized versus nonvascularized bone grafts			*VBG*	*NVBG*	*VBG*	*NVBG*	
Braga-Silva 2008	RCT	80 (1) 2.6–3.1	91%	100% p = u	-	-	VBG: 1,2 ICSR NVBG: iliac crest
Caporrino 2014	RCT	75 (1) 2.4	89%	80% p > 0.05	-	-	VBG: 1,2 ICSR NVB: distal radius
Ribak 2010	RCT	46 (1) 2	89%	73% p < 0.05	-	-	VBG: 1,2 ICSR NVBG: distal radius
Ferguson 2015	Systematic review	5465 (144) u	84%	80% p = u	*In the presence of AVN* 72%	62% p = u	44 studies including 528 patients reported on outcomes in the presence of AVN
Pinder 2015	Systematic review	1602 (48) u	92%	88%* p = u	*Proximal pole fractures* 97% (range: 82–100%)	93% (range: 61–100%)	* VBG group poor prognostic factors 7 studies including 125 patients reported on outcomes in proximal pole fractures
Overall complication rate			*Graft source*	*Graft source*			
Pinder 2015	Systematic review	679 19 > 0.5	DR 1%	IC 9% p = u			DR grafts constituted both VBG and NVBG.

Pts: patients; F/U: follow up (years); AVN: avascular necrosis; RCT: randomized controlled trial; VBG: vascularized bone graft, NVBG: non vascularized bone graft; u = unknown; 1,2 ICSR: 1,2, intercompartmental supraretinacular artery pedicle.

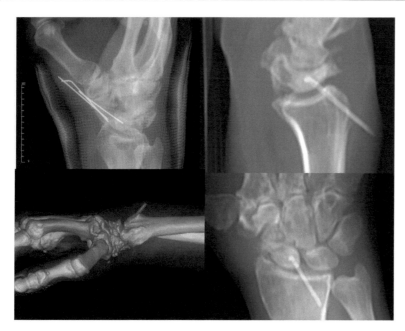

Fig. 9.13 Example of K-wire migration following anterior wedge bone grafting of a scaphoid waist nonunion. Note the potential role of the cast (upper left corner) ending at the base of the first metacarpal. Perhaps, prolonging a cast up to the interphalangeal joint of the thumb can limit this problem. © Dr. Buijze 2020.

3

Commonly reported complications following PRC include synovitis and edema (3.1%) versus nonunion (4.9%) following 4CA. Mulford et al described a higher incidence of osteoarthritis in patients treated with PRC (3.7%) compared to 4CA (1.4%), although the correlation with clinical symptoms is uncertain.

Caution is required for use of bone substitutes. Application of recombinant human bone morphogenetic protein (rhBMP) in case of scaphoid nonunion is an off-label use. Its use has not shown a reproducible superior rate of union in patients with scaphoid nonunion. Moreover, patients should be counseled that when rhBMP is used for the treatment of scaphoid nonunion, there are risks of heterotopic ossification and reoperation as reported by multiple authors.

9.3.3 Tips and Tricks

- In case of delayed union, doubt can exist regarding the union status of a percutaneously fixed scaphoid, especially when there was initial displacement. In the presence of hardware, CT may lose its accuracy to determine union due to artifacts. Arthroscopic evaluation may be considered as this offers an in vivo and dynamic assessment of the union status for the surgeon to decide whether to wait and see or to take down the nonunion.[17]
- In case of screw loosening with circumferential bone loss (radiographic lucency), the screw can be easily removed and an iliac peg corticocancellous strut can be placed in the screw channel with an anterior wedge graft.[18]
- For nonunion without loosening of the screw, simple debridement of the nonunion site, ABG without removing the screw is another option. Intraoperative screw stability can be evaluated on-site.

- Advantages of multiple K-wire use in well-stuffed grafting are less "humpback" compression, less risk of graft extrusion, and no hardware removal trouble in case of revision.
- In case of a humpback deformity with concomitant DISI, the radiolunate interval is reduced with the Linscheid maneuver (▶ Fig. 9.14). In the presence of an intact SL ligament, dorsiflexion deformity of the proximal pole of scaphoid is corrected by firstly passive wrist flexion to realign the extended lunate with the radius.
- In aiming retrograde K-wires, the nondominant hand of the surgeon can maintain the patient's wrist in extension, hypersupination, and ulnar deviation by intertwining the surgeon's first webspace with that of the patient and keeping the surgeon's index finger on patient's Lister's tubercle. The dominant hand can then aim for the index finger while extending the scaphoid and avoiding humpback deformity.
- When palliative surgery is indicated, consider distal scaphoid resection before PRC or 4CA. For established SNAC 2–3 wrists PRC and 4CA yield comparable pain relief and function, while complications are higher following 4CA. Be mindful that SNAC 3 may not always be good indication for PRC as the capitate articulating surface has been involved. Some surgeons may still use this but modifying with osteochondral grafting of the proximal capitate using the intact lunate surface or a proximal capitate implant.
- With regard to rehabilitation, immobilize the wrist following scaphoid nonunion surgery for as long as "radiographically" necessary, generally much longer than acute fracture fixation. In well-compliant patients, early active wrist mobilization could be considered.
- Great caution must be taken as the increased wrist forces involved in weightbearing on standard crutches

Table 9.3 Salvage procedures—PRC versus 4CA and Distal Scaphoid Resection: range of motion, grip strength, function, pain

Outcome	Study design	Pts (studies)	Outcome					Comments
Range of Motion				*PRC*	*4CA*	*DSR*	p-value	
Aita 2016*	RCT	27 (1)	Total ROM	69%	58%	-	>0.05	Total ROM, relative to contralateral unaffected side
Malerich 2014	Retrospective	19 (1)	Total ROM	-	-	139°	-	Total arc of motion
Saltzman 2014*	SR	u (5)	FE UR	75° 32°	64° 30°	-	<0.01 >0.05	No significant difference in *change* in FE arc between PRC and 4CA
Mulford 2009*	SR	2143 (52)	FE UR	75° 32°	64° 41°.	-	u u	
Grip strength (relative to unaffected side)				*PRC*	*4CA*	*DSR*		
Aita 2016	RCT	27(1)		79%	65%	-	>0.05	
Saltzman 2014*	SR	240 (7)		67%	74%	-	<0.01	No significant difference in *change* in gripstrength PRC and 4CA
Mulford 2009*	SR	u (44)		70%	75%	-	u	
Malerich 2014	Retrospective	19 (1)				85%	-	
Function				*PRC*	*4CA*	*DSR*		
Aita 2016	RCT	27 (1)		11	13	-	>0.05	Dash score
Saltzman 2014*	SR	u (2)		21	28	-	>0.05	Dash score
Brinkhorst 2016	Retrospective	48 (1)		87	69	-	<0.01	MHQ score
Pain				*PRC*	*4CA*	*DSR*		
Aita 2016	RCT	27 (1)		2.3	2.9	-	>0.05	VAS score
Brinkhorst 2016	Retrospective	48 (1)		10	48	-	<0.01	MHQ scale
Mulford 2009*	SR	977 (26)		16%	15%	-	u	Percentage of patients reporting pain as "poor" versus "good"
Malerich 2014	Retrospective	19 (1)		-		0.9	-	VAS score (0-10)
Overall complication rate				*PRC*	*4CA*	*DSR*		
Saltzman 2009*	SR	101 (6)		14%	29%	-	0.01	

(Continued)

Table 9.3 *(Continued)* Salvage procedures—PRC versus 4CA and Distal Scaphoid Resection: range of motion, grip strength, function, pain

Outcome	Study design	Pts (studies)	Outcome						Comments
									Most common: PRC: synovitis and edema (3.1%) 4CA: nonunion (6.9%)
Risk of osteoarthritis			*PRC*	*4CA*	*RR*	*DSR*			
Mulford 2009*	SR	231(6)	3.7%	1.4%	2.6	-	<0.05	Follow-up
Malerich 2014	Retrospective	19 (1)	-	-	-	72%		Mean follow-up: 15 years
Risk of conversion to fusion			*PRC*	*4CA*	*RR*	*DSR*			
Mulford 2009*	SR	261 (7)	3.9%	2.9%	1.3	-	>0.05	
Salltzman 2014*	SR	u (2)	7.1%	10%	0.71	-	>0.05	
Malerich 2014	Retrospective	19 (1)				5.3%	-	Additionally 1 conversion to PCR (=5.3%)

F/U: follow up in years; PRC: proximal row carpectomy; 4CA: 4 corner arthrodesis; DSR: distal scaphoid resection; ROM: range of motion; FE: flexion-extension arc; UR: ulnar-radial deviation arc; u: unknown; VAS: visual analogue scale; Dash score: lower score indicated better hand function; MHQ: Michigan Hand outcome Questionnaire (function: higher score indicates better hand function; pain: higher score indicates more pain); RR: relative risk of specified outcome PRC vs 4CA. Pts (studies): number of patients (and studies) in which the specified outcome was measured.
*Studies included patients with scaphoid nonunion advanced collapse and scapholunate advanced collapse.

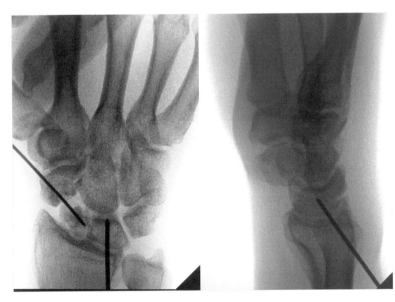

Fig. 9.14 Transfixation is done with a 1.1-mm K-wire inserted from the scaphoid tubercle. © Dr. Ho 2020.

can destabilize reduction and fixation and potentially lead to nonunion.[11] Forearm gutter crutches or axillary crutches are safe functional alternatives.

9.4 Recalcitrant Scaphoid Nonunion

When surgery for nonunion is unsuccessful, bone stock and bone quality are further compromised, which may undermine conditions for further corrective surgery. Another attempt to gain healing may be considered if there is felt to be adequate bone and minimal arthritis.

Recalcitrant nonunion is defined as absent consolidation on CT 6 months after bone grafting of a scaphoid nonunion. Reported rates are highly variable and range from 0 to 60%. The rate of nonunion is not associated to the type of bone graft, whether nonvascularized, vascularized, or arthroscopic-assisted (▶ Table 9.2). Risk factors reducing the chance of successful nonunion surgery include smoking, longer time to surgery, and fractures located at the proximal pole. Dinah and Vickers reported an 82% success rate following internal fixation and bone grafting of scaphoid nonunion among nonsmokers versus 40% among smokers. As such, patient-associated factors (e.g., nonabstinence from smoking) and parameters associated to the primary surgery should be analyzed with scrutiny before launching oneself into any revision as the global rate of union is likely inferior to 80%, even in specialized centers.[19]

At this stage of chronicity and multiple previous procedures, palliative procedures may be recommendable in some cases. For example, a heavy smoker who did not succeed in abstinence at first surgery may be a better candidate for a distal pole resection instead with quicker recovery.

If another attempt for achieving union is decided upon in the treatment of recalcitrant nonunion, most surgeons will shift toward either a vascularized bone graft or an arthroscopic bone graft attempting to spare the local vascularity.

Currently, the most popular vascularized graft seems to be the technique described by Zaidemberg in 1991.[20] This graft is pedicled from the radial aspect of the distal radius including the 1,2 intercompartmental supraretinacular artery (1,2-ICSRA). Its main advantage is its relative technical ease in proximal and waist nonunion without humpback deformity.

An advantage of both the free vascularized iliac crest and the volar-sided distal radius graft pedicled on the volar carpal artery, as described by Kuhlmann in 1987, is the correction of a humpback deformity by a wedge shape through the same volar approach.[21] To our knowledge, the largest series reported to date on recalcitrant nonunion of the scaphoid is described by Arora et al.[19] They studied the use of a free vascularized iliac bone graft in the treatment of 21 patients with an avascular nonunion of the scaphoid in which conventional bone grafting had previously failed. With a minimal follow-up of 2 years, the union rate was 76% (16/21). Dodds and Halim achieved union with this technique supplemented by volar buttress plating in eight of nine recalcitrant nonunions.[22]

A major advantage of the free medial femoral condyle graft is its chimeric properties creating the possibility of reconstructing an avascular proximal pole with an osteochondral graft.[23] However, donor site morbidity at the knee is not negligible and should be (carefully) discussed with the patient. Treatment by ABG has the advantage to reduce devascularization of the site and optimizing healing potential with minimal scarring. Moreover, it allows a comprehensive staging of articular degeneration which can make conversion to a salvage procedure preferable in some cases. However, as any extensive minimally invasive surgical procedure, it is technical and one should be aware of the learning curve.

Rehabilitation generally involves below-elbow cast immobilization with or without thumb immobilization for 8 up to 12 weeks to diminish risk of K-wire migration. K-wires are removed upon radiographic confirmation of early bony consolidation.

9.4.1 Tips and Tricks

- Recalcitrant nonunion does not per se imply salvage. An attempt at repeat bone grafting can be performed and stabilized by a volar plate or K-wires, although union rates are inferior.
- If ABG was previously performed, the procedure can be repeated although the success rates are yet to be established.

9.5 Scaphoid Malunion

The malunited scaphoid waist fracture usually results in a humpback deformity and is rarely symptomatic. Although suspicion can be raised on radiographs showing increased scapholunate (>70 degrees) and radiolunate (>20–30 degrees) angles after consolidation of a scaphoid fracture, a definitive diagnosis is based on a CT scan in the coronal and sagittal planes of the longitudinal axis of the scaphoid. It consists of flexion of the distal fragment in the sagittal plane, ulnar deviation of the distal fragment in the frontal plane, and pronation of the distal fragment (▶ Fig. 9.12). Various parameters have been studied to quantify abnormal angles on CT: a lateral intrascaphoid angle superior to 35 degrees and/or height to length ratio superior to 0.73.

Scaphoid malunion after operative fixation is nearly exclusively related to technical error. Anecdotal preventable technical imperfections include avoiding humpback deformity caused by either insufficient reduction and/or volar-eccentric compression screw placement (▶ Fig. 9.12). The latter creates unbalanced overcompression forces on the volar cortex with distraction of the dorsoradial ridge. Controlling central screw placement with four adequate views and/or a second stabilizing K-wire can prevent torsional and angular forces. Arthroscopic control of step-off and gaps can be performed in specialized centers but has no proven benefit over careful fluoroscopy.

The exact relationship between malaligned scaphoid fragments and disability or pain remains debatable as most malunions are asymptomatic. However, in combination with carpal instability, it may produce pain, early arthritis, and wrist dysfunction. In other words, abnormal scaphoid morphology has not yet been shown to correlate with outcome, unless associated with DISI which is associated with poorer outcomes.

Therefore, debate continues regarding treatment. Although prior case series report favorable results with surgical correction, recent studies demonstrate similar outcomes with conservative treatment.[24] It is, therefore, important to obtain a detailed history and perform a meticulous and repeated physical examination to ascertain the degree of disability experienced by a scaphoid malunion. There seems to be a humble consensus to reserving correction osteotomy for patients with scaphoid malunion and clearly associated symptomatic carpal malalignment. In case of impingement between the distal scaphoid tubercle and the radial styloid—typically with radial deviation—without symptomatic carpal instability, local debridement with a radial styloidectomy and limited dorsal rim resection may be indicated.

Rehabilitation is comparable to scaphoid nonunion surgery. In case of correction of carpal malalignment, carpal kinematics can only be fully restored if eventual concomitant ligamentous injury has been addressed at the same time.

9.5.1 Tips and Tricks

- Avoiding "humpback eccentric screw position" of the screw is best checked using four scaphoid specific views under fluoroscopy (▶ Fig. 9.1).
- Leaving the first placed K-wire in situ—which is generally not perfectly central—will help guide the second K-wire for cannulated screw fixation and avoid distraction/malrotation forces when applying the screw.
- When using the Slade technique of antegrade screw insertion, excessive flexion of the wrist should be avoided to displace a volarly flexed distal fragment. Alternatively, the fragment can be aligned and temporarily transfixed with a fine K-wire in a retrograde manner before antegrade pinning and screwing is attempted.
- In planning a corrective osteotomy of the scaphoid, obtaining bilateral CT scan with 3D reconstructions can be valuable.

9.6 Miscellaneous Complications

9.6.1 Nerve/Tendon Lesions/Infection

Other complications following fixation of scaphoid fractures include those related to the scar, to the surrounding structures related to the approach and infection.

Complications related to scarring are quite common in open approaches. These were best highlighted in the prospective series of 44 patients treated for ORIF of scaphoid waist fractures by Dias et al.[2] A total of 10/44 patients had minor complications related to the scar. One patient had a superficial wound infection, three a sensitive scar, four a hypertrophic scar, three a sensitive and hypertrophic scar. Percutaneous approaches seem to limit these, though may be more prone to complications of subcutaneous structures.

Structures at risk with volar percutaneous approaches include the flexor carpi radialis tendon, the palmar cutaneous branch of the median nerve, and the superficial branch of the radial artery. For the dorsal approach, structures at risk include the radial-sided wrist and finger extensors and the posterior interosseous nerve.

Infection after scaphoid screw fixation can be categorized as superficial (local swelling, pain, erythema, delayed wound healing) or deep (wrist pain and edema with or without purulent discharge, elevated infection parameters). In a meta-analysis comparing operative versus conservative treatment for nondisplaced scaphoid waist fractures, there were only two cases of postoperative infection among all 207 patients who were allocated to surgical treatment in seven primary trials.[4] Superficial infections can be treated by local wound care, immobilization, and antibiotics, whereas deep infections are best aspirated with eventually open/arthroscopic lavage and debridement as necessary of both the radiocarpal and midcarpal joints. Seldom indications for hardware removal include recurrent infection, osteomyelitis, osteonecrosis, and fungal infections, notably in immune-compromised patients. A 20-year delayed presentation of isolated hardware-associated scaphoid osteomyelitis has been reported,[25] which was successfully treated by total scaphoidectomy and intravenous antibiotics, followed by a secondary PRC.

9.7 Take-Home Message

Getting scaphoid fractures to heal after operative fixation without any complication is challenging. If all minor healing disturbances and secondary procedures are taken in account, the true complication rate after is likely closer to 30% than the commonly reported 1 to 10%. One thing is certain, a vast percentage is preventable. Prevention starts with awareness of the most common pitfalls such as inadequate screw length or positioning as well as insufficient fixation construct stability or overenthusiastic unprotected rehabilitation. Solid indications, meticulous surgical technique, technical pearls, and cautious rehabilitation can limit many unforeseen problems. When unpreventable, revision surgery to resolve complications is nearly always feasible and satisfactory, functional outcomes can be expected.

3

References

[1] Bushnell BD, McWilliams AD, Messer TM. Complications in dorsal percutaneous cannulated screw fixation of nondisplaced scaphoid waist fractures. J Hand Surg Am. 2007; 32(6):827–833

[2] Dias JJ, Wildin CJ, Bhowal B, Thompson JR. Should acute scaphoid fractures be fixed? A randomized controlled trial. J Bone Joint Surg Am. 2005; 87(10):2160–2168

[3] Saedén B, Törnkvist H, Ponzer S, Höglund M. Fracture of the carpal scaphoid. A prospective, randomised 12-year follow-up comparing operative and conservative treatment. J Bone Joint Surg Br. 2001; 83 (2):230–234

[4] Buijze GA, Doornberg JN, Ham JS, Ring D, Bhandari M, Poolman RW. Surgical compared with conservative treatment for acute nondisplaced or minimally displaced scaphoid fractures: a systematic review and meta-analysis of randomized controlled trials. J Bone Joint Surg Am. 2010; 92(6):1534–1544

[5] Patel S, Giugale J, Tiedeken N, Debski RE, Fowler JR. Impact of screw length on proximal scaphoid fracture biomechanics. J Wrist Surg. 2019; 8(5):360–365

[6] Moatshe G, Godin JA, Chahla J, et al. Clinical and radiologic outcomes after scaphoid fracture: injury and treatment patterns in National Football League Combine Athletes between 2009 and 2014. Arthroscopy. 2017; 33(12):2154–2158

[7] Singh HP, Taub N, Dias JJ. Management of displaced fractures of the waist of the scaphoid: meta-analyses of comparative studies. Injury. 2012; 43(6):933–939

[8] Clementson M, Jørgsholm P, Besjakov J, Björkman A, Thomsen N. Union of scaphoid waist fractures assessed by CT scan. J Wrist Surg. 2015; 4(1):49–55

[9] Kang KB, Kim HJ, Park JH, Shin YS. Comparison of dorsal and volar percutaneous approaches in acute scaphoid fractures: a meta-analysis. PLoS One. 2016; 11(9):e0162779

[10] Rettig AC, Weidenbener EJ, Gloyeske R. Alternative management of midthird scaphoid fractures in the athlete. Am J Sports Med. 1994; 22(5):711–714

[11] Buijze GA, Goslings JC, Rhemrev SJ, et al. CAST Trial Collaboration. Cast immobilization with and without immobilization of the thumb for nondisplaced and minimally displaced scaphoid waist fractures: a multicenter, randomized, controlled trial. J Hand Surg Am. 2014; 39 (4):621–627

[12] Wong WC, Ho PC. Arthroscopic management of scaphoid nonunion. Hand Clin. 2019; 35(3):295–313

[13] Ferguson DO, Shanbhag V, Hedley H, Reichert I, Lipscombe S, Davis TR. Scaphoid fracture non-union: a systematic review of surgical treatment using bone graft. J Hand Surg Eur Vol. 2016; 41(5):492–500

[14] Pinder RM, Brkljac M, Rix L, Muir L, Brewster M. Treatment of scaphoid nonunion: a systematic review of the existing evidence. J Hand Surg Am. 2015; 40(9):1797–1805.e3

[15] Malerich MM, Catalano LW, III, Weidner ZD, Vance MC, Eden CM, Eaton RG. Distal scaphoid resection for degenerative arthritis secondary to scaphoid nonunion: a 20-year experience. J Hand Surg Am. 2014; 39(9):1669–1676

[16] Saltzman BM, Frank JM, Slikker W, Fernandez JJ, Cohen MS, Wysocki RW. Clinical outcomes of proximal row carpectomy versus four-corner arthrodesis for post-traumatic wrist arthropathy: a systematic review. J Hand Surg Eur Vol. 2015; 40(5):450–457

[17] Liu B, Wu F, Ng CY. Wrist arthroscopy for the treatment of scaphoid delayed or nonunions and judging the need for bone grafting. J Hand Surg Eur Vol. 2019; 44(6):594–599

[18] Fernandez DL, Kakar S, Buijze GA. Non-vascularized bone grafts. In: Buijze GA, Jupiter JB, eds. Scaphoid fractures: Evidence-based management. 1st ed. St. Louis: Elsevier; 2018:303–320

[19] Arora R, Lutz M, Zimmermann R, Krappinger D, Niederwanger C, Gabl M. Free vascularised iliac bone graft for recalcitrant avascular nonunion of the scaphoid. J Bone Joint Surg Br. 2010; 92(2):224–229

[20] Zaidemberg C, Siebert JW, Angrigiani C. A new vascularized bone graft for scaphoid nonunion. J Hand Surg Am. 1991; 16(3):474–478

[21] Kuhlmann JN, Mimoun M, Boabighi A, Baux S. Vascularized bone graft pedicled on the volar carpal artery for non-union of the scaphoid. J Hand Surg [Br]. 1987; 12(2):203–210

[22] Dodds SD, Halim A. Scaphoid plate fixation and volar carpal artery vascularized bone graft for recalcitrant scaphoid nonunions. J Hand Surg Am. 2016; 41(7):e191–e198

[23] Pulos N, Kollitz KM, Bishop AT, Shin AY. Free vascularized medial femoral condyle bone graft after failed scaphoid nonunion surgery. J Bone Joint Surg Am. 2018; 100(16):1379–1386

[24] Gillette BP, Amadio PC, Kakar S. Long-term outcomes of scaphoid malunion. Hand (N Y). 2017; 12(1):26–30

[25] Burns J, Moore E, Maus J, Rinker B. Delayed Idiopathic Hardware-Associated Osteomyelitis of the Scaphoid. J Hand Surg Am. 2019 ;44 (2):162.e1–162.e4

10 Management of Complications in Lunate Facet Fracture Fixation

Simon B.M. MacLean and Greg I. Bain

Abstract

The lunate facet represents the "critical corner" of the distal radius, and the main load-bearing area. The injury may be overlooked by an inexperienced surgeon. Lunate facet fractures can be one of five types: (1) a volar ulnar corner fracture (VUC) as an isolated fragment, (2) VUC fragment with extension radially to involve the radiocarpal ligaments (the entire volar rim), (3) VUC fragment as one component of a metaphyseal fracture, (4) VUC fragment as part of a high-energy "pilon-type" fracture, or (5) in combination with a greater arc injury. Standard locking volar distal radius plates often provide inadequate support to and fixation of this fragment and each subtype requires separate consideration for management.

In this chapter we will outline the anatomy of the fracture. We will discuss treatment principles including imaging, surgical approach, and fixation techniques. We will cover salvage procedures, rehabilitation, and tips and tricks to ensure satisfactory treatment of this injury.

Keywords: lunate facet fracture, volar marginal rim fractures, distal radius, volar plate, fragment-specific fixation, complications

10.1 Definition and Problem

The volar marginal rim of the distal radius owes its importance to both loadbearing function as well as the attachment of the radiolunate ligaments, which prevent volar subluxation and ulnar translocation of the carpus.[1,2] The centroid of force application is volarly on the lunate facet, and because it is offset in a palmar direction relative to the radial shaft, this area transmits high loads and is difficult to stabilize.[2] The volar marginal rim, or "lunate facet" fracture, therefore, is an important subset of frac-

tures, which may not be adequately fixed with traditional volar-locking plate technology. Specific volar rim plates have been designed to sit distal to the watershed line of the radius and contain this critical fragment. Despite fragment-specific technology however, hardware positioning can be challenging, and fixation may be inadequate to stabilize this challenging injury. The lunate facet fracture may be only one component of a more extensive distal radius or carpal injury, and poor outcomes may result from treatment of this fracture in isolation.

10.2 Anatomy of the Fracture

The importance of the ligamentous attachments of the distal radius was described by Melone and Medoff.[3,4] Melone specifically described the role of the two medial fragments for articular function, and their strong ligamentous attachments.[3,5] Medoff recognized the contribution of these ligaments to fracture displacement, radiocarpal instability, and the contribution of ligament avulsion to the creation of "rim" fragments leading to catastrophic failure of fixation.[4]

All low-energy injuries occur between ligaments on the distal radius, and each fragment is likely to have an attached ligament.[6] We describe this as the "osteoligamentous concept of distal radius fracture" (▶ Fig. 10.1).

Physiological extension of the wrist creates tension on the volar radiocarpal ligaments and acts as a tension band, increasing contact pressure on the lunate facet. Following impact on an outstretched hand, forced hyperextension and axial compression causes a fracture of the subchondral bone plate and avulsion of the lunate facet with the attached short radiolunate ligament (SRLL). The wrist settles in volar subluxation with this fragment. If the force propagates radially to include the scaphoid facet, then the long radiolunate ligament (LRLL) will also avulse, leading to ulnar translocation.[8]

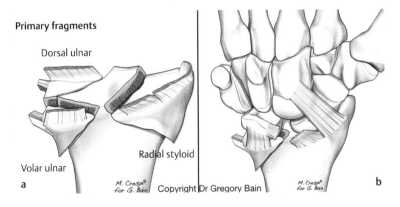

Primary fragments

Dorsal ulnar

Volar ulnar

Radial styloid

M. Crespo for G. Bain Copyright Dr Gregory Bain

a

b

Fig. 10.1 Osteoligamentous concept.[7] **(a)** Diagram of osteoligamentous unit, **(b)** Isolated volar ulnar corner fracture. Copyright Dr. Gregory Bain, with permission.

3

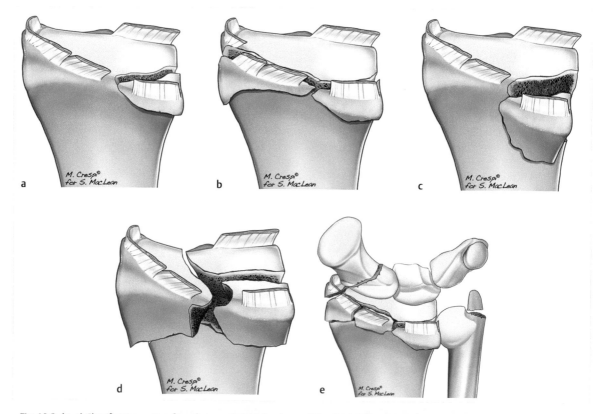

Fig. 10.2 (a–e) Classification system for volar marginal rim fractures of the distal radius. Copyright Mr. Simon MacLean, with permission.

10.3 Treatment: Management of Volar Rim Fractures

All patients require computed tomography (CT) scanning as well as plain radiographs. Critical review of these is imperative to identify other fractures of the carpus and ulnar styloid, as well as assessment for carpal alignment and carpal instability.

Volar rim fractures of the lunate facet may occur in isolation or may be one component of a distal radius fracture with comminution. Identifying this will aid in determining the fixation system required. We have a low threshold for performing diagnostic and/or therapeutic arthroscopy at the time of fixation if preoperative imaging suggests this may be beneficial.

Before deciding on management, the type of volar rim fracture should be determined. From our clinical experience, we have determined five main fractures of the distal radius involving the volar rim (▶ Fig. 10.2).

10.3.1 Surgical Approach

Surgical approach is determined by the type of fracture. If the lunate facet fracture is an isolated injury we prefer a volar ulnar approach. This allows direct access to the lunate facet. We then proceed with fragment-specific fix-

ation. This approach can also be extended into the palm, past the distal transverse wrist crease if concomitant carpal tunnel decompression is required.[9,10]

If the lunate facet fracture is one component of a distal radius fracture or there is more radial extension of the marginal rim fracture, we prefer a distal flexor carpi radialis (FCR) approach with oblique extension past the distal wrist crease, which allows excellent access to the radial metaphysis, as well as *both* the scaphoid and lunate facets.

Volar-Ulnar Approach

An incision is made between FCU and palmaris longus to the distal transverse wrist crease. The interval between the ulnar neurovascular bundle and the carpal tunnel contents is used, and these structures are protected with right-angled retractors. If an extensile incision is used, the distal wrist crease is crossed obliquely and extended longitudinally in line with the ring finger. The flexor retinaculum is released completely. The pronator quadratus (PQ) is elevated from the radial aspect of the distal radius. The volar-ulnar fragment is then exposed. Small K-wires can be used as a joystick, then temporarily secure the fragment. Alternatively, sutures at the bone-ligament junction can be used to reduce the fracture (▶ Fig. 10.3).

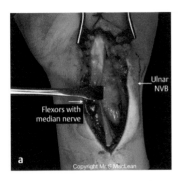 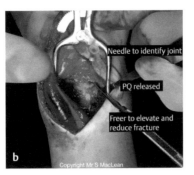 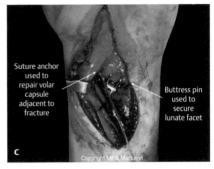

Fig. 10.3 The extended volar-ulnar approach to the distal radius used to fix a type 2 fracture. **(a)** The ulnar neurovascular bundle is retracted ulnarly, and the flexors with median nerve are retracted radially. The pronator quadratus (PQ) is exposed. **(b)** The PQ is released from radial to ulnar. A fine needle is used to identify the radiocarpal joint. **(c)** A buttress pin is used to fix the lunate facet fragment. Small all-suture anchors are used to repair the adjacent radial capsule with the long radiolunate ligament (LRLL), which has avulsed from the marginal rim of the distal radius. Copyright Mr. Simon MacLean, with permission.

Distal FCR Approach

The incision is based over the FCR tendon, and the skin incision proceeds obliquely for 1 cm over the distal wrist crease in a radial direction. The sheath of the tendon is opened and the FCR tendon retracted ulnarly. The posterior bed of the sheath is released to expose the deep volar compartment. We do not specifically identify the median nerve but retract the flexors with the nerve ulnarly. A right-angled retractor is used to protect the radial artery. The PQ is released. We routinely release the distal insertion of brachioradialis by sharp dissection. This allows pronation of the distal fragment to aid anatomical reduction. The components of the distal radius fracture are identified, and each separate component reduced. We proceed with reduction of the intermediate column, including the lunate facet. Next the radial column is reduced. These components are held with K-wires or buttressed with the chosen plate for fixation. Lastly, the ulnar column is reduced and fixed if required.

10.3.2 Fixation Techniques

Lunate facet fractures represent avulsion of an osteoligamentous unit in the "critical corner" of the distal radius.[11] Strain energy from wrist hyperextension causes progressive lengthening of the SRLL before avulsion of the fragment, as the ultimate tensile strength of the distal radius bone is usually reached before that of the ligament. Radiocarpal dislocations *can* occur without fracture however, and these injuries represent failure at the junction of the bone and the ligament (osteoligamentous junction). A marginal rim fracture therefore can occur together *with* avulsion of the adjacent radiocarpal ligaments, including the LRLL and radioscaphocapitate ligament (RSCL) (type 2). The size of the fragment and any adjacent injury to the radiocarpal ligaments determine the type of fixation used.

Direct vision and fluoroscopy are used to determine anatomical reduction. In isolated type 1 fractures we prefer a fragment-specific plate. If the fragment is particularly small, a volar buttress pin (▶ Fig. 10.4) provides rigid fixation without the risk of further comminution to the fragment. If the fragment is larger, we prefer a fragment-specific volar buttress plate. If there is adjacent capsular injury (type 2), this should be repaired. Our preference is to use two to three all-suture anchors. These are positioned along the marginal rim, under subchondral bone, and the capsule is repaired (▶ Fig. 10.5).

If the lunate facet fracture is part of a comminuted intra-articular distal radius fracture with metaphyseal components (type 3), we prefer the Geminus distal radius plate (LMT Surgical, Florida, USA) with a hook plate extension to secure the volar rim[2] (▶ Fig. 10.6). The Geminus plate has fixed and variable angle capability, and is recessed on the radial column to avoid irritation of the flexor pollicis longus (FPL) tendon. After plate application, the relation of the lunate facet fragment to the distal edge of the plate is examined to decide if sufficient fixation is provided. If insufficient, a hook plate is used. A reduction tool and guide is used to facilitate application of the hook plate, which is secured with a set screw to the volar plate.

The volar marginal rim fracture may be a component of a greater carpal injury (type 5). In these cases, a combination of fixation techniques is required (▶ Fig. 10.7).

Fluoroscopy is essential throughout the procedure. Provocative maneuvers should be used following lunate facet fixation to ensure radiocarpal stability. If fixation is inadequate the carpus may translocate ulnarly if radial-ulnar translation is performed. The radius may sublux or dislocate over the rim of the distal radius if a dorsal-volar force is applied.

If there is concern regarding stability of the construct, fixation should be revised or a bridge plate added to neutralize forces on the fragment and the repaired radiocarpal ligaments.

3

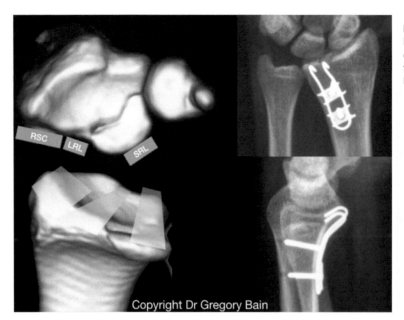

Fig. 10.4 Type 1 injury involving an isolated avulsion fracture to the volar ulnar corner. Stability is achieved by stable fixation to the fragment. Copyright Dr. Gregory Bain, with permission.

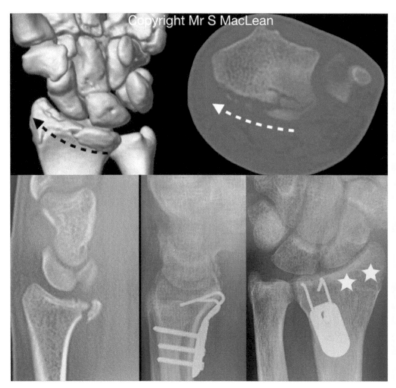

Fig. 10.5 Type 2 injury—the force has propagated in the radial direction, and the long radiolunate ligament (LRL) and radioscaphocapitate ligament (RSCL) have avulsed with small rim fragments (*dashed arrows*). Three all-suture anchors were used to repair the capsule after fixation to the volar ulnar rim fragment (*stars*). Copyright Mr. Simon MacLean, with permission.

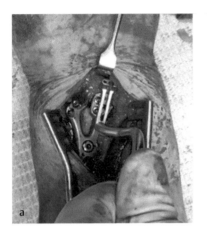
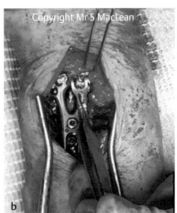
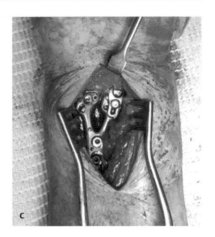
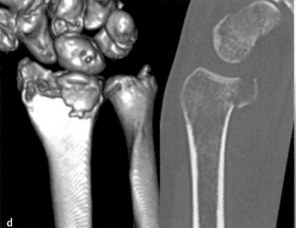
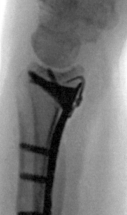
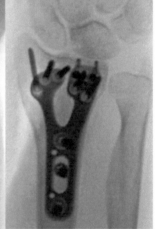

Fig. 10.6 The use of the hook plate extension on the Geminus distal radius plate. **(a)** The reduction guide is used to reduce the lunate facet fracture distal to the plate. **(b)** Two K-wires are used through the guide to provide provisional fixation to the fragment. **(c)** The hook plate is inserted after removal of the wires and secured to the Geminus plate with a set screw. **(d)** Preoperative imaging and fluoroscopy images showing final fixation. Copyright Mr. Simon MacLean, with permission.

Bridge Plating

Bridge plating can be used for primary fixation of the wrist in cases with marked comminution to the metaphysis or in "pilon-type" fractures (types 3 or 4).[12] Bridge plating can act as temporary fixation in the setting of "damage-control orthopaedics" in a patient with multiple other injuries.[13] We usually use a bridge plate as an *adjunct* to our primary fixation as required. Bridge plating off-loads the fragment-specific fixation of the lunate facet (▸ Fig. 10.8 and ▸ Fig. 10.9). It is also of use in patients with marked comminution at the lunate facet, or in patients with osteoporosis, when there is a higher chance of fixation failure with fragment-specific fixation in isolation. In cases of polytrauma, when bed transfer and rehabilitation is essential, placement of a bridge plate

as an "internal external fixator" allows early load transfer through the affected limb. We prefer to use an 8- or 10-hole 3.5-mm metaphyseal limited contact dynamic compression plate (LC-DCP). The tapered end sits distally to avoid extensor tendon irritation over the metacarpal. The plate can be inserted using "MIPO" technique. A longitudinal incision is made over the third metacarpal and the extensor tendon is retracted. The plate is slipped below the extensor tendons, over periosteum to the metadiaphysis of the distal radius. An incision is made dorsally over the proximal part of the plate and tendons from dorsal compartments 1 and 2 retracted as required. The position is checked under fluoroscopy. Fixation is achieved with six cortices of cortical fixation proximally and distally, or with locking screws as required. The plate is removed at 3 months postoperatively.

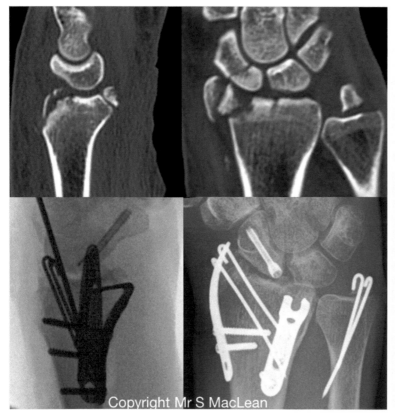

Fig. 10.7 The volar marginal rim fracture may be a component of a greater carpal injury (type 5). This patient sustained a trans-styloid, trans-scaphoid perilunate injury with a marginal rim fracture of the lunate facet. The *intermediate column* was reduced and fixed with a volar buttress plate. The radial styloid (*radial column*) was fixed with a styloid-specific plate. The proximal pole scaphoid fracture was fixed. A lunotriquetral wire was used to stabilize the lunotriquetral joint. This same wire was advanced into the distal radius to stabilize the radiocarpal joint and off-load the volar rim fixation. Lastly, the basal ulnar styloid fracture (*ulnar column*) was reduced and fixed. Copyright Mr. Simon MacLean, with permission.

10.4 Arthroscopy

Magnetic resonance imaging (MRI) scanning is often impractical or inconclusive in patients with distal radius fractures. We have a high suspicion of other carpal injuries in patients with a fracture involving the volar marginal rim. Arthroscopy can be used prior to and after fixation of the lunate facet. Arthroscopy serves a number of important roles, both diagnostic and therapeutic:

1. Scapholunate ligamentous injuries are a common finding in distal radius fractures.[14,15] If there is marked diastasis and involvement of the entire SLL complex, consideration should be made to acutely stabilizing/repairing the joint.
2. Triangular fibrocartilaginous complex (TFCC) injuries may involve the foveal insertion. If there is clinical distal radioulnar joint (DRUJ) instability following fixation and evidence of a significant foveal insertion tear, the TFCC can be repaired (open or arthroscopic-assisted).
3. Loose fragment of bone and other chondral injuries can be identified and excised/treated.
4. An anatomical reduction of the lunate facet can be determined. With placement of hardware distal to the watershed line of the distal radius, there is a risk of

joint penetration with screws, pins, or anchors. Fluoroscopy may not always identify this complication, and arthroscopy allows the best visual inspection of the radiocarpal joint.

10.5 Lunate Facet Fractures: The Tip of the Iceberg

We have performed a retrospective review of 25 lunate facet fractures, comparing them to a control group of 25 intra-articular fractures *not* involving the volar rim. There was a significantly increased number of other carpal injuries in the volar rim group including carpal and ulnar styloid fractures, scapholunate diastasis, and ulnar translocation of the carpus (▶ Fig. 10.10). The lunate facet fracture may therefore be part of a greater spectrum of injury to the wrist.

10.6 Rehabilitation

Patients are placed in a backslab at the time of surgery. We proceed cautiously with these injuries, as fixation may be precarious, and prefer to keep a short arm cast on

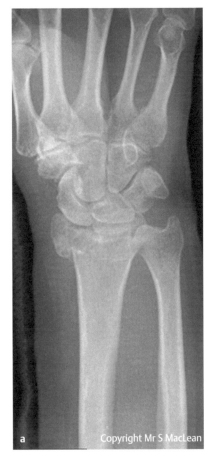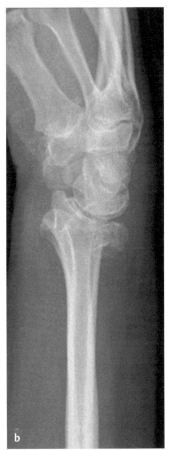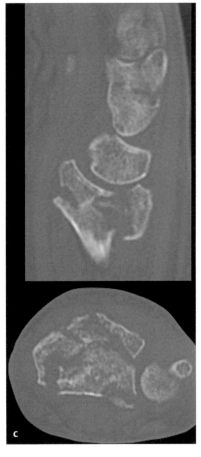

Fig. 10.8 (a–c) Preoperative radiographs and computed tomography (CT) images: Case of an osteoporotic patient with a pilon-type fracture (type 4) involving the volar ulnar rim, dorsal ulnar rim, and radial styloid. Copyright Mr. Simon MacLean, with permission.

for 6 weeks postoperatively. With adequate reduction and fixation of the lunate facet, osseous union is usually evident at 6 weeks, and full range of motion and strengthening encouraged with physiotherapy.

If there has been an extensive capsular injury requiring fixation in addition to the lunate facet fracture, we encourage the patient to avoid heavy loading/manual labor until 3 months postoperatively.

Most of these implants sit distal to the watershed line, and may irritate the flexor tendons as a result. If the implant is prominent or the patient develops symptoms of flexor irritation, we advise removal of the implant once the injury has fully healed.

10.7 Salvage

Salvage techniques are determined by patient factors, time from index surgery, the status of the lunate facet fragment, the status of the carpus, and the alignment of the radiocarpal joint. The lunate facet fragment may be avascular as its blood supply may be retrograde through its distal capsular attachments. Nonunion and resorption of the fragment may occur.

In acute cases, where inadequate index support of the lunate facet fracture has occurred, fixation can be revised to support this fragment.

In delayed cases, when resorption of the fragment and radiocarpal malalignment has occurred, other salvage techniques should be considered.

Orbay et al described a distal radius volar opening wedge technique, to redirect joint forces to the dorsal aspect of the radial articular surface and unload the volar lunate facet.[2] The volar tilt of the distal radius is corrected to at least neutral, and a volar-locking plate is bent to match the distal radius tilt. Olecranon autograft is added as bone graft. In three cases in his study, all patients achieved satisfactory concentric joint reduction and functional outcome.

In late presentations, radiolunate degeneration and static instability occur. Volar approach and radioscapholunate

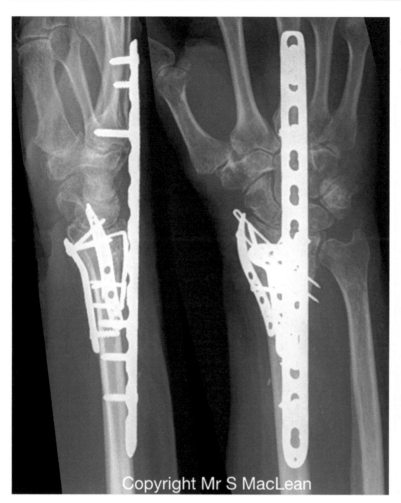

Fig. 10.9 Postoperative images: Primary fixation of the rim fragments was neutralized with a bridge plate as an adjunct. Copyright Mr. Simon MacLean, with permission.

fusion should be considered to maintain dart-thrower's motion. In cases with more advanced degeneration, total wrist fusion may be required.

10.8 Tips and Tricks

1. Careful review of preoperative imaging, as this will determine the fracture subtype, appropriate surgical approach, and selection of implants.
2. We advise always having suture anchors available in cases with massive capsular disruption *in addition* to the lunate facet fracture.
3. For an isolated lunate facet fracture, the volar-ulnar approach allows a safe direct approach to the fracture, without over-retraction of the median nerve.
4. Choose fragment-specific fixation carefully to avoid comminuting the fragment. Placement is well past the watershed line and often more distal than expected.

5. These fractures may be one of a number of injuries to the wrist—we advise a low threshold for the use of arthroscopy to aid diagnosis and treatment.
6. A bridge plate should be available as a back-up in all cases.

10.9 Take-Home Message

Lunate facet fractures are a challenging distal radius fracture subtype. They are associated with a higher rate of fixation failure and other carpal injuries. Management begins with appropriate radiographs and CT scanning. Selection of surgical approach and fixation techniques is crucial. The surgeon should take a step-by-step approach —with judicious use of fluoroscopy and arthroscopy to ensure satisfactory fixation. If primary fixation is tenuous or if in any doubt, a bridge plate should be added to neutralize forces and allow fracture healing.

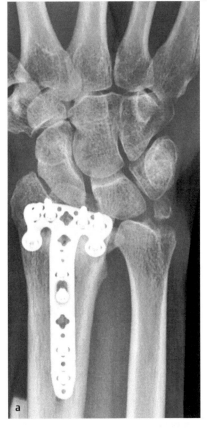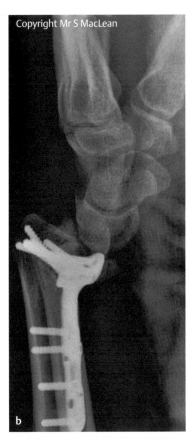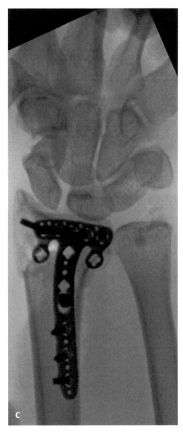

Fig. 10.10 There is a high association with volar marginal rim fractures of failure of fixation and other carpal injuries. **(a)** Ulnar translocation of the carpus. **(b)** Volar carpal subluxation. **(c)** Scapholunate ligament injury. Copyright Mr. Simon MacLean, with permission.

References

[1] Berger RA, Landsmeer JMF. The palmar radiocarpal ligaments: a study of adult and fetal human wrist joints. J Hand Surg Am. 1990; 15 (6):847–854

[2] Orbay JL, Rubio F, Vernon LL. Prevent collapse and salvage failures of the volar rim of the distal radius. J Wrist Surg. 2016; 5(1):17–21

[3] Melone CP, Jr. Articular fractures of the distal radius. Orthop Clin North Am. 1984; 15(2):217–236

[4] Medoff RJ. Essential radiographic evaluation for distal radius fractures. Hand Clin. 2005; 21(3):279–288

[5] Melone CP, Jr. Distal radius fractures: patterns of articular fragmentation. Orthop Clin North Am. 1993; 24(2):239–253. 0030–5898 (Print)

[6] Mandziak DG, Watts AC, Bain GI. Ligament contribution to patterns of articular fractures of the distal radius. J Hand Surg Am. 2011; 36 (10):1621–1625

[7] Bain GI, Alexander JJ, Eng K, Durrant A, Zumstein MA. Ligament origins are preserved in distal radial intraarticular two-part fractures: a computed tomography-based study. J Wrist Surg. 2013; 2(3):255–262

[8] MacLean SBM, Bain G. Anatomy of the fracture. In: del Piñal F, ed. Distal radius fractures and carpal instabilities. IFSSH 2019 Instructional Book. Thieme Medical Publishers Inc; 2019:1–11

[9] Pourgiezis N, Bain GI, Roth JH, Woolfrey MR. Volar ulnar approach to the distal radius and carpus. Can J Plast Surg. 1999; 7(6):273–278

[10] Bain GI, Pourgiezis N, Roth JH. Surgical approaches to the distal radio-ulnar joint. Tech Hand Up Extrem Surg. 2007; 11(1):51–56

[11] Harness NG, Jupiter JB, Orbay JL, Raskin KB, Fernandez DL. Loss of fixation of the volar lunate facet fragment in fractures of the distal part of the radius. J Bone Joint Surg Am. 2004; 86(9):1900–1908

[12] Mithani SK, Srinivasan RC, Kamal R, Richard MJ, Leversedge FJ, Ruch DS. Salvage of distal radius nonunion with a dorsal spanning distraction plate. J Hand Surg Am. 2014; 39(5):981–984

[13] Richard MJ, Katolik LI, Hanel DP, Wartinbee DA, Ruch DS. Distraction plating for the treatment of highly comminuted distal radius fractures in elderly patients. J Hand Surg Am. 2012; 37(5):948–956

[14] Richards RS, Bennett JD, Roth JH, Milne K, Jr. Arthroscopic diagnosis of intra-articular soft tissue injuries associated with distal radial fractures. J Hand Surg Am. 1997; 22(5):772–776

[15] Forward DP, Lindau TR, Melsom DS. Intercarpal ligament injuries associated with fractures of the distal part of the radius. J Bone Joint Surg Am. 2007; 89(11):2334–2340

11 Management of Complications Following Open Reduction and Plate Fixation of Distal Radius Fractures

Niels W.L. Schep

Abstract

Most guidelines advise nonoperative treatment in the form of plaster cast immobilization for patients with adequately reduced distal radius fractures.[1,2] However, open reduction and plate fixation has become more popular, as it improves quality of reduction and fracture stability allowing for early postoperative mobilization and quicker return to work.[3,4]

Nevertheless, most of the radiological parameters correlate poorly with functional outcome.[5,6] Patient-reported outcome measures (PROMs) have gained importance in studies concerning fracture treatment, and clinical decision-making is more often based on studies that use these outcomes.[7] The patient-rated wrist evaluation (PRWE) and disabilities of the arm, shoulder, and hand (DASH) are two specific PROMs related to wrist function, and are valid and reliable outcome measures in patients with distal radius fractures.[8] A meta-analysis by Vannabouathong et al concluded that open reduction and plate fixation offers the best results for adult patients with a DRF, in terms of radiological-functional outcome and fracture healing.[9]

Yet, open reduction and plate fixation comes with a trade-off of complications. The complication percentage following plate fixations of DRFs ranges between 10 and 50%, depending whether implant removal is considered as a complication. In 2014 Bentohami et al published a systematic review showing 9% minor and 8% major complications.[10,11,12]

Complications can be categorized into tendon-, nerve-, reduction or hardware-related, and general complications such as deep and superficial infections. The aim of this chapter is to share our experience in preventing or treating these complications.

Keywords: distal radius fracture, complications, surgical approach, neuromas, reduction, malunion, infection

11.1 Complications Related to the Surgical Approach

11.1.1 Neuromas due to the Volar Approach

A modified Henry approach is our working horse to approach the volar side of the distal radius. The surgeon sits at the head of the patients, which enables a good view on the ulnar part of the radius. Dissection is performed radially from the FCR (flexor carpi radialis) leaving the tendon-sheath intact. This may help avoid adhesions of the FCR to the skin. Moreover, this may also evade accidental damage to the palmar cutaneous branch of the median nerve (PCBMN). The PCBMN originates from the medial side of the median nerve 3 to 8 cm proximal to the wrist palmar crease. It follows a path parallel and medial of the FCR tendon and the palmaris longus. However, it may also run inside the FCR sheath or perforate the sheath. A painful neuroma may be formed postoperatively following retraction of the FCR, opening the FCR sheath or because of aggressive dissection. By dissecting on the radial side of the FCR instead of going next to the tendon sheath, injury of the PCBMN may be avoided.

Subsequently, the pronator quadratus (PQ) is L-shaped incised along the radial radius border and below the watershed line. Avoid damaging the volar ligaments while exposing the distal radius. The brachioradialis insertion is released from the distal radial fracture fragment until we encounter the first extensor compartment. This will aid reducing the distal radial fragment, especially if there is a long delay between trauma and surgery. The fracture is reduced, dictated by the fracture pattern and temporarily fixed with K-wires. If fracture reduction is problematic, Orbay's maneuver is performed; the proximal radius shaft is pronated with a reduction clamp while the patient's hand is fixated with your other hand. This exposes the dorsal side of the distal radius and lifting off the extensor tendons subperiosteally and enables fracture debridement and therefore reduction. Once adequate reduction is reached, the plate is positioned. During closure, the PQ is not reinserted because there is no functional advantage in repairing this muscle and may even lead to less pronation strength.[13,14] (Only the skin is closed using absorbable monofilament.) Pressure bandage is applied (making sure MCP joints are free) for 48 hours. The patient will start non-weightbearing wrist motion exercises the same day to avoid stiffness and swelling. Weightbearing is allowed 6 weeks postoperatively.

During K-wires fixation, the sensory branch of the radial nerve (RSN) should be protected as neuromas can result from a (blind) percutaneous approach (▶ Fig. 11.1). Treatment of RSN neuroma includes resection. The proximal RSN is dissected free of the surrounding tissues in such a way that it allows relocation of the nerve. Subsequently, an opening is made in the proximal mobile wad and the nerve is buried without tension. A single absorbable suture between the epineurium and the muscle fascia is used to hold the nerve in place. The nerve may also be relocated in the radius; therefore, a cortical hole is

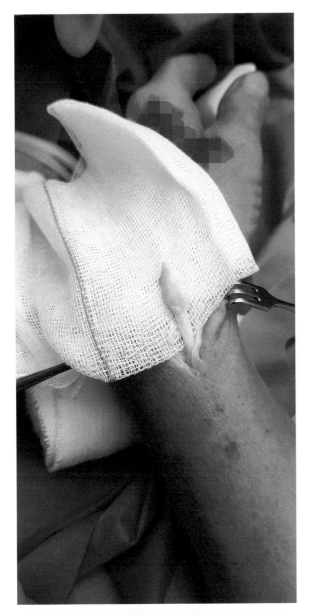

Fig. 11.1 A painful neuroma due to transection of a branch of the superficial radial nerve (RSN) at the level of the styloid process of the radius following temporary K-wire fixation.

drilled obliquely to a size larger than the nerve. The nerve is held in place with a absorbable suture between the epineurium and periosteum.

11.1.2 Posterior Interosseous Nerve and Tendon Problems due to the Dorsal Approach

For the dorsal approach we make an incision just ulnar of Lister's tubercle. When this anatomic structure is difficult to palpate due to edema or fracture anatomy, a longitudi-

nal line just radial of the third finger is chosen to mark the incision. Next, the extensor retinaculum is incised at the level of the third extensor compartment and the tendon of the extensor pollicis longus (EPL) is elevated to the radial side.

On the bottom of compartment four, the terminal branch of the posterior interosseous nerve is found and excised for 2 cm. We do not bother its proprioceptive properties because nerve division does not appear to be associated with decreased proprioception of the wrist.[15] Moreover, we encountered multiple patients with a painful dorsal wrist following dorsal plate fixation in which the nerve was trapped under the plate or where a symptomatic neuroma had formed just at the wrist capsule.

Next, subperiosteal dissection is performed under compartment four to release the common extensor tendons. The dissection is continued until the distal radioulnar joint (DRUJ) but be careful not to open the DRUJ. We try to leave the dorsal capsule closed; however, when deemed necessary the dorsal capsule may be opened to inspect the intra-articular anatomy by a mini-Berger flap.

When the dorsal plate is positioned on the dorsal part of the lunate facet, the plate is covered with a flap of the extensor retinaculum to protect the extensor tendons. The EPL is left out of its compartment and sits dorsally to the extensor retinaculum. The skin is closed using absorbable monofilament.

11.2 Complications Related to the Quality of Reduction

The AAOS guidelines advise operative treatment for fractures with postreduction radial shortening > 3 mm, dorsal tilt of > 10 degrees or intra-articular step off of more than 2 mm. On the contrary, the Dutch guidelines are more liberate: more than 10 degrees tilt in any direction, more than 5 mm radial shortening or intra-articular step off of more than 2 mm.

As stated in the introduction the commonly used radiographic parameters seem not to perfectly correlate with patient-related outcome measures. However, most surgeons will agree that when an open reduction and plate fixation is chosen as treatment modality we should aim for a perfect anatomic reduction.

Therefore, accurate assessment of intraoperative fluoroscopic images is essential. First, the surgeon should assess the posterior anterior fluoroscopic view instead of the anterior posterior view. Otherwise, the position of the ulnar styloid and the length of the radius may not be judged accurately.

11.2.1 Posterior Anterior View

- Radial inclination: Measures from the tip of radial styloid process (PSR) to the center point of the ulnar side of the distal radius. This center point (CRP) is located

3

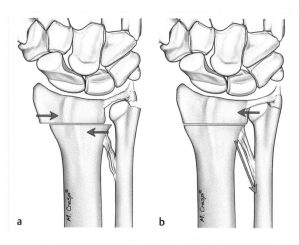
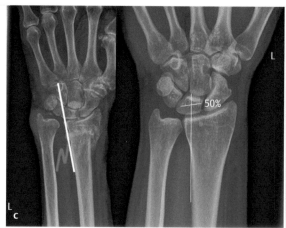

Fig. 11.2 (a–c) Coronal plane translation can be measured by drawing a line on the ulnar side of the radius which intersects the lunate. This line should bisect the lunate in an anatomic situation.

between the volar and dorsal rim which can easily be identified on the PA fluoroscopic image. Radial inclination is normally 20 to 25 degrees.

- Ulnar variance: The distance between the CRP and distal articular surface of the ulna. Normally + 0.9 mm (range −4.2 to 2.3 mm).
- Radial length: It is defined by the length measured between the tip of the radial styloid and the distal articular surface of the ulna. Normally 10 to 13 mm.

Next we will address the coronal plane translation, which we consider a significant parameter. This term is used to describe radial displacement of the distal fragment. Radial translation of the distal fragment might be associated with DRUJ instability due to lack of tension on the distal oblique bundle (the most distal part of the distal interosseous membrane) and the PQ. As we noted earlier, the surgeon sits at the head of the patient because the ulnar side of the radius can be accurately assessed from that side. To avoid coronal plane translation fracture reduction should be perfect at the ulnar side of the radius (▶ Fig. 11.2).

11.2.2 Lateral View

- Volar or dorsal dislocation of the ulna in relation to the radius can only be assessed in a pure lateral view of the wrist. In a pure lateral fluoroscopic image, the pisiform projects between the distal pole of the scaphoid and the capitate.
- Volar tilt: It is the angle between a line drawn through the center of the radial shaft and a line drawn through the apices of the palmar and dorsal rims of the radius. The normal volar tilt is between 5 and 11 degrees.[16]
- Carpal malalignment: Carpal malalignment is correlated with poor functional outcome.[17] It is measured by drawing a line along the inner rim of the volar cortex of

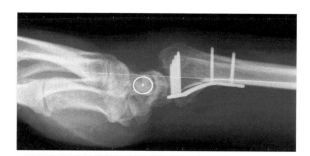

Fig. 11.3 The carpus is malaligned when the line along the inner rim does not transect the center of the capitate. By measuring the perpendicular distance to the center of the capitate, the degree of carpal malalignment can be quantified.

the radius (marginal line of Lewis) and determining the center of the capitate. (The center of the capitate is at the center of a circle drawn around the base of the capitate.) The carpus is aligned when the line along the inner rim transects the center of the capitate. By measuring the perpendicular distance to the center of the capitate, the degree of carpal malalignment can be quantified. Based on the study by Selles et al,[18] a margin of 0.5 cm of dorsal and 0.5 cm of volar displacement would be within the range of normal alignment[18] (▶ Fig. 11.3). When there is loss of carpal alignment this can be due to an extra- or intra-articular problem.

Malunions

Nonunion following distal radius fractures other than an infected defect is very rare and will not be addressed in this chapter. Treatment of infections are covered in Chapter 11.4. Malunions however occur in approximately 11% of operatively treated patients and may cause considerable disability. Commonly reported symptoms are func-

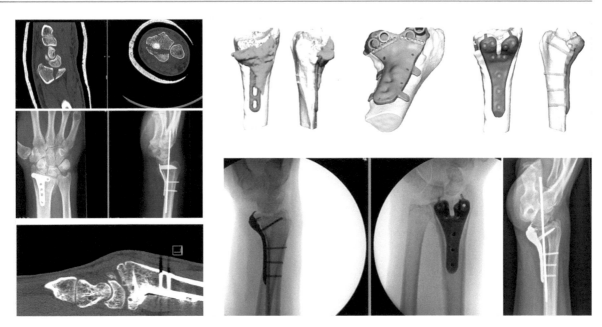

Fig. 11.4 In this case the volar rim of the lunate facet was not fixed. Therefore, the carpus dislocates to the volar side. Patient-specific saw and drilling guides were fitted on the distal part of the radius and next a 3D printed titanium plate was used for fixation.

tional impairment, loss of grip strength, and pain. Moreover, patients are frequently unsatisfied with the aesthetics of the wrist due to the malunion. We tend to correct malunions as soon as possible even between 4 and 6 weeks of follow-up. Some authors advise to let the fracture maturate; however, we do not encounter any problems performing a corrective osteotomy during the remodeling phase. The decision whether to surgically correct distal radial malunions is primarily based on functional demand and wrist pain. Contraindications for surgery are poor health, severe osteoporosis, and advanced arthrosis.

Malunions can be classified in extra-articular, intra-articular, or combinations. An extra-articular malunion is defined as a healed radius which does not comply to the reduction criteria as stated above with a special emphasis of carpal alignment and coronal plane translation. For extra-articular malunions we prefer an open wedge osteotomy over closed wedge osteotomies because they improve radial length and can be used to correct angular deformities in multiple directions. Bone grafts are only used in rare cases where there is a considerable gap or in revision cases. Mulders et al published long-term outcomes of extra-articular corrective osteotomies in 48 patients. The median age was 54.5 years (IQR 39–66) and 71% was female with a median time to follow-up of 27 months. The median DASH and PRWE scores showed good results and were respectively 10.0 (IQR 5.8–23.3) and 18.5 (6.5–37.0).[19]

The indication to correct an intra-articular malunion is less straightforward. However, intra-articular arthrosis of the radiocarpal joint or DRUJ is not an absolute contraindication in our institute. Only symptomatic patients with a functional limitation, pain, and radiological parameters confirming the deformity are offered surgery which means that we do not intend to perform prophylactic corrections to prevent symptomatic arthrosis in the future, e.g., patients with asymptomatic intra-articular step offs. Nowadays, most cases are performed with patient-specific implants, including saw and drilling guides combined with 3D printed titanium plates (▶ Fig. 11.4).

11.3 Complications due to Plate and Screw Position

11.3.1 Volar Plating

Soong et al developed a classification system to determine plate prominence in relation to the watershed line. Plates that do not extend volar to the critical line are classified as Grade 0, those volar to the line but proximal to the volar rim as Grade 1, and plates directly on or distal to the volar rim as Grade 2. In a group of patients where Grade 2 volar prominence was present, the increased incidence of flexor tendon ruptures approached statistical significance.[20]

Volar plates can be classified as extra-articular plates, volar column plates, juxta-articular plates, and volar rim plates. The type of plate dictates an ideal placement relative to the watershed line. Therefore ideal placement of an extra-articular plate will be classified as Soong 0, a volar column plate as Soong 0, a juxta-articular plate as Soong 1, and a volar rim plate as Soong 2. Selles et al found that the Soong classification was significantly higher in patients who had plate removal compared with

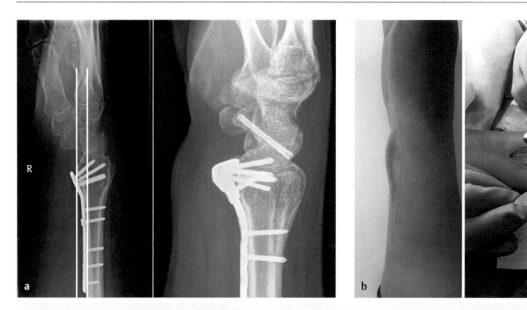

Fig. 11.5 (a) An extra-articular plate extending the watershed line and with a nonanatomic reduction of the volar rim resulting in a Soong grade 2. **(b)** An example of flexor tendinitis due to a volar rim plate. Highlight the volar soft tissue swelling on the X-ray.

those who did not. For patients with plate positioning classified as Soong grade 2, the incidence of plate removal was almost six times higher than those classified as Soong grade 0, most likely due to flexor tendon irritation. The relationship between volar plate removal and a higher Soong grading stresses the importance of accurate plate positioning (▶ Fig. 11.5). Consequently, we advise to remove all volar plates graded as Soong 2 eight weeks following surgery.[21]

The distal screws are aimed at the subchondral bone plate just proximal to the radial carpal joint. Whereas, here the load of the scaphoid and lunate is transmitted to the metaphyseal area and the multilayer subchondral plate offers the optimal stability for the screws. When the screws are too proximal and aimed in the metaphysis, the reduced radius may collapse under physiologic forces, especially in the elderly and osteoporotic patients. Drilling and positioning the distal screws should be *uni*cortical to protect the extensor tendons and especially the EPL tendon. Once an EPL rupture occurs this is treated with an extensor indicis proprius (EIP) tendon to EPL transfer. When judging the length of the distal screws on the lateral fluoroscopic image, be aware of Lister's trap. Lister's tubercle sits like a shark fin on the dorsal part of the distal radius. Therefore, inexperienced surgeons may judge

that the distal tip of the screws do not penetrate the far cortex; however, in reality Lister's tubercle is falsely mistaken for the dorsal cortex (▶ Fig. 11.6).

The loadbearing area of the lunate is volar. Therefore when confronted with a Type C intra-articular fracture involving the volar or dorsal lip of the lunate facet, the surgeon should accurately assess the sagittal and transverse CT reconstructions.

Brink and Rikli published the four-corner concept. This concept shows us to define "the key fragment."[22] The lunate facet is assessed on the sagittal CT reconstruction. The adage is "follow the lunate." When the lunate subluxes together with a dorsal or volar corner fragment, the fragment which is related to the direction of the subluxation is the key fragment. This fragment should be treated with a stable fixation and dictates whether a dorsal, volar, or combined approach is mandatory. Moreover, in most cases the volar key fragment is regularly not only one large fragment but consists of more fragments. All these fragments should be fixated to avoid the devastating effect of volar dislocation of the carpus following plate fixation (▶ Fig. 11.4).

Following plate fixation, intraoperative fluoroscopy is used to check the Soong classification and screw lengths on the PA and lateral images. Moreover, we recommend

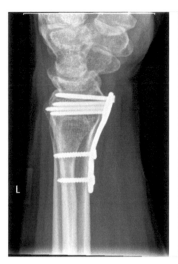

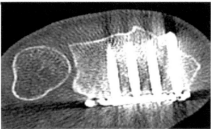

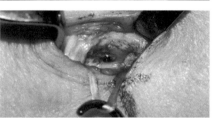

Fig. 11.6 Dorsal screws are penetrating in extensor tendon compartment one and three (not in the picture), resulting in an extensor pollicis longus (EPL) rupture. The penetrating screw is shown at the bottom of compartment three whereas the hook holds the remaining EPL.

additional fluoroscopic skyline (dorsal tangential) views or carpal-shot-through views. An image perpendicular to distal part of the plate and articular surface of the radius may help to judge screw lengths and to avoid penetration of the dorsal cortex and therefore injury to the extensor tendons. Occasionally better visualization of the dorsal radial cortex is achieved with the wrist in flexion (skyline view) and sometimes in extension (carpal shot through). Pitfall is to confuse the scaphoid and lunate for dorsal radial cortex in these images.

11.4 Complications due to Infections

The incidence of deep infections following plate fixation is less than 1%.[10] However, once a deep infection occurs the consequences may be devastating. For treatment, we prefer the Masquelet technique. It is important to stop all antibiotics at least 2 weeks before surgery. First a thorough surgical debridement is performed and at least five deep tissue/implant specimens are collected. Next, a temporary cement spacer (with gentamycin and vanco-mycin) is fitted in the defect. Stability is the cornerstone of treatment and this may best be provided by a spanning plate, a conventional DRF plate, or external fixator. After a synovial-like membrane is formed after 5 weeks, the spacer is removed and the defect is treated with a bone graft from the iliac crest or with a Reamer Irrigator Aspirator system. In elderly patients we sometimes perform a one-stop procedure by filling the void with a resorbable ceramic bone graft substitute intended to fill bone gaps and voids to promote bone healing. The antibiotic susceptibility of the pathogens will guide antimicrobial treatment for at least 6 weeks (▶ Fig. 11.7).

11.5 Take-Home Message

- Avoid accidental damage to the palmar cutaneous branch of the median nerve (PCBMN) by dissecting on the radial side of the FCR (flexor carpi radialis) instead of going through the tendon sheath when using a modified Henry approach to the distal radius.
- When using radial-sided (temporary) K-wires, protect the sensory branch of the radial nerve as neuromas can result from a (blind) percutaneous approach.
- Release of the brachioradialis insertion on the distal fracture fragment aids in achieving anatomical reduction.
- There is no benefit in repairing the pronator quadratus muscle after volar plate fixation. It might actually reduce pronation strength.
- Carpal alignment and coronal plane translation are unfamiliar but important reduction criteria for distal radius fractures.
- Dorsal screw protrusion is common due to Lister's trap. Avoid drill and screw penetration of the dorsal cortex.
- Do not position volar plates distally from the watershed line. For it can cause flexor tendon irritation or rupture.
- Treat deep infections with surgical debridement and Masquelet technique and stable fixation.

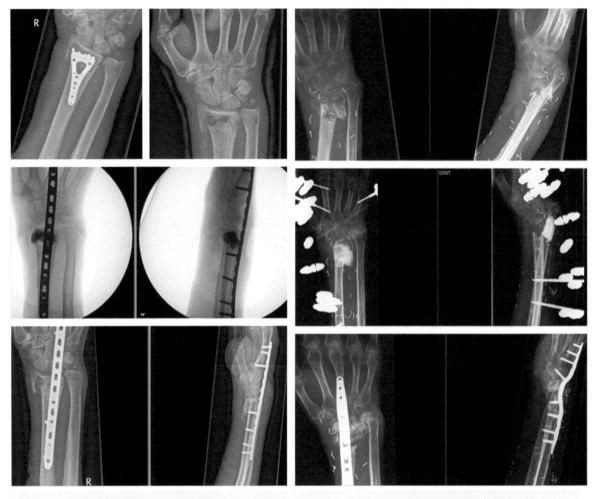

Fig. 11.7 Left: the volar plate was removed due to the deep infection and a plaster was provided. Due to the lack of stability the infection continued. A one-step procedure was performed; following debridement the void was filled with a resorbable ceramic bone graft. Right: this patient had a deep infection which was only treated with a radial forearm flap and an external fixator which was removed. Next a Masquelet procedure was performed with temporary fixation and ultimately with a wrist cushion.

References

[1] Lichtman DM, Bindra RR, Boyer MI, et al. Treatment of distal radius fractures. J Am Acad Orthop Surg. 2010; 18(3):180–189

[2] Handoll HH, Madhok R. Closed reduction methods for treating distal radial fractures in adults. Cochrane Database Syst Rev. 2003(1): CD003763

[3] Levin SM, Nelson CO, Botts JD, Teplitz GA, Kwon Y, Serra-Hsu F. Biomechanical evaluation of volar locking plates for distal radius fractures. Hand (N Y). 2008; 3(1):55–60

[4] Dias JJ, Wray CC, Jones JM, Gregg PJ. The value of early mobilisation in the treatment of Colles' fractures. J Bone Joint Surg Br. 1987; 69 (3):463–467

[5] Ng CY, McQueen MM. What are the radiological predictors of functional outcome following fractures of the distal radius? J Bone Joint Surg Br. 2011; 93(2):145–150

[6] Mulders MAM, Detering R, Rikli DA, Rosenwasser MP, Goslings JC, Schep NWL. Association between radiological and patient-reported outcome in adults with a displaced distal radius fracture: a systematic review and meta-analysis. J Hand Surg Am. 2018; 43(8):710–719.e5

[7] Fitzpatrick R, Davey C, Buxton MJ, Jones DR. Evaluating patient-based outcome measures for use in clinical trials. Health Technol Assess. 1998; 2(14):i–iv, 1–74

[8] van Eck ME, Lameijer CM, El Moumni M. Structural validity of the Dutch version of the disability of arm, shoulder and hand questionnaire (DASH-DLV) in adult patients with hand and wrist injuries. BMC Musculoskelet Disord. 2018; 19(1):207

[9] Vannabouathong C, Hussain N, Guerra-Farfan E, Bhandari M. Interventions for distal radius fractures: a network meta-analysis of randomized trials. J Am Acad Orthop Surg. 2019; 27(13):e596–e605

[10] Bentohami A, de Burlet K, de Korte N, van den Bekerom MP, Goslings JC, Schep NW. Complications following volar locking plate fixation for distal radial fractures: a systematic review. J Hand Surg Eur Vol. 2014; 39(7):745–754

[11] Lutz K, Yeoh KM, MacDermid JC, Symonette C, Grewal R. Complications associated with operative versus nonsurgical treatment of distal radius fractures in patients aged 65 years and older. J Hand Surg Am. 2014; 39(7):1280–1286

[12] Rampoldi M, Marsico S. Complications of volar plating of distal radius fractures. Acta Orthop Belg. 2007; 73(6):714–719

[13] Mulders MAM, Walenkamp MMJ, Bos FJME, Schep NWL, Goslings JC. Repair of the pronator quadratus after volar plate fixation in distal

radius fractures: a systematic review. Strateg Trauma Limb Reconstr. 2017; 12(3):181–188

[14] Sonntag J, Woythal L, Rasmussen P, et al. No effect on functional outcome after repair of pronator quadratus in volar plating of distal radial fractures: a randomized clinical trial. Bone Joint J. 2019; 101-B (12):1498–1505

[15] Patterson RW, Van Niel M, Shimko P, Pace C, Seitz WH, Jr. Proprioception of the wrist following posterior interosseous sensory neurectomy. J Hand Surg Am. 2010; 35(1):52–56

[16] Medoff RJ. Essential radiographic evaluation for distal radius fractures. Hand Clin. 2005; 21(3):279–288

[17] McQueen MM, Hajducka C, Court-Brown CM. Redisplaced unstable fractures of the distal radius: a prospective randomised comparison of four methods of treatment. J Bone Joint Surg Br. 1996; 78(3):404–409

[18] Selles CA, Ras L, Walenkamp MMJ, Maas M, Goslings JC, Schep NWL. Carpal alignment: a new method for assessment. J Wrist Surg. 2019; 8(2):112–117

[19] Mulders MA, d'Ailly PN, Cleffken BI, Schep NW. Corrective osteotomy is an effective method of treating distal radius malunions with good long-term functional results. Injury. 2017; 48(3):731–737

[20] Soong M, Earp BE, Bishop G, Leung A, Blazar P. Volar locking plate implant prominence and flexor tendon rupture. J Bone Joint Surg Am. 2011; 93(4):328–335

[21] Selles CA, Reerds STH, Roukema G, van der Vlies KH, Cleffken BI, Schep NWL. Relationship between plate removal and Soong grading following surgery for fractured distal radius. J Hand Surg Eur Vol. 2018; 43(2):137–141

[22] Brink PR, Rikli DA. Four-corner concept: CT-based assessment of fracture patterns in distal radius. J Wrist Surg. 2016; 5(2):147–151

3

12 Management of Distal Radius Malunion

Abstract

Distal radius malunion is a common complication after distal radius fracture. About 5% of these malunions are symptomatic. The surgical treatment of a symptomatic distal radius malunion is an osteotomy aimed at restoring the distal radius articular surfaces in the radiocarpal and distal radioulnar joints as anatomically as possible.

Traditional 2D imaging techniques consist of radiographs in posterior-anterior (PA) and lateral views. The relationship between the classical evaluation criteria such as radial inclination, ulnar variance, volar tilt, and the symptoms of the patient is generally very limited because dorsovolar translation, radioulnar translation, and rotation deformation are not taken into account. The conventional evaluation criteria are therefore far from optimal in pre-, intra-, and postoperative imaging of radius malunion.

With the advent of 3D imaging techniques in recent decades, new opportunities have emerged in the areas of preoperative planning, navigation, and 3D printing.

The aim of Part A of this chapter is to provide an overview of the existing literature on the advantages, disadvantages, and future prospects of current computer-aided technology for correction osteotomy. Patient-specific 3D printed guides and implants are currently the most promising technology to transfer the preoperative plan to the patient.

In Part B, the focus will be on surgical aspects itself.

Keywords: distal radius, osteotomy, malunion, computer-assisted surgery, plate fixation, patient-specific plate, surgical guides, virtual planning, navigation, complications, radial inclination, ulnar shortening osteotomy

12.1 Part A: Planning: From Educated Guess toward Computer-Assisted Correction Osteotomies; Pitfalls and Complications

S.D. Strackee and J.G.G. Dobbe

12.1.1 Introduction

The most common complication following a distal radius fracture is a malunion. This occurs in approximately 11% of fractures treated surgically and in 23% of fractures treated conservatively. The distal radius has a relatively thin dorsal cortex, and in the great majority of cases a distal radius fracture is extra-articular. The weightbearing distal segment of the bone is tilted roughly dorsally and

radially, and near the fracture line the radial shaft shifts toward the ulna. Due to its strong attachment to the brachioradial tendon, the distal radius rotates in supination, which may cause the proximal part of the affected forearm to pronate more. There is often some shortening of the radius, and due to this, the relatively longer ulna will come into contact with the proximal ulnar carpal bone. In extra-articular fractures, the palmar cortex is often a simple transverse fracture, so the rotation of the forearm will be limited, particularly in supination.[1,2] However, limitation of movement of the forearm is dependent on a number of factors. Contraction and later fibrosis of the pronator quadratus muscle can also strongly limit supination. The same applies to the fibrosis of the palmar distal-radioulnar (DRU) joint capsule and the interosseous membranes.[3] Approximately 5% of all distal radius fractures that have healed in an abnormal position with altered anatomical relationships between proximal radius, ulna, and the carpals will lead to symptoms.[4] These can vary from pain on exertion, pain on movement (flexion, radioulnar deviations in extension, and rotation of the forearm), limitation of movement of the radial and ulnar carpals and the DRU joint, deformities of the forearm with dorsal prominence of the ulna, deviation of the hand dorsally and radially in relation to the forearm, carpal tunnel syndrome, and loss of strength.

12.1.2 Diagnostics

The first step in the correction of a malunion is to make an unequivocal diagnosis that explains the relationship between the symptomology and the anatomical changes. Ideally, by quantifying the abnormality, the boundary between acceptable and nonacceptable symptoms can be defined.

Only a small proportion of patients with a malunion have major symptoms. Generally, a slight limitation in range of movement does not lead to the wish for a correction. However, if the limitation of range of movement is accompanied by pain or a strong restriction in load-bearing capacity, then the wish for a correction is greatly increased. Pain on rotation of the forearm is a substantial problem as it leads to loss of function in the entire upper limb. Diagnostic assessment thus focuses on pain in the wrist and/or limitations of rotation in the forearm.

Conventional Diagnostic Assessment

The analysis of the malunion always starts with conventional two-dimensional (2D) radiology with posterior-anterior (PA) and lateral views. A carefully carried out radiological investigation is of the greatest importance in order to obtain reproducible results.[5,6,7]

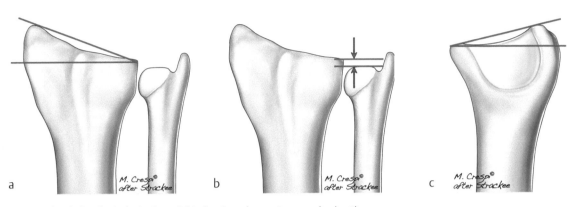

Fig. 12.1 (a–c) The classical criteria: radial inclination, ulnar variance, and volar tilt.

The radiographic images are evaluated in accordance with the classical criteria such as radial inclination, ulnar variance, and volar tilt (▶ Fig. 12.1).

In PA projection, the radial inclination is the angle between the line perpendicular to the long axis through the radius and the line through the distal radial surface. Normal values are between 16 and 28 degrees with an average of 25 degrees.

In lateral view, volar (or palmar) tilt is also the angle between the line perpendicular to the long axis of the radius and the line through the distal radial surface. Normal values are between 0 and 22 degrees with an average of 15 degrees.

Ulnar variance is the difference measured in PA projection between the horizontal line at the level of the ulno-distal border of the lunate fossa perpendicular to the long axis of the radius and the horizontal line through the end of the ulna.[5]

These 2D measurements are of limited reliability. The technique of taking radiographic images is often less than optimal, and their evaluation is also subjective. As far back as 1996, Kreder et al[7] concluded: "In view of our inability to measure deformity more accurately, the concept of a specific relationship between a given degree of deformity and outcome must be questioned."

The relationship between the measured parameters and the symptoms of the patient is generally very limited, certainly if on radiograph the 2D parameters differ very little from normal. This is due to the fact that the malunion is a three-dimensional (3D) deformity which cannot be quantified adequately from two plain orthogonal radiographic images. Overprojection and hidden rotations around the long axis of the bone are the two main limitations of using 2D imaging.[8,9,10,11]

An important attendant problem is that chronic pain in the wrist due to malunion is multifactorial. Cheng et al[12] found that four factors contributed to the symptoms of pain: ulna carpal abutment, ulnar styloid nonunion, tri-angular fibrocartilage complex (TFCC) tears whether or not they were associated with instability, intercarpal ligament lesions, and cartilage damage. Thus, symptoms following consolidation in malunion are the result of both bony and soft tissue factors, which brings evaluation purely on bony parameters into question. Haase[13] identified the problem, i.e., there is little correlation between symptomology and the severity of the radiological abnormalities. However, this did not deter him from postulating criteria for "unacceptable healing" (▶ Table 12.1).

Diagnosis from 2D to 3D

Active experimentation with 3D techniques began in the early 1990s. First with lithographic or printed models,[14] followed later by 3D computer simulations, usually using the healthy contralateral side as a reference.[15]

The scans of both the affected and the healthy radii are segmented, thereby creating virtual models for visualization. By aligning the proximal section of the mirrored healthy radius with the affected radius using registration techniques, the deformity can be made clearly visible on the computer screen. It is also possible to assess the best site for the osteotomy. If desired, the virtual bone models, or a model of the corrected bone, can be printed using a 3D printer (▶ Fig. 12.2).

The abnormality can also be expressed quantitatively in size and number. For this purpose, a distal and proximal section of the affected virtual bone is clipped, and this is then aligned with the healthy side by means of registration. The positioning required for this can be described by means of a transformation matrix. Therefore, the alignment of each of the segments of bone results in a transformation matrix for the distal segment (**Mdist**), and one for the proximal segment (**Mprox**). These matrices are combined in a correction matrix **Mcorr** (Mcorr = Mprox^{-1}. Mdist) for the reduction (correction) of the affected distal segment with respect to the

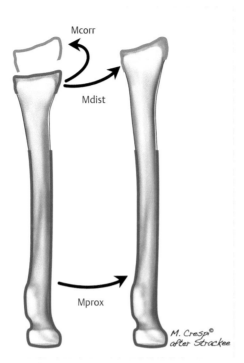

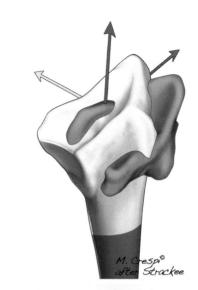

Fig. 12.3 The six asymmetry parameters Δx, Δy, Δz, $\Delta\varphi x$, $\Delta\varphi y$, and $\Delta\varphi z$ are expressed in terms of the anatomical coordinate system (3 translations along and 3 rotations around the orthogonal axes x (red), y (yellow), and z (blue).

Fig. 12.2 Distal segment (red) and the proximal segment (blue) of the 3D model of the affected bone (left) are registered on the mirrored 3D model of the healthy contralateral bone (right). Each registration results in a transformation matrix (**Mprox**, **Mdist**). These matrices are combined in a correction matrix (**Mcorr = Mprox⁻¹. Mdist**).

proximal segment. The reduction can be expressed as translations along, and rotations around, the axes of a 3D coordinate system with three axes X, Y, and Z. The axis system for the radius is usually chosen as follows: the longitudinal axis is the Z-axis, the X-axis is perpendicular to it and oriented toward the radial styloid process. The Y-axis is again perpendicular to the X and Z axes. Here, the evaluation of the malunion is done using six parameters: three displacements and three rotations around three orthogonal axes (▶ Fig. 12.3).

Using this technique, it is possible to plan in 3D preoperatively. However, it should be noted that when using the mirrored contralateral side, there is a physiological difference between left and right. Both radii and ulnae are longer in the dominant arm than in the nondominant arm (2.63 ± 2.03 mm and 2.08 ± 2.33 mm, respectively). This is particularly important in terms of translation along the Z (longitudinal) axis, as errors in the direction of this axis can result in an ulnar variance that is positive and can thus give rise to an ulnocarpal abutment. If necessary, this must be checked and corrected in the preoperative phase or during the procedure.[16]

Vroemen et al[10] retrospectively examined 25 patients who had undergone correction on the basis of conventional diagnostics with 2D parameters. The results were

radiologically evaluated postoperatively, using both the 2D technique and the 3D CT technique described above, and three validated patient outcome questionnaires (DASH, PRWHE, and MHOQ). In both patient groups, the corrected wrists were compared with the healthy, nonoperated contralateral wrists. Interestingly, no correlations were found in the 2D evaluation, but significant correlations between the rotational abnormalities and the clinical outcome measures were found in the 3D assessment.

Clearly, it is not possible to give one single unequivocal criterion for the indication for treatment of an extra-articular malunion on the basis of 2D parameters. In partial or complete intra-articular fractures, the standard radiological evaluation is limited to obtaining an overview of the situation and further evaluation will have to take place by means of CT examination, preferably with a 3D reconstruction. Similarly, after segmentation, a qualitative image can then be obtained which can be assessed on the computer screen or printed out as a visual model. After mirroring and registration, the same dataset can also be used for a quantitative assessment and further be applied in the virtual planning of an operative correction.

12.1.3 Treatment

The best way to prevent a malunion is to make the right choices at the time that the fracture is diagnosed. In the past, several classifications of distal radius fractures have been proposed. One of the most commonly used is the AO classification. In this, fractures of the wrist are divided into three types: Type A is extra-articular where the distal part has shifted dorsally (Colles type), or has shifted to palmar

(Smith type). Bentohami et al regarded more than half of the fractures in 494 patients as being Type A. The remaining fracture types were either Type B partial intra-articular fractures, or Type C fully intra-articular fractures: each accounting for approximately 24% of the total.[17]

In approximately two-thirds of cases there is a displaced fracture where there may or may not be an indication for open reduction and fixation. Based on the type of fracture, an estimate is made of the degree of instability and thus the risk of developing a malunion. Based on this expectation, a certain treatment strategy is chosen. In 2015, Walenkamp et al showed that 143 different definitions of fracture instability were used in 479 studies. In only one study the definition of instability was based on clinical research (level IIIb).[18]

This lack of consensus makes it difficult to compare treatment strategies on the basis of current studies. As a result, it is not possible to make a proper assessment of the risk of a malunion based on the fracture classification.

The surgeon is often confronted with a preexisting malunion. The treatment strategy then involves making a plan to correct the malunion after an analysis of the abnormal position has been carried out. This plan must then be applied to the patient, using a form of navigation to place the bone segments correctly in the physical space, after which fixation takes place. Fixation can be carried out using screws/plates or wedges of various materials, potentially custom-made.

Conventional Treatment Strategies

Using data on the average values of classical criteria obtained from the literature, i.e., radial inclination, radial height, ulnar variance, and volar tilt, the degree of abnormality of the malunion is determined. Of course, this can also be obtained by comparison with the contralateral healthy side of the patient. Usually, the dimensions of the required bone graft are calculated on the basis of a cutting plane determined on the radiograph; as Von Campe observed back in 2006, "We conclude that a distal radius osteotomy using a precisely planned and measured interpositional corticocancellous graft does not restore distal radius alignment in most patients, and that failure to restore length is associated with continued pain and stiffness."[19] In their investigations into the long-term results of corrective osteotomy for malunion, Lozano-Calderon et al found the results in the area of function to be changeable. Among other things, this was attributed to the occurrence of posttraumatic osteoarthritis as a result of an imperfect anatomical position.[20] The reproduction of bones from virtual 3D models based on segmented 3D computed tomography (CT) images has been possible for a long time, but has rarely been used because production using a numerically controlled milling machine is very costly and time-consuming.

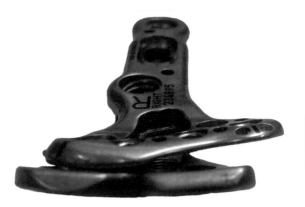

Fig. 12.4 Comparison between two different makes of distal radius fracture fixation plates.

The arrival of 3D printers has made it possible to create life-sized plastic replicas of bones. Using the models of the affected side and the mirrored contralateral side, it is possible to gain insight into the abnormality. Reproducing a planned correction using these models proved less successful in the study by Walenkamp et al.

A variant of this approach is the use of physical models on which to model standard fixation plates preoperatively. In the study by Kataoka et al, this resulted in corrections that deviated less than 3 mm (total translation error) and 2 degrees (total rotational error) from the preoperative planning.[21]

Nowadays, a popular approach is the use of the so-called anatomical plates. These plates are considered to fit the average patient anatomy and are currently used as standard osteosynthesis material. However, the shapes of the plates differ considerably (▶ Fig. 12.4), and it is logical that they have been shown to lead to considerable positioning error in individual patients.[22]

Treatment Based on Computer-Aided 3D Planning

One of the earliest attempts to visualize a malunion of the radius was Bilic's 1994 wire model. This model, based on two orthogonal 2D images of the radius, was compared with a wire model which was based on the average values of healthy volunteers. From this, the dimensions of a corrective graft were calculated. The biggest disadvantage of this was that a way to transfer the plan to the patient was missing.

Over the past 15 years, the use of high-resolution CT scans and the development of accurate segmentation techniques have made it possible to obtain accurate 3D patient-specific models of patient bone. The same segmentation technique is now used for preoperative position planning, and for further 3D planning of the location and orientation of the osteotomy.

As mentioned in the diagnostics section, there is a physiological difference in length between the dominant and nondominant arm. If this is not taken into account, there is a risk of under- or overcorrection of the radius, resulting in discongruity in the DRU joint and/or ulnocarpal abutment. When planning, Dobbe used a linear regression model to compensate for this difference in length.[16]

Initially, the repositioning of bone segments was assessed and planned almost exclusively by means of 2D imaging. An early exception was Croitoru's work in 2001.[8] Generally, 2D techniques are still being used postoperatively to evaluate the positioning of bone segments. This is extremely odd, as the literature has shown that 2D imaging provides only a moderate reflection of 3D positioning. Evaluation using the conventional parameters, therefore, does not contribute (or only marginally so) to finding a relationship between the positioning error and the clinical signs.[23,24,25]

There are now several commercially available software packages for preoperative planning that use computer-assisted 3D techniques in which the unaffected contralateral radius serves as a reference for restoring the affected side.

However, if the contralateral side is also affected or unavailable, the use of a 3D statistical shape model is an option. This technique predicts the pretrauma healthy shape of the pathological bone using a static shape model of the radius. This shape model is aligned as carefully as possible with the nondeformed parts of the affected radius using characteristic local shapes such as thicknesses, curves, etc. Mauler et al used 59 scans of healthy forearms in which three scenarios to predict radial shape were simulated: 50% of the proximal segment, 50% of the distal segment, or the shape of the whole radius. The result was compared with the original shape as a reference. The differences found were on average to be less than 1 mm in translation and with the rotations over the X, Y, and Z axes being 0.6, 0.5, and 2.9 degrees, respectively, and thus better than what is known from the literature about techniques where the contralateral radius is the reference. The experiments with ulnae showed similar results.[26]

In the preoperative virtual planning phase, the fixation method should also be taken into account. Usually, commercially available fixed-angle locking plates and screws are used. A virtual replica of these plates is sometimes supplied by the manufacturer or the shape of the plates is scanned in. The plate is placed virtually on to the reconstructed radius model where it fits best. Certainly, if there is a severe deformation in the region of the malunion, this can lead to a substantial space or mismatch between plate and bone. Adjusting the plate on the basis of a printed model and then scanning the plate may be a solution to this. The position and direction of the screw holes in the fixed-angle locking plate are taken into account in the virtual planning. If it is not possible to use a standard plate (with possible adjustments), then a patient-specific plate can be made using the additive manufacturing process; the plate is usually made of a biocompatible titanium alloy (Ti-6A1–4V). The location, direction, and size of the screw holes can be freely determined.

12.1.4 Navigation and Fixation

The next step is the transfer of the preoperative plan to the patient. In this process, the virtual space and the physical space are linked to each other (registration). Actions in the physical space can thus be made visible in the virtual space (on the computer), and vice versa. To link the virtual and physical spaces, especially dedicated instruments with trackers are traced in the physical space using a tracking system. By using this instrument to point out certain landmarks on the physical bone, and by using the computer mouse on the virtual bone, the computer establishes the link between the bone in the physical and virtual spaces. In practice, a tracker is also applied to the bone so that the extremity can move in the physical space without losing the link with the virtual space. Croitoru et al[8] were one of the first to use an infrared tracking system in the correction of a radius malunion. The disadvantage of this technique is that placing a tracker on the bone is an additional invasive action. Also, the equipment is quite large and expensive.

An alternative way to navigate is to create patient-specific templates. Such a template is only able to fit on the bone in one way. The specific placement of the template thus forms the link between the physical and virtual spaces. Defining a saw cut "relative to the template" in virtual space is the same as defining a saw cut "relative to the template" in physical space. The transfer of a plan from virtual to physical space in the operating theater is therefore very simple. The template with saw guide and drill-hole guide is designed for the volar or dorsal surface of the malunited radius and fits exactly over the shape of the specific piece of bone that requires correction. A biocompatible and sterilizable plastic (polyamide) is used for printing. Various methods have been described for navigating the bone segments to the correct relative position.

Using a Reduction Guide that Fits the Bone Segments

After the osteotomy, the distal radius must be positioned in the physical space. This can be done with a second (reduction) template. This template is modelled over the volar or dorsal surfaces of the corrected radius in the planning phase. The printed repositioning template is placed on the proximal radius during the operation and temporarily fixed with K-wires. The distal radius section is then positioned in the template and also temporarily fixed with K-wires.

Despite releasing the insertion of the brachioradialis tendon, it often takes a lot of effort to maneuver the distal radial section exactly into the reduction template. This mainly depends on the degree of proximal displacement of the parts of the fracture and the amount of scarring at the dorsal side of the wrist.

Using Pins in a Reduction Guide

In practice, it is often difficult to apply a fixation plate as well as the above-mentioned reduction template. A solution to this problem was suggested by Murase et al in 2008.[27] In their technique, holes are cut out of the drilling/sawing template to accommodate four 3-mm width pins or K-wires grouped as a distal and a proximal pair. During planning, the pins are placed parallel in the corrected radius. The reduction template, actually a bar with four parallel holes, is used during the operation to temporarily hold the pins in the planned position. Pin placement is chosen in such a way that there is room to place a fixation plate of the surgeon's preference. After fixation, the reduction template and the pins are removed. In the planning method described above, the pins were placed in the corrected radius. Because the drilling/sawing template is placed on the affected bone, the distal pins must first be transformed to the affected position before they are included in the saw template. The inverse correction matrix Mcorr can be used for this purpose.

Using a Standard or Modified Plate

In this method, a 3D model of a fixation plate is placed over the virtually corrected bone segments during the virtual planning procedure. Next, the orientation of the screws, the screw length, and the location/orientation of the osteotomy can be determined. Using this information, a drilling/sawing template can then be made, which contains holes that can be predrilled in the correct direction. A slot in the template guides the saw blade for making the osteotomy. Just as described in the previous method, the fixation plate is placed over the corrected segments and the screw holes are set in the planned position. Because the drilling/sawing template is placed on the affected bone, these distal drill holes must first be transformed to the affected position before they are included in the saw template. The inverse correction matrix Mcorr can again be used for this purpose. During the surgical procedure, and after removal of the drilling/sawing template, the fixation plate can be fixed using fixation screws in the predrilled holes. Since the distance between the plate and the bone surface is not taken into account during the planning, a translation error may persist. This can be resolved by using a patient-specific plate.

The Patient-Specific Plate

This plate is a custom plate that combines fixation and patient-specific placement. The plate is modeled on a corrected virtual bone model. Further preoperative planning is similar to the method described above. After using a drilling/sawing template for predrilling screw holes and making the osteotomy, the template is removed and the patient-specific plate is fixed with screws in the predrilled holes. The specific shape ensures placement of the bone segments as planned. The plate is usually produced in titanium and can also be provided with holes suitable for fixed-angle screws. The curved shape of patient-specific plates will render these plates very rigid, which offers the opportunity to manufacture these plates much thinner. The first experiences with this method are of recent date, and no large series have yet been described.

The use of templates or a custom-made plate also has its disadvantages. A lot of dissection is needed as the periosteum has to be dissected from large parts of the radius to make a template fit exactly. If this is not done, then the template does not lie well on the bone, which makes it unstable. The result is that the alignment of the osteotomy plane and screw-hole positions does not match the planning. With shaft corrections, it is difficult to position the template, because there are too few characteristic local landmarks. This can partly be solved by draping the template slightly over the contour of the bone, which increases accuracy.

A commonly occurring problem in drilling and sawing is that too much oblique pressure is exercised. Also, if there is too much play in the saw or drill-guided openings, there is a good chance that errors will occur in the osteotomy, and that the screws will not fit in the appropriate holes. In addition, there is a risk that a lot of tension will develop in the plate or screws, which may cause them to break. If the screws are screwed into the plate at the wrong angle, damage to the plate/screw connection is possible, which may make it difficult to remove the screws. This is especially true of titanium fixation material.

If templates are used, there is virtually no possibility of adjusting the planning during the procedure, making a length adjustment for example.

One frequently mentioned advantage of using a template is that it saves time. However, this is partially cancelled out by the longer preoperative preparation time required. Localization of the soft tissues, and the origins and insertions of muscles and ligaments in particular, is not included in the virtual correction. It is recommended that an experienced surgeon should help the planning engineer in designing a practical and useable template. This is also applicable to the surgical approach to the operative field. There are a number of synthetic materials that satisfy the requirements for sterilization and that also maintain their shape and can be easily printed. The cost of these materials is low, but the development of patient-specific tools requires experienced staff and is therefore relatively expensive.

12.1.5 Take-Home Message

Careful preoperative diagnosis of the radius malunion and careful preoperative planning of the correction osteotomy are the prerequisites for an optimal outcome. With the help of high-resolution 3D CT scans and accurate segmentation techniques, precise 3D planning of the location and orientation of the osteotomy is possible. There are several commercially available software packages for preoperative planning that use computer-assisted 3D techniques in which the unaffected contralateral radius serves as a reference for restoring the affected side. Take care to correct for length differences between the dominant and nondominant side. If the contralateral side is also affected or unavailable, the use of a 3D statistical shape model is an option. In the preoperative virtual planning phase, the fixation method should also be taken into account. Usually, commercially available fixed-angle locking plates and screws are used. If it is not possible to use a standard plate (with possible adjustments), then a patient-specific plate can be manufactured. Make sure that you are aware of the advantages and disadvantages of the standard- and patient-specific plate.

12.2 Part B: Practical Guideline: Malunion of Distal Radius

Thomas Verschueren and Frederik Verstreken

12.2.1 Timing: Early versus Late

There are no general guidelines to decide on the best moment for corrective surgery. The indications are primarily based on patient complaints and not on radiographic criteria. Although a significant correlation between radiographic malalignment and symptoms has been shown, it is greatly mitigated in elderly patients.[28] So it is perfectly acceptable to wait for sufficient time, and to only treat patients with persistent symptoms. However, there is a group of younger patients with malunion and unacceptable deformity that will benefit from early correction. The procedure is technically easier as less soft tissue contracture (tendons, nerves, and ligaments) has developed. When intervening within 4 to 8 weeks, early callus is more easily distinguished from the cortical bone and can be removed as needed. The original fracture plane can be identified, different fragments can be mobilized with restoration of anatomical alignment. Not only is correction achieved more easily, early intervention can also eliminate the need for a structural bone graft.[29]

Jupiter and Ring found that the results of early intervention (average 8 weeks from injury) were comparable to the results of late intervention (average 40 weeks from injury). Grip strength, however, averaged 42 kg after early, compared with 25 kg after late intervention. They

Table 12.1 Criteria for malunion

Parameter	Malunion
Radial inclination	< 10 degrees
Radial tilt	Volar tilt > 20 degrees, dorsal tilt > 20 degrees
Radial length	< 10 mm
Ulnar variance	> + 2 mm
Intra-articular step or gap	> 2 mm

confirmed that early reconstruction is also technically easier and reduces the overall disability time in patients who meet radiographic criteria predictive of functional impairment.[30]

Haase et al have proposed criteria for "unacceptable" healing (▶ Table 12.1), not compatible with normal pain-free function of the wrist.[13]

Another argument for early intervention is the fact that malunion can be a prearthritic condition, due to adaptive carpal malalignment or an intra-articular step off. Early correction of these deformities will prevent further degenerative changes.

When the decision for intervention has been made, surgery should be performed as soon as possible, provided there are no trophic changes, soft tissues have sufficiently recovered from the original trauma, and bone quality is acceptable.

12.2.2 How to Do It

Approaches, Fixation, and Grafts

The goal of surgical treatment for distal radius malunion should be to restore normal anatomy as precisely as possible with focus on reorientation of the articular surfaces to restore normal load transmission and reestablish normal radiocarpal kinematics and DRUJ function.

To achieve this, both a dorsal and a volar approach are possible options. The dorsal approach has historically been used by many surgeons, specifically for the most common type of deformity, dorsally tilted malunions. It uses the interval between the third and fourth extensor compartment to gain access to the deformed bone. An opening wedge osteotomy can easily be made with restoration of volar tilt and radial inclination. Bone graft can be inserted, followed by internal fixation. To maintain reduction, rigid fixation with plates and screws is preferred over K-wire fixation, as some bone resorption and collapse may occur due to revascularization. When indicated, the dorsal wrist capsule can be incised and direct visualization of the articular surface of the wrist joint is possible. One of the major drawbacks of this approach is the risk of extensor tendon-related complications.[31,32]

Newer plating systems that are more anatomical and low profile have tried to address this risk of hardware-induced tendon problems. Tiren et al reported zero hardware removals in their series on 11 patients treated with a dorsal opening wedge osteotomy. Schurko et al however found a 38% removal rate of dorsal plates due to tendon irritation.[32,33] With the introduction of fixed-angle and anatomical volar-locking plates, the volar approach has become increasingly popular and is now the preferred approach for most extra-articular corrections. This approach has the advantage of a better soft tissue envelope and less tendon irritation. Schurko et al compared 37 volar and 16 dorsal corrective osteotomies. Improvement of the QuickDASH scores and range of motion was found in both groups, but a volar approach and plating resulted in better QuickDASH scores and range of motion with fewer complications compared with dorsal plating.[32]

Our preferred technique is an opening wedge osteotomy through a classic volar Henry approach. A distal release of the brachioradialis tendon is performed to facilitate later reduction and insertion of bone graft. The pronator quadratus muscle is incised near its most radial and distal insertion and the volar cortex of the radius is exposed. A fixed-angle locking plate is provisionally fixed on the distal malunited segment with K-wires. The position and orientation of the plate takes the desired correction of volar tilt and radial inclination into account. The angle between the plate and the radial shaft is checked on lateral and AP fluoroscopy images, to confirm it corresponds with the preplanned correction (▶ Fig. 12.5). Many systems now have tools to facilitate positioning of the plate in the appropriate preplanned position. When correct positioning is confirmed, at least two distal screws are drilled, and their length is measured. The plate is then temporarily removed, or rotated out of position, so that an osteotomy can be made. The osteotomy is typically made at the level of the previous fracture, and parallel to the joint line in the sagittal plane. A lamina spreader is used to open the osteotomy site, and soft tissues are further released as needed to avoid undue stress on the bone fragments. The plate is then refixed on the distal fragment as planned and further fixation on the shaft should provide the planned correction. The goal is to correct anatomy as precisely as possible and besides correction of malangulation in all directions, restoration of malrotation and ulnar variance needs to be taken into account. Derotation and additional lengthening of the radius is often indicated. Following correction and fixation, cancellous chips of allograft or autologous iliac crest bone graft are brought into the osteotomy site. As the brachioradialis tendon is released off the radius, the grafts can easily be inserted through the same approach.

The use of the dorsal approach in our practice is now reserved for the correction of intra-articular malunions or to cases where a previous osteosynthesis has been performed by means of dorsal plating.[34] The major advantage of the dorsal approach is that the joint capsule can be opened for inspection of joint congruency following correction of an intra-articular deformity.

3D Technology

In 3D-guided cases, the complete procedure is preplanned using 3D computer software and patient-specific instruments are designed. Anatomical models of the malunited and corrected radius as well as patient-specific drilling and cutting guides are 3D printed and sterilized. The surgical approach is similar and the patient-specific drilling guide fits precisely onto the deformed volar surface of the distal radius and is secured with K-wires. It is evident that exact positioning of the guide is essential to obtain the planned correction, and fluoroscopy as well as the printed bone model can be used to facilitate and confirm this. Using the drilling guide, all the trajectories for later screw insertion are predrilled into the bone of the distal radius. Next, the drill guide is removed and replaced by the cutting guide, over the retained parallel K-wires. An oscillating bone saw is used to perform the osteotomy at the correct site and along the preplanned plane. When correcting an intra-articular deformity, the fragments are separated by making multiple drill holes along the previous fracture plane (▶ Fig. 12.6). A standard plate or, when indicated, a 3D printed custom-made plate is fixed with locking screws, first distally, then proximally.

Arthroscopy

Arthroscopy is a very valuable tool to assist with corrective surgery for the correction of intra-articular malunions. It allows for better visualization of intra-articular deformity, compared to standard techniques and fluoroscopy. Osteotomies can be performed "inside-out" to precisely separate and mobilize intra-articular malunited fragments. Following reduction and fixation, articular congruency can be confirmed. Del Pinal et al found good midterm (12 to 48 mo) clinical and radiological results in 11 patients with their technique of dry arthroscopic guidance.[35]

12.2.3 How to Deal with the Gap?

The correction of a malunited fracture will almost invariably lead to the formation of a gap and the way to deal with this problem is a point of debate. For smaller defects, especially when some cortical contact has been maintained and rigid fixation is obtained, studies have shown that the gap does not need to be filled to obtain bony healing. Disseldorp et al reported on a series of 132 corrective osteotomies without bone grafting with a minimum follow-up of 12 months. All osteotomies healed, and in only two cases, healing took more than 4 months. They stated that, when cortical contact at one side of the osteotomy is maintained, leaving the gap open without the insertion of bone graft is a reliable technique.[36] This finding was confirmed in a paper by Ozer et al when

3

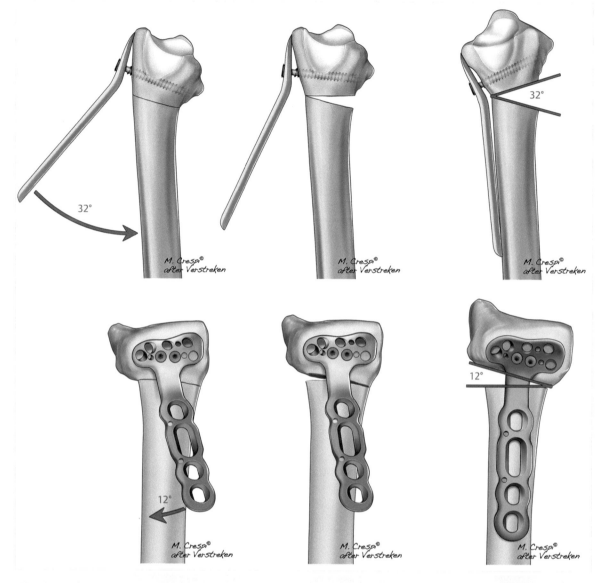

Fig. 12.5 Locking screw technology allows prefixaton of the plate on the distal radius in the appropriate angle to obtain the preplanned correction.

comparing the outcome of two groups of patients following corrective osteotomies with remaining volar cortical contact. The first group (n = 14) underwent a corrective osteotomy without any bone graft, and in the second group (n = 14), allograft bone chips were inserted at the osteotomy site. The osteotomies in both groups healed uneventfully, without loss of surgical correction. There were no significant differences in time to union and final outcome between the two groups.[37]

The need for cortical contact to use this technique is important, as has been confirmed in a study by Scheer et al. The study, initially planned to include 25 cases of corrective osteotomy without bone grafting, was discontinued when three nonunions occurred in six patients

following osteotomy and the formation of a trapezoid void without bone contact.[38]

The advent of locking plates has eliminated the need for structural cortical bone graft to fill and support the defect. Even for larger defects, cancellous bone grafts are positioned in the defect with a similar outcome compared to structural bone graft when rigid angular stable fixation is used. Ring et al compared two groups of ten patients, one group received a corticocancellous bone graft and the other group received a nonstructural autologous cancellous graft, both from the iliac crest. All osteotomies healed within 4 months without the loss of surgical correction. Radiographic and functional results were comparable between both groups.[39]

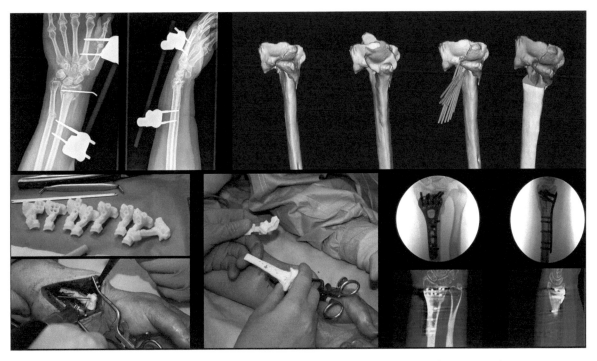

Fig. 12.6 Correction of a complex intra-articular deformity, with use of 3D preperative planning and patient specific instrumentation.

Bone substitutes have been proposed as a less invasive alternative for bone graft. Their use eliminates potential donor site morbidity and reduces surgical time compared to the use of autografts. Scheer et al performed a series of seventeen osteotomies with the use of tricalcium phosphate bone substitute. Clinically, they found a significant improvement in forearm rotation and DASH scores. Radiographic outcomes, however, showed a mean loss of radial height of 1.1 mm (SD 1.0 mm), with unknown impact on clinical outcomes. In 10 out of 14 patients, there were radiolucent zones around the bone substitute after 6 to 8 weeks. They concluded that instead of supporting the osteotomy, tricalcium phosphate bone substitutes can delay osteotomy healing and their use is not ideal for corrective osteotomy of the distal radius.[40] Luchetti studied the use of carbonated hydroxyapatite in a small series of six patients undergoing a distal radius corrective osteotomy, fixed with K-wires. Postoperative range of motion and grip strength improved significantly. Radiographs showed complete osseointegration of the carbonated hydroxyapatite. Radiographic parameters were restored but at 6 months and final follow-up, the volar tilt showed a minimal loss from its original correction.[41]

12.2.4 Ulna Shortening Osteotomy

Ulna shortening osteotomy (USO) can be the preferred treatment option for a selected group of distal radius malunions, when shortening of the radius is present without marked angular deformity (▶ Fig. 12.7). It is a straightfor-

ward procedure with a low complication rate and high clinical success rate when done technically well. Srinivasan et al reported a successful outcome of USO in patients with up to 20 degrees of dorsal angulation and radial inclination as low as 2 degrees.[42] Ulna shortening can also be combined with corrective surgery of the radius to avoid the possible complications of extensive lengthening of the radius, such as soft tissue contractures, delayed healing, loss of correction, and complex regional pain syndrome (▶ Fig. 12.8). Angular deformity is corrected at the distal radius with a closing or opening wedge osteotomy, combined with a USO to restore ulnar variance.[43] The plate can be positioned on the dorsal, medial, or palmar surface of the ulna. Each has its advantages and disadvantages and there is no consensus in the literature to guide on the optimal position.[44] The authors prefer a direct ulnar approach with the elbow positioned in a flexed position. This allows easy and unrestricted access to the medial surface of the ulna where the plate is positioned. A 8-cm incision is made just palmar and parallel to the subcutaneous ridge (margo posterior) of the ulna, starting 4 cm proximal to the ulnar styloid. The fascia of the flexor carpi ulnaris and flexor digitorum profundus muscle is incised just palmar to its insertion on the ulna. The medial surface is exposed by dissecting the muscle of the bone, without damaging the periosteum. Only at the site of the osteotomy, an incision in the dorsal extensor carpi ulnaris fascia is made and the ulna is exposed circumferentially. Several commercial systems are available that facilitate precise preplanned shortening of the ulna

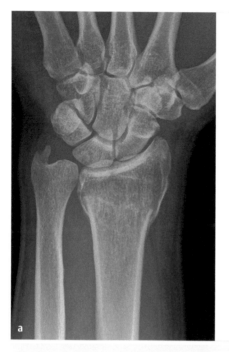
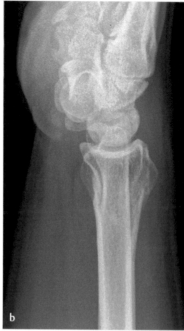
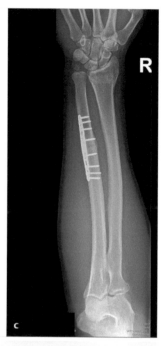

Fig. 12.7 Ulna shortening osteotomy as a treatment for a distal radius malunion with acceptable alignment.

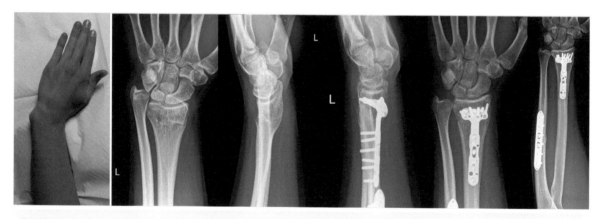

Fig. 12.8 Corrrection of deformity of the distal radius combined with ulna shortening osteotomy to avoid the risks of extensive distraction and gap formation.

and rigid plate fixation. This incorporates a guide to pre-drill the fixation holes, guide the shortening osteotomy, and allow compression of the bony fragments and stable fixation with a low-profile plate. The authors prefer a transverse osteotomy over an oblique osteotomy as it is easier to make; it allows precise preplanned shortening without the risk of bony fragments sliding over each other, and similar healing rates have been reported when compared to oblique osteotomies in a recent meta-analysis.[45] Ice cold saline (4 °C) is used to rinse and cool the bone when making the osteotomy. The bone fragments are then compressed and the appropriate plate is applied and fixed using the predrilled holes. Fluoroscopy is used to check the position of the bony fragments, the plate

position and screw length, and the ulnar variance at the wrist joint. The fascia can easily be closed over the plate, followed by skin closure. A compressive dressing is applied, and patients are encouraged to mobilize immediately as pain and swelling allows. Radiographic signs of healing with bony trabeculae bridging the osteotomy site are typically seen at around 10 weeks postoperatively.

12.2.5 Outcome

Extra-Articular Deformities

Diego Fernandez pioneered corrective surgery for malunion of the radius as we know it today. Already in 1982, he published on a series of 20 young patients treated with an opening wedge corrective osteotomy, bone graft insertion, stable plate fixation, and early motion. Results were satisfactory when preoperative range of motion was adequate and no degenerative changes were present. Since then, several studies have been published on the outcome following corrective osteotomy for distal radius malunion. Huang et al published on their results in 10 patients treated with a volar plate and bone graft. They found significant improvement in QuickDASH and Mayo Wrist scores. All 10 osteotomies healed within 3 months of surgery and radiographic parameters were restored.[46] Prommersberger et al reported on a series of 29 patients in 2004 who underwent an osteotomy for extra-articular deformity. They found significant improvement in range of motion, pain scores, grip strength, and radiographic parameters after correction through a volar approach.[47] De Smet et al studied the restoration of carpal malalignment in a series of 31 osteotomies. The patients were divided into two groups: one group with midcarpal malalignment and the other with radiocarpal malalignment. They found that corrective osteotomy for the distal radius malunion restored the alignment in both groups with low complication rates.[48] Andreasson et al published on a series of 37 patients who underwent corrective osteotomy through a combined volar and dorsal approach. They found significant improvement in radiographic parameters and functional outcomes as grip strength and range of motion.[49]

Pillukat et al performed a prospective study on 17 patients who underwent an opening wedge osteotomy for extra-articular malunion of the distal radius. Sixteen out of the 17 procedures were performed through a volar approach and iliac crest bone grafts were used. They compared short-term to long-term clinical and radiological results and found no deterioration in the long term. Grip strength was even found to improve significantly over time. All osteotomies showed bony union.[50] It is important, however, to note that not all long-term outcome reports are excellent and that further improvements in treatment technique may be indicated. Krukhaug et al reported that 24% of patients in their study of 33 patients reported a poor functional outcome at a mean follow-up of 7 years after corrective osteotomy.[51] In their series of 22 patients, Lozano-Calderon et al performed a long-term outcome analysis of clinical and radiographical results with a mean follow-up of 13 years. Although wrist alignment was maintained over time, 13 out of 22 patients developed mild-to-moderate symptomatic wrist arthritis, indicating that clinical result may deteriorate over time.[52] Gradl et al performed a long-term follow-up study (mean follow-up of 7 years) in 18 patients. Ten out of 18 patients had a good clinical outcome, 2 patients had a fair outcome but 6 patients had a poor clinical result according to the scale of Fernandez.[53]

Intra-Articular Deformities

While surgical correction for extra-articular malunion is widespread and thoroughly studied, there are not many reports on interventions focused on intra-articular malunions of the distal radius. In 2005, Ring et al published on their results of surgery in 23 patients with intra-articular malunions. They found that the results of surgery for these deformities are comparable to those for extra-articular malunion and concluded that it is a useful procedure to improve wrist function in symptomatic, healthy, and active patients.[14]

Del Pinal et al performed arthroscopically guided osteotomies in 11 patients with fair to good functional results and good correction of intra-articular step-offs.[35] Buijze et al evaluated 18 patients after corrective osteotomy for a combined intra- and extra-articular malunion of the distal radius. All patients healed without problem and final range of motion and grip strength improved significantly. They reported 72% good to excellent functional scores.[54]

3D-Guided Osteotomies

Michielsen et al reported on a series of 30 patients with extra-articular or combined intra- and extra-articular deformities, performed at our institution in 2018. The patients were prospectively reviewed and were found to have an overall improvement of function, grip strength, and pain, with a significant improvement in the DASH score. Radiographical evaluation of final correction showed that restoration of preset radiographic parameters was achieved in 73% of cases. This compares favorably with the reported outcome following conventional planning.[19,36] Schweizer et al performed a corrective osteotomy on six patients with a symptomatic intra-articular malunion of the distal radius using 3D-printed patient-specific guides. At 8 weeks, all osteotomies showed radiographic signs of consolidation and there were no signs of intra-articular step-offs. All patients showed a clear improvement in wrist function and four out of six patients reported no pain at 1 year follow-up.[55] Buijze et al compared a 3D-planned technique with conventional 2D planning in a randomized controlled trial of 40 patients. They found a trend toward better patient-reported outcome scores for 3D technique, but these differences did not reach statistical significance, because of (post hoc) insufficient power of the study. Radiographic analysis, however, showed significant differences in the mean residual volar angulation and radial inclination in favor of the 3D group.[56]

12.2.6 Complications

Possible complications following a corrective osteotomy of the distal radius are numerous and comparable to

133

those seen following operative treatment of acute fractures. As these procedures are often more complex, the reported complication rate is higher. Haghverdian et al reported complications in 25 of 60 patients (42%) who underwent an extra-articular osteotomy over a period of 8 years. There were seven cases of nonunion, all of which occurred in the distraction-type osteotomy (no cortical contact at osteotomy site with intervening bone graft). Three patients had a delayed extensor pollicis longus (EPL) rupture, treated with an extensor indicis proprius (EIP) to EPL transfer. Other minor complications comprised flexor and extensor tendon irritation necessitating hardware removal in three patients.[57]

Rivlin et al reported on six patients with EPL rupture after osteotomy and volar plate fixation for malunited distal radius fractures. The average time to tendon rupture was 10 weeks after surgery. Etiological factors were, besides screw prominence, dorsal callus, prominent osteotomy edges, and osteophytes.[58]

Mulders et al found 18 complications in their series of 48 corrective osteotomies. Five patients suffered from implant failure (screw or plate breakage). Four patients had a tendon rupture: the extensor pollicis longus (EPL) in three patients treated with an EIP transfer and the extensor digitorum communis (EDC) of the third digit in one patient. Superficial wound infection was found in three patients and subsequently treated with antibiotics.[59]

Another complication after osteotomy for distal radius malunion is incomplete correction. Von Campe et al have shown that, with conventional planning, only 40% of patients obtained the planned radiographic correction. The clinical impact of this finding is currently unclear as it was merely the failure to restore correct ulnar variance that caused persistent pain and stiffness.[19] Studies have shown that with advanced 3D planning and the use of patient-specific guides, a better radiographic outcome can be obtained.

12.2.7 Rehabilitation

The rehabilitation program needs to be adapted for each specific case and close communication between surgeon and therapist is needed in each phase of the healing process. Important factors to be taken into account when deciding on the rehabilitation protocol include postoperative inflammatory response, pain, soft tissue state, type of correction, bone quality, and fixation strength. Immediately postoperative, pain and swelling need to be addressed with cooling, splinting, elevation, and anti-inflammatory medication. In most cases a splint is provided for the first 2 weeks, followed by a removable cast or brace for another 4 weeks. Patients should be encouraged to start shoulder, elbow, and finger mobilization the day after surgery. Active and passive range of motion exercises of the wrist, flexion/extension, and pronation/supination can be started within pain limits after 2 weeks

when rigid fixation of the osteotomy is obtained. Throughout the rehabilitation process, hand therapists should closely monitor excessive inflammatory reactions and adjust the training program accordingly. Compensation strategies of the upper limb such as exaggerated internal rotation of the shoulder instead of pronation should be corrected. Early signs of a possible CRPS reaction need to be addressed with additional pain medication and an adapted physiotherapy program. Provoking factors for CRPS, such as hardware problems, nerve compression, or other causes of pain, need to be looked for and addressed appropriately. When pain, soft tissue state, and bone-healing tendency allow it, progressive loading exercises can be started after 6 weeks. Further follow-up is arranged every 4 weeks until complete bony union and maximal return of function is obtained.

12.2.8 Tips and Tricks

- The indication for corrective surgery is primarily based on clinical symptoms, where pain and loss of forearm rotation are the most important complaints.
- Ulnar-sided wrist pain is the most common complaint following a distal radius malunion. This needs to be addressed by correction of ulnar variance and restoration of DRUJ congruency.
- Associated bony or ligamentous injuries to the carpus and distal radioulnar joint can present and need to be addressed when symptomatic.
- A degree of malrotation is often part of distal radius malunion and directly affects forearm rotation. Correction of this aspect of the malunion will improve clinical outcome.
- For the correction of complex multidirectional and/or intra-articular deformities, the use of 3D technology can be an essential tool.
- Release of soft tissues, specifically the contracted brachioradialis insertion, will facilitate the correction of deformity.
- When large correction is needed, combining a corrective osteotomy of the radius with a shortening osteotomy of the ulna is an option. It avoids the creation of a large gap and extensile distraction of soft tissues.
- Osteotomies can take longer to heal than acute fractures, so to avoid hardware failure, the use of strong plate and additional fixation is indicated.

12.2.9 Take-Home Message

Malunion remains the most common serious complication of distal radius fractures and surgical correction is indicated when it causes pain or functional problems. The goal of corrective surgery is to restore anatomy as precisely as possible, which is your best option to restore normal pain-free function. Therefore, precise preoperative planning, often based on imaging of the contralateral side, is essential. New techniques based on 3D technology allow better evaluation of deformity and planning of correction when indicated. The use of patient-specific surgical guides will facilitate surgical correction, especially for multidirectional and intra-articular deformity correction. Despite the advances in planning and fixation techniques, the reported complication rate remains high. Most commonly reported complications are nonunion, malunion, hardware failure, and tendon rupture. Many of these complications can be avoided by precise surgical technique, attention to detail at each step of the procedure, and the use of new technology when indicated.

References

[1] Kihara H, Palmer AK, Werner FW, Short WH, Fortino MD. The effect of dorsally angulated distal radius fractures on distal radioulnar joint congruency and forearm rotation. J Hand Surg Am. 1996; 21(1):40–47

[2] Crisco JJ, Moore DC, Marai GE, Laidlaw DH, Akelman E, Weiss AP, et al. Effects of distal radius malunion on distal radioulnar joint mechanics: an in vivo study. J Orthop Res. 2007; 25(4):547–555

[3] Moore DC, Hogan KA, Crisco JJ, III, Akelman E, Dasilva MF, Weiss APC. Three-dimensional in vivo kinematics of the distal radioulnar joint in malunited distal radius fractures. J Hand Surg Am. 2002; 27(2):233–242

[4] Cooney WP, III, Dobyns JH, Linscheid RL. Complications of Colles' fractures. J Bone Joint Surg Am. 1980; 62(4):613–619

[5] Mann FA, Wilson AJ, Gilula LA. Radiographic evaluation of the wrist: what does the hand surgeon want to know? Radiology. 1992; 184(1):15–24

[6] Pennock AT, Phillips CS, Matzon JL, Daley E. The effects of forearm rotation on three wrist measurements: radial inclination, radial height and palmar tilt. Hand Surg. 2005; 10(1):17–22

[7] Kreder HJ, Hanel DP, McKee M, Jupiter J, McGillivary G, Swiontkowski MF. X-ray film measurements for healed distal radius fractures. J Hand Surg Am. 1996; 21(1):31–39

[8] Croitoru H, Ellis RE, Prihar R, Small CF, Pichora DR. Fixation-based surgery: a new technique for distal radius osteotomy. Comput Aided Surg. 2001; 6(3):160–169

[9] Cirpar M, Gudemez E, Cetik O, Turker M, Eksioglu F. Rotational deformity affects radiographic measurements in distal radius malunion. Eur J Orthop Surg Traumatol. 2011; 21(1):13–20

[10] Vroemen JC, Dobbe JGG, Strackee SD, Streekstra GJ. Positioning evaluation of corrective osteotomy for the malunited radius: 3-D CT versus 2-D radiographs. Orthopedics. 2013; 36(2):e193–e199

[11] Miyake J, Murase T, Yamanaka Y, Moritomo H, Sugamoto K, Yoshikawa H. Comparison of three dimensional and radiographic measurements in the analysis of distal radius malunion. J Hand Surg Eur Vol. 2013; 38(2):133–143

[12] Cheng HS, Hung LK, Ho PC, Wong J. An analysis of causes and treatment outcome of chronic wrist pain after distal radial fractures. Hand Surg. 2008; 13(1):1–10

[13] Haase SC, Chung KC. Management of malunions of the distal radius. Hand Clin. 2012; 28(2):207–216

[14] Ring D, Prommersberger KJ, González del Pino J, Capomassi M, Slullitel M, Jupiter JB. Corrective osteotomy for intra-articular malunion of the distal part of the radius. J Bone Joint Surg Am. 2005; 87(7):1503–1509

[15] Vroemen JC, Dobbe JGG, Jonges R, Strackee SD, Streekstra GJ. Three-dimensional assessment of bilateral symmetry of the radius and ulna for planning corrective surgeries. J Hand Surg Am. 2012; 37(5):982–988

[16] Dobbe JG, Vroemen JC, Strackee SD, Streekstra GJ. Corrective distal radius osteotomy: including bilateral differences in 3-D planning. Med Biol Eng Comput. 2013; 51(7):791–797

[17] Bentohami A, Bosma J, Akkersdijk GJM, van Dijkman B, Goslings JC, Schep NWL. Incidence and characteristics of distal radial fractures in an urban population in The Netherlands. Eur J Trauma Emerg Surg. 2014; 40(3):357–361

[18] Walenkamp MMJ, Vos LM, Strackee SD, Goslings JC, Schep NWL. The unstable distal radius fracture: how do we define it? A systematic review. J Wrist Surg. 2015; 4(4):307–316

[19] von Campe A, Nagy L, Arbab D, Dumont CE. Corrective osteotomies in malunions of the distal radius: do we get what we planned? Clin Orthop Relat Res. 2006; 450(450):179–185

[20] Lozano-Calderón SA, Brouwer KM, Doornberg JN, Goslings JC, Kloen P, Jupiter JB. Long-term outcomes of corrective osteotomy for the treatment of distal radius malunion. J Hand Surg Eur Vol. 2010; 35(5):370–380

[21] Kataoka T, Oka K, Miyake J, Omori S, Tanaka H, Murase T. 3-Dimensional prebent plate fixation in corrective osteotomy of malunited upper extremity fractures using a real-sized plastic bone model prepared by preoperative computer simulation. J Hand Surg Am. 2013; 38(5):909–919

[22] Vroemen JC, Dobbe JGG, Sierevelt IN, Strackee SD, Streekstra GJ. Accuracy of distal radius positioning using an anatomical plate. Orthopedics. 2013; 36(4):e457–e462

[23] Stockmans F, Dezillie M, Vanhaecke J. Accuracy of 3D virtual planning of corrective osteotomies of the distal radius. J Wrist Surg. 2013; 2(4):306–314

[24] Byrne AM, Impelmans B, Bertrand V, Van Haver A, Verstreken F. Corrective osteotomy for malunited diaphyseal forearm fractures using preoperative 3-dimensional planning and patient-specific surgical guides and implants. J Hand Surg Am. 2017; 42(10):836.e1–836.e12

[25] Vlachopoulos L, Schweizer A, Graf M, Nagy L, Fürnstahl P. Three-dimensional postoperative accuracy of extra-articular forearm osteotomies using CT-scan based patient-specific surgical guides. BMC Musculoskelet Disord. 2015; 16:336

[26] Mauler F, Langguth C, Schweizer A, et al. Prediction of normal bone anatomy for the planning of corrective osteotomies of malunited forearm bones using a three-dimensional statistical shape model. J Orthop Res. 2017; 35(12):2630–2636

[27] Murase T, Oka K, Moritomo H, Goto A, Yoshikawa H, Sugamoto K. Three-dimensional corrective osteotomy of malunited fractures of the upper extremity with use of a computer simulation system. J Bone Joint Surg Am. 2008; 90(11):2375–2389

[28] Young BT, Rayan GM. Outcome following nonoperative treatment of displaced distal radius fractures in low-demand patients older than 60 years. J Hand Surg Am. 2000; 25(1):19–28

[29] Evans BT, Jupiter JB. Best approaches in distal radius fracture malunions. Curr Rev Musculoskelet Med. 2019; 12(2):198–203

[30] Jupiter JB, Ring D. A comparison of early and late reconstruction of malunited fractures of the distal end of the radius. J Bone Joint Surg Am. 1996; 78(5):739–748

[31] Prommersberger KJ, Pillukat T, Mühldorfer M, van Schoonhoven J. Malunion of the distal radius. Arch Orthop Trauma Surg. 2012; 132(5):693–702

[32] Schurko BM, Lechtig A, Chen NC, et al. Outcomes and complications following volar and dorsal osteotomy for symptomatic distal radius malunions: a comparative study. J Hand Surg Am. 2020; 45(2):158.e1–158.e8– [Internet]

[33] Tiren D, Vos DI. Correction osteotomy of distal radius malunion stabilised with dorsal locking plates without grafting. Strateg Trauma Limb Reconstr. 2014; 9(1):53–58

[34] Michielsen M, Van Haver A, Bertrand V, Vanhees M, Verstreken F. Corrective osteotomy of distal radius malunions using three-dimensional computer simulation and patient-specific guides to achieve anatomic reduction. Eur J Orthop Surg Traumatol. 2018; 28(8):1531–1535 [Internet]

[35] del Piñal F, Cagigal L, García-Bernal FJ, Studer A, Regalado J, Thams C. Arthroscopically guided osteotomy for management of intra-articular distal radius malunions. J Hand Surg Am. 2010; 35(3):392–397– [Internet]

3

3

[36] Disseldorp DJ, Poeze M, Hannemann PF, Brink PR. Is bone grafting necessary in the treatment of malunited distal radius fractures? J Wrist Surg. 2015; 4(3):207–213

[37] Ozer K, Kiliç A, Sabel A, Ipaktchi K. The role of bone allografts in the treatment of angular malunions of the distal radius. J Hand Surg Am. 2011; 36(11):1804–1809 [Internet]

[38] Scheer JH, Adolfsson LE. Non-union in 3 of 15 osteotomies of the distal radius without bone graft. Acta Orthop. 2015; 86(3):316–320

[39] Ring D, Roberge C, Morgan T, Jupiter JB. Osteotomy for malunited fractures of the distal radius: a comparison of structural and non-structural autogenous bone grafts. J Hand Surg Am. 2002; 27(2):216–222

[40] Scheer JH, Adolfsson LE. Tricalcium phosphate bone substitute in corrective osteotomy of the distal radius. Injury. 2009; 40(3):262–267

[41] Luchetti R. Corrective osteotomy of malunited distal radius fractures using carbonated hydroxyapatite as an alternative to autogenous bone grafting. J Hand Surg Am. 2004; 29(5):825–834

[42] Srinivasan RC, Jain D, Richard MJ, Leversedge FJ, Mithani SK, Ruch DS. Isolated ulnar shortening osteotomy for the treatment of extra-articular distal radius malunion. J Hand Surg Am. 2013; 38(6):1106–1110– [Internet]

[43] Wada T, Isogai S, Kanaya K, Tsukahara T, Yamashita T. Simultaneous radial closing wedge and ulnar shortening osteotomies for distal radius malunion. J Hand Surg Am. 2004; 29(2):264–272

[44] Das De S, Johnsen PH, Wolfe SW. Soft tissue complications of dorsal versus volar plating for ulnar shortening osteotomy. J Hand Surg Am. 2015; 40(5):928–933– [Internet]

[45] Owens J, Compton J, Day M, Glass N, Lawler E. Nonunion rates among ulnar-shortening osteotomy for ulnar impaction syndrome: a systematic review. J Hand Surg Am. 2019; 44(7):612.e1–612.e12– [Internet]

[46] Huang HK, Hsu SH, Hsieh FC, Chang KH, Chu HL, Wang JP. Extra-articular corrective osteotomy with bone grafting to achieve lengthening and regain alignment for distal radius fracture malunion. Tech Hand Up Extrem Surg. 2019; 23(4):186–190

[47] Prommersberger KJ, Lanz UB. Corrective osteotomy of the distal radius through volar approach. Tech Hand Up Extrem Surg. 2004; 8(2):70–77

[48] De Smet L, Verhaegen F, Degreef I. Carpal malalignment in malunion of the distal radius and the effect of corrective osteotomy. J Wrist Surg. 2014; 3(3):166–170

[49] Andreasson I, Kjellby-Wendt G, Fagevik-Olsén M, Aurell Y, Ullman M, Karlsson J. Long-term outcomes of corrective osteotomy for malunited fractures of the distal radius. J Plast Surg Hand Surg. 2020; 54(2):94–100 [Internet]

[50] Pillukat T, Gradl G, Mühldorfer-Fodor M, Prommersberger KJ. Die fehlverheilte distale Radiusfraktur - Langzeit-ergebnisse nach extraartikulärer Korrekturosteotomie. [Malunion of the distal radius: long-term results after extraarticular corrective osteotomy]. Handchir Mikrochir Plast Chir. 2014; 46(1):18–25

[51] Krukhaug Y, Hove LM. Corrective osteotomy for malunited extra-articular fractures of the distal radius: a follow-up study of 33 patients. Scand J Plast Reconstr Surg Hand Surg. 2007; 41(6):303–309

[52] Lozano-Calderon SA, Brouwer KM, Doornberg JN, Goslings JC, Kloen P, Jupiter JB. Long-term outcomes of corrective osteotomy for the treatment of distal radius malunion. J Hand Surg Am. 2010; 35E(5):370–380

[53] Gradl G, Jupiter J, Pillukat T, Knobe M, Prommersberger KJ. Corrective osteotomy of the distal radius following failed internal fixation. Arch Orthop Trauma Surg. 2013; 133(8):1173–1179

[54] Buijze GA, Prommersberger KJ, González Del Pino J, Fernandez DL, Jupiter JB. Corrective osteotomy for combined intra- and extra-articular distal radius malunion. J Hand Surg Am. 2012; 37(10):2041–2049– [Internet]

[55] Schweizer A, Fürnstahl P, Nagy L. Three-dimensional correction of distal radius intra-articular malunions using patient-specific drill guides. J Hand Surg Am. 2013; 38(12):2339–2347– [Internet]

[56] Buijze GA, Leong NL, Stockmans F, et al. Three-dimensional compared with two-dimensional preoperative planning of corrective osteotomy for extra-articular distal radial malunion: A multicenter randomized controlled trial. J Bone Joint Surg Am. 2018; 100(14):1191–1202

[57] Haghverdian JC, Hsu JY, Harness NG. Complications of corrective osteotomies for extra-articular distal radius malunion. J Hand Surg Am. 2019; 44(11):987.e1–987.e9– [Internet]

[58] Rivlin M, Fernández DL, Nagy L, Graña GL, Jupiter J. Extensor pollicis longus ruptures following distal radius osteotomy through a volar approach. J Hand Surg Am. 2016; 41(3):395–398– [Internet]

[59] Mulders MAM, d'Ailly PN, Cleffken BI, Schep NWL. Corrective osteotomy is an effective method of treating distal radius malunions with good long-term functional results. Injury. 2017; 48(3):731–737– [Internet]

Section 4

Bone Surgery: Arthritis

4

13 Treatment of Complications after Surgery for Finger Joint Arthritis

Daniel B. Herren

Abstract

Joint arthroplasty and joint fusion are the most popular surgical treatment options for destroyed, painful, and nonfunctional finger joints. The complication rate of these procedures is significant and the challenges are diverse. A thorough analysis should identify the cause of the problem and an individual treatment plan needs to be established. General complications like infection and wound-healing problems need to be treated according to the usual treatment guidelines in hand surgery. More specific, procedure-related complications should be addressed at the source of the dysfunction. According to the author's experience and the studies published, a good reason for revision of finger joint arthroplasty is residual pain, while stiffness and especially joint instability are more unpredictable in their postoperative results. Implant change, in given situations, to another type of implant, with or without soft tissue corrections, is demanding. An overview of the different treatment options will be given in this chapter.

In small joint fusion, the most common complications are nonunion and malunion. Nonunion might occur due to biological reasons, mainly difficult bone conditions or be a result of technical problems with the bone fixation. Revision includes hardware removal and re-arthrodesis with a bone graft. Malunion can give functional problems especially in the coordination with the other fingers of the hand. Corrective osteotomy is to be considered in disabling situations.

Keywords: complications, revision, arthroplasty, arthrodesis, finger joints

13.1 Introduction

Surgical treatment options for destroyed finger joints include joint replacement and joint arthrodesis. The ideal goal for reconstruction of end-stage joint arthritis is, if possible, a pain-free restoration of sufficient mobility and stability, providing adequate functionality. The metacarpal phalangeal (MCP) joint is one of the main targets in rheumatoid arthritis but rarely affected in degenerative osteoarthritis. The distal interphalangeal (DIP) joint and the proximal interphalangeal (PIP) joint are, together with the thumb saddle joint, the main affected joints in degenerative disease of the hand. The two joints have different functional tasks. While the DIP is responsible for grasping smaller objects and coordinates fine-tuning of finger function, the PIP joint is the main mobile motor for the finger. It has been shown that the PIP joint mobility has an important functional value within the scope of the entire hand depending on the position.[1] On the ulnar rays, in particular, mobility has a great functional importance since it is only possible to grasp small objects while maintaining mobility of this joint. While on the radial side of the hand, especially in the index finger, stability is crucial for a stable pinch with the thumb and a forceful grip. However, a stiff index finger PIP joint is often a functional obstacle.[2] Therefore, arthroplasty of the PIP joint has become a predominant treatment of option for a painful PIP destruction even in the index finger. PIP joint arthrodesis in a functionally good position provides adequate function, although fine motor skills, in particular, may be affected.

On the other hand, arthrodesis is widely accepted as the standard treatment of DIP joint problems. Reliable pain relief is a well-documented outcome of DIP arthrodesis and the obtained stability achieved primarily in the radial rays for pinching with the thumb is of importance. However, DIP joint arthroplasty is able to provide reasonable functional results, especially in the ulnar finger rays.[3,4]

For a systematic discussion, it is meaningful to categorize revision surgery of these two standard procedures by the cause of revision. It can be classified into general complications, soft tissue–driven complications, and implant-related complications. ▶ Table 13.1 gives an overview of the different postsurgical complications after PIP arthroplasty and PIP/DIP fusion.

From a patient's perspective, the main reasons for revision include pain, functional disability due to joint stiffness or instability, and aesthetic complaints.

13.2 Complications in PIP and DIP Arthroplasty: Review of the Literature

In 2019 Yamamoto and Chung[5] published a meta-analysis for complications following primary PIP arthroplasty with different implants. The revision rate for silicone implants was overall 6 to 11%. They also compared different approaches (volar, lateral, dorsal) and could find that the lowest number of revisions was found for the volar approach whereas the lateral and dorsal approaches showed a slight higher revision rate of 10 to 11%. In contrast, the revision rate for surface replacement with the first-generation implants was much higher with 18 to 37%. They concluded that the placement of the surface-replacing components from volar is more difficult, since

Table 13.1 Synopsis of the possible complications in the surgical treatment of finger arthritis including arthroplasty and joint fusion

	Cause	Therapeutical options	Salvage
General complications			
Wound-healing problems	Biological	Revision	
Infection	Biological	Revision debridement Antibiotics	Amputation
CRPS	Dystrophic reaction	Therapy Medication Vitamin C	Amputation
Bone nonunion	Biological	Revision with bone graft	
Bone malunion	Surgical mistake/Fixation	Revision osteotomy	
Soft tissue–driven complications			
Tendon adhesions	Biological Inadequate therapy/noncompliance Pain	Therapy Tenolysis	
Ossifications: Around tendons Joint capsule	Biological Surgical technique	Often nothing Steroid injection Removal ossification/ ±Arthro-/tenolysis	
Tendon rupture/insufficiency	Preexisting imbalances/insufficiency Tendon scarring Surgical technique	Tendon reconstruction Tendon transfer	Implant tensioning Ligament insufficiency Implant characteristics
Tendon imbalances/insufficiency: Swan neck deformity Boutonniere deformity	Tendon imbalances/insufficiency: Swan neck deformity Boutonniere deformity	Tendon rebalancing Implant characteristics	Joint fusion
Joint instability	Implant tensioning Ligament insufficiency Implant characteristics (Silicone)	Implant revision Ligament reconstruction Implant change (two-component implant)	Joint fusion
Implant-driven complications			
Joint instability/dislocation	Implant tensioning Ligament insufficiency Adequate trauma	Implant revision ± Ligament reconstruction Revision according to the damage	Joint fusion
Implant loosening	Biological Insufficient primary fixation Implant wear	Implant revision ±bone grafting Implant change (Silicone)	Joint fusion
Joint deformation	Implant malposition Lateral deviation Anteropostero subluxation	Implant revision/change Ligament insufficiency	Joint fusion
Joint stiffness	Scarring Tendon Joint capsule Inadequate therapy /noncompliance Pain Implant overstuffing	Therapy Arthro-/tenolysis Implant revision/change	Joint fusion

4

4

the anatomical orientation is different and the implant alignment is difficult to control. Implant placement in silicone implants is more forgiving and through its material elastic properties a self-alignment is observed.

In 1995 Foliart[6] published a literature review of 70 articles summarizing reasons for implant-related revision in a total of 15,556 Swanson original silicone arthroplasties for all different finger joints. Overall, the prevalence rate of complications after silicone implants was very low. Implant fractures were reported in only 2%. Systemic problems due to silicone particle wear, like synovitis or even lymphadenopathy, were rather anecdotal with a prevalence of around 0.6%.

Herren et al[7] analyzed in a retrospective study the results after silicone revision arthroplasty. In 27 cases the outcome for revision procedures of silicone implants were evaluated. The main reason for revision was pain in 35% and stiffness in 26% of the patients. It could be showed that the revision procedure was best indicated in stiff joints with or without pain. The range of motion could be increased to a functional level, which satisfied most patients. Also, the pain could be improved to a substantial amount. However, joint instability and axis deviation in silicone implants could not be corrected sufficiently.

In a series from the Mayo Clinic, the results after PIP-revision arthroplasty with silicone interposition arthroplasty and surface replacement with pyrocarbon implants and metal on polyethylene (PE) implants were analyzed.[8] From the revised silicone implants, 84% were converted into a surface replacement in order to achieve better joint stability. The 10-year survival rate after the revision procedure was overall 70%. However, 25% of all revised replacements needed an additional procedure. Also in their series, instability as a revision reason remained an unsolved problem with the worst results of all revision procedures.

Aversano and Calfee described in their publication a significant revision rate for PIP arthroplasty. Revision is associated with a significant complication rate and subsequent reinterventions.[9] An analysis of the complications of the different implants in more detail helps to understand the individual problems and subsequent revision options. While the main problems of silicone devices are implant failure and cystic bone formation with time,[10] two component implants show implant loosening and joint dislocation.

Overall, recurrence of pre-existing PIP joint deformity is high.[11,12]

In summary, the different published studies on the results of PIP revision arthroplasty showed a similar picture: Revision of failed or problematic PIP arthroplasty is challenging and often gives unsatisfactory results. It seems that a good reason for revision is residual pain, while stiffness and especially instability are unpredictable in their postoperative results.

For the DIP joint, there are much less reports about arthroplasty replacement. In the series by Sierakowski et al[3] the overall complication rate was 5%. Four out of 131 joints had a general complication and developed infection or soft tissue irritation requiring implant removal and subsequent fusion. Two joints were fused because of instability and marked ulnar deviation and one had a persistent mallet-type deformity corrected by tendon shortening. In the series by Neukom et al,[4] 21% of the DIP arthroplasties underwent reoperation. Five out of 39 joints had to be fused due to instability. Three other arthroplasties were operated again, either due to an implant breakage (revised with a new silicone implant), a granuloma, which needed excision or for a painful osteophyte.

13.3 Indication for Revision Surgery of Finger Arthroplasty

As outlined, the reasons for a revision arthroplasty in failed primary implants are different and depend not only on the cause and symptoms but also on the type of implant. Silicone implants act as a spacer only and do not replicate the joint biomechanics. As a mono-block implant, it offers a certain primary stability in the different joint axes. The secondary stability relies on the scarring around the implant during the healing process.

13.3.1 Implant Fracture or Loosening

Silicone implant fracture does not automatically imply a revision intervention. Often implant fracture remain undetected since it is not always obvious to see implant fractures on regular X-rays. However, the fibrous capsule preserves the joint function even if the implant is not intact.

Silicone implant fracture and abrasion leads to a synovial reaction.[13,14,15] Erosive osteolysis can be seen on X-ray and remarkable bone defects may occur (▶ Fig. 13.1). The severity of this inflammatory reaction depends on the particle size and is much more often seen in silicone wrist implants than in finger arthroplasties.

Since the implant stem has no firm connection to the bone, over time the silicone stems create an endomedullary reaction, which can be seen on the X-rays as a fine sclerotic line between the implant and the surrounding bone.[16] In revision cases, it appears as an endomedullar synovial layer. This reaction is provoked by the so-called pistoning effect, a movement of the implant in the bones during flexion and extension. The nonbinding character of the implant facilitates its replacement and makes it technically easy.

In *two-component implants*, often quoted as surface replacement devices, the fixation of the device follows the principles of other joint replacement surgeries. Either through a press-fit cementless fixation or a classical bone cementation with polymethyl methacrylate (PMMA) the

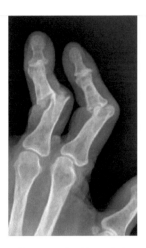

Fig. 13.1 Broken silicone proximal interphalangeal (PIP) implants. The joints are completely dislocated and unstable. There is a significant endomedullary inflammatory bone reaction to the interaction with the silicone.

implant is secured to the bone. The cementing has the advantage of immediate primary stability while the osteointegrative binding takes usually 6 to 8 weeks for definitive implant fixation. Despite the better primary fixation of the implant, the cementation has substantial disadvantages. The revision of a cemented implant reveals more difficulties. Well-fixed implant components, which need to be removed, leave a rather big defect in the endomedullary bone. Sometimes even a phalanx osteotomy needs to be applied, similar as described for the removal of well-fixed femur components in the hip, in order to take out the implant. In addition, bone cement leaves biological bone damage through its exothermic reaction. This impedes fixation for a revision implant and even secondary cementation is of lesser quality. Osteointegration, on the other hand, is provided by materials, which allow bony integration. In finger implants this is mainly titanium with or without hydroxyapatite coating. These materials have proven their capacity for a solid bone fixation in millions of dental implants. Other materials include ceramics and pyrocarbon. Both materials have shown, in different series, problems in implant fixation.[11,17,18] High rates of loosening and implant migration are reported. It is stated that neither ceramics nor pyrocarbon is able to create osteointegration.

13.3.2 Implant Malalignment

Another indication for revision is malalignment of the implant. Obviously, this is less of a problem in flexible silicone implant arthroplasty. In two-component implants, which aim to mimic the biomechanics of the joint, the positioning of the components is crucial for the function. Malalignment can happen in the different axis, but the disturbing effect on functionality depends on the plane of

malalignment. For proper joint function restoration of the joint, center of rotation should be re-established. There are biomechanical considerations about the ideal prosthetic placement but in vivo studies are lacking.

Almost always a problem is joint overstuffing or overtensioning. A tight joint replacement creates pain and difficulties especially for extension.

Implantation errors lead to maltracking of the joint motion and soft tissue can hardly compensate for it. It is important to check after implantation and tendon reposition the tenodesis movement of the finger on the OR table. Most deformities become obvious in flexion. It is difficult to correct implant maltracking during rehabilitation. The ligaments can hardly compensate the wrong movement planes.

13.3.3 Other Causes of Revision

Joint dislocation happens almost exclusively in two-component implants (▶ Fig. 13.2), but can be rarely seen in incorrect placed silicone implants as well. The cause of dislocation is either a wrong implant placement, such as insufficient primary or secondary stability and/or trauma.

Implant fractures are rare and often caused iatrogenic through incorrect implant handling, especially in more brittle materials as ceramics or pyrocarbon.

Bone fractures are mainly seen during implantation. The press-fit character of most endomedullary stems has a potential of bone blasting.

Infection as an indication for revision in general is rare. However, impending or established infection in finger arthroplasty or fusion is serious and needs attention. Superficial wound infection can often be handled conservatively with antibiotics only. Deeper and more extensive infections require revision surgery with debridement and often implant removal. In severe cases, even finger amputations have been described.[8,19]

13.4 Solutions for Failed Finger Arthroplasty

Principally, there are four different possibilities to revise a problematic finger arthroplasty (▶ Table 13.1). These include:
1. Soft tissue procedure according to the reason for revision.
   a) Tendon procedure in tendon insufficiency or imbalance.
   b) Ligament reconstruction or release.
2. Implant change and replacement with the same implant.
3. Implant removal and revision with a different implant.
4. Implant removal and conversion to a fusion.

The choice of the procedure depends mainly on the reason for revision, the local requirements, and the patient's need, and it also depends on which finger is affected. It is obvious that the soft tissue situation is crucial for the decision and additional soft tissue procedures are often required in revision arthroplasty.

In revision implant arthroplasty, the primary implant, or parts of it, is removed and replaced with a new implant. It can be the same prosthesis type in a different shape or size or with a complete new implant. The reason for revision dictates the major direction of the type of possible intervention. The local bone and soft tissue condition refines then the final choice of intervention. Together with the patient the individual solution needs to be defined. It has to be taken into consideration that

every new intervention at the PIP joint has an even bigger risk of additional scarring and thus stiffness and/or pain.

▶ Fig. 13.3 shows a decision tree for revision in PIP arthroplasty depending on the bone situation and the joint stability regardless of the primary implant.

13.4.1 Soft Tissue Revisions

Tendon Adhesions/Ossifications

Joint stiffness is multifactorial but tendon adhesions are always at least a concomitant reason for unsatisfactory joint mobility. Adhesions may occur together with ossifications, either along the tendons or around the joint capsule. Depending on the surgical approach used either a scarring of the extensor or the flexor tendons can be indicated. The collateral ligaments play an important role in the stiffness and according to the orthopaedic teaching of joint release, they need to be sequentially cut from inside-out. After each step of release, joint play needs to be controlled. Ideally the intervention is done in local anesthesia or the WALANT technique. This allows intraoperative control of the tendons and joint release. In addition, it can be visualized to the patients, how much of mobility gain could be reached intraoperatively. The results of these interventions are mixed and depend highly on the patient's motivation for postoperative mobilization.

Tendon Imbalance

The cause of tendon imbalance after PIP joint arthroplasty is often not apparent. Joint deformity as Swan neck or Boutonniere can be seen in all different approaches and often appear with a remarkable delay after the primary intervention. The joint tightness seems to play an important role. Loose joints tend to hyperextension deformity and can create a Swan neck position, while too tight joints have the tendency to create a Boutonniere deformity. In addition, soft tissue scarring or central slip insufficiency might be present.

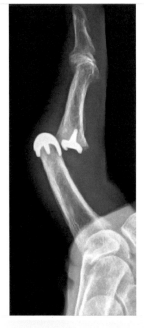

Fig. 13.2 Trauma-induced implant dislocation of surface replacement prosthesis. There are no signs of implant loosening.

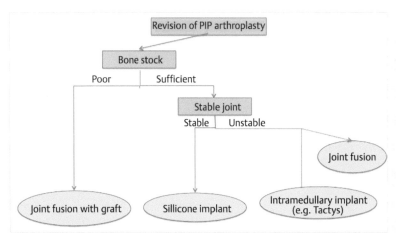

Fig. 13.3 Simplified decision tree for proximal interphalangeal (PIP) revision arthroplasty. With the assessment of the remaining bone quality and the joint stability, the different solutions might be defined, regardless of the primary implant.

It is, therefore, important before planning a revision intervention to evaluate the possible contribution of the implant itself to the tendon imbalance.

The reconstruction of the deformity follows the usual techniques described for this problem. In Swan neck deformities we prefer to perform a flexor digitorum superficials (FDS) tendon hemisling.

The correction of a Boutonniere deformity is more challenging and its indication should be discussed critically. The usual techniques of Boutonniere correction may be applied, including central slip reconstruction and lateral band reconstruction with release of the transverse retinacular ligament. An experienced therapist needs to take care of the after treatment and flexion loss should be avoided.

Collateral Ligament Insufficiency

Collateral ligamentous insufficiency without any relation to the type of implant is mainly seen in trauma cases after arthroplasty joint replacement.

In these cases, a formal collateral ligament reconstruction, almost always with a free tendon graft, can be offered. However, it is crucial to have here as well an individual tailored rehabilitation program. Other than that, the joints tend to develop stiffness. In cases of severe instability and joint dislocation, salvage to joint fusion might be reasonable drawback.

13.5 Implant-Related Revisions

13.5.1 Silicone Implants

Revision of failed Silicone implants has slightly different options, since the amount of bone resection is more extensive and in any surgical solution this has to be taken into consideration. In addition, the quality of the endomedullar bone is limited due to the interaction with the silicone stem. As described, there is a local synovial reaction to the implant material. This is an issue as well in implant replacement as for fusion procedures. Since only endomedullary fixed revision implants can be used due to the primary bone resection, it must be guaranteed that the bone is able to host a new implant accordingly. Especially uncemented revisions need a decent endomedullary bone quality. But even arthrodesis needs good bone, which is able to secure bone healing, even in presence of a bone graft.

We gain more and more experience to convert an unstable situation after a silicone arthroplasty with a two-component implant. For example, the Tactys prosthesis (Stryker USA) has an extreme modularity which allows mixing the different implant components in such a way that even bigger bone defects might be compensated. ▶ Fig. 13.4 demonstrates a conversion of an unstable broken silicone implant into a Tactys arthroplasty. Through its more constrained characteristics it has a good

potential to correct the deformity and to provide more intrinsic stability to the joint. The broad endomedullary stem allows secure primary fixation without the use of cement.

To replace a Silicone implant with another silicone implant makes only sense if the primary implant is broken and creates problems, for example, bone impingement. Then a secondary resection of the bone and a replacement of the implant with a new spacer have a good potential. In cases of instability or deformity, it is virtually impossible to improve the situation with an implant change to another silicone prosthesis, even if additional soft tissue stabilization measures are undertaken.[7]

13.5.2 Two-Component Implants

Two-component implants, if they are modular and the parts exchangeable, can be adapted to the revision needs. Especially unstable situations can be solved if one or more components can be changed in such a way that there is more stability in the joint. However, overstuffing, also in revision situations, is not advisable and leads to bad clinical results.

In situations of mainly stiffness, either a soft tissue procedure alone or a joint fusion is often advisable. If the joint motion needs to be preserved, the change to a

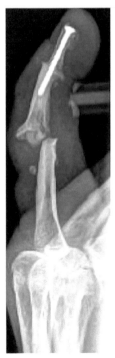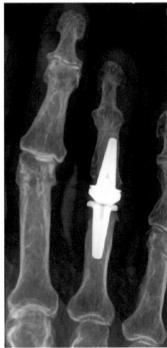

Fig. 13.4 Fracture and instability of a silicone proximal interphalangeal (PIP) arthroplasty and distal interphalangeal (DIP) fusion. Revision with a two-component implant after DIP screw removal.

silicone spacer may be a good solution, together with a meticulous soft tissue release and balancing. The silicone implant has the advantage to be flexible and create less tension in a joint just by its material properties.

13.6 Joint Fusion for Failed Implant Arthroplasty

Joint fusion is often a reliable solution to revise a difficult residual situation after primary arthroplasty implantation.[9] If the joint to be reoperated on is already stiff, the decision to go for this intervention has a low threshold. In cases of severe instability with some functional mobility, the decision to convert the situation into a fusion is more difficult and needs to be evaluated with the patient.

The two main challenges in joint fusion after arthroplasty are bone healing and positioning of the arthrodesis. As already outlined, any type of implant arthroplasty leaves a significant bone defect and alters the local biological situation and thus the healing potential. The worst situation is after a cemented arthroplasty where, besides the bone defect, which tends to be relatively large, the endomedullary bone has been partially replaced by the bone cement. The situation is similar with Silastic implants. The bone has at the interface with the implant a synovial layer, which needs to be removed before viable bone is present. In addition, there is a significant bone defect at the entrance of the implant into the bone through the rather voluminous shape of the stems. So, the surface of the bone, which is needed for joint fusion, is limited.

In any type of implant a bone graft is often needed to bridge the defect otherwise the finger can get unacceptably short. Either homologous or autologous grafts or a mix of them can be used. We prefer bone grafts from the radius; if several fingers are affected, bone graft from the iliac bone crest or homologous bone might be needed. The volar side of the radius provides a more solid graft and the scar is less visible. The cancellous bone can be used to fill the endomedullary cavity in order to provide some healthy bone for healing and additional primary stability. After the removal of the prosthesis, the local situation is unstable and it is technically not easy to fix the joint in the planned position. Either the graft is placed between the bone ends and preliminarily fixed with a wire. Alternatively, the graft can be fixed to the plate first and then placed together on the bone ends (▶ Fig. 13.5). Most critical is the position of rotation. It is absolutely necessary to check the three-dimensional position of the finger in flexion, especially in relation to the neighbor fingers. Already minimal rotational deformity may be functionally disabling. The fusion angle depends on the position of the finger in the hand and the other PIP joints. The ulnar fingers, especially the small finger, need more functional flexion than the index finger, which is mainly pitching with the thumb.[20]

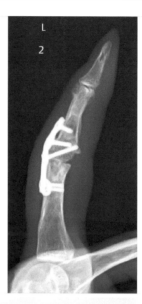

Fig. 13.5 Proximal interphalangeal (PIP) revision fusion after implant removal. The fixation is provided with a dorsal plate and a structural autologous bone graft to bridge the defect.

Especially with homologous bone grafts, healing might be prolonged and protection splints are needed often up to 3 months.

Finger amputation as a salvage intervention must be discussed in cases of multiple revision and unsolvable problems including infection or significant soft tissue deficiency.

13.7 Complications of PIP and DIP Fusion

In small joint fusion the most common complications are nonunion and malunion.[15,20,21] Stern and Fulton reported a complication rate of 20% for major complications which needed reintervention and 16% of minor complications like cold intolerance or paraesthesia.[20] Nonunion might occur due to biological reasons, mainly in difficult bone conditions or be a result of technical problems with the bone fixation. Bone conditions for joint fusion might be compromised after infection, in the course of an inflammatory disease or in posttraumatic joints with severe bone defects with or without previous bone grafting. Since bone defects overall are relatively low in volume and some shorting is functionally acceptable, conventional grafting with a rigid fixation often solves the problem. Prolonged immobilization might be needed in some cases, until bone healing is confirmed radiographically.

Malunion can be functional disabling especially in the coordination with the other fingers of the hand. This includes malrotation and lateral deviation. It is therefore mandatory to check during the procedure these parameters carefully. This is best done in lifting the hand of the

OR table and check the orientation of the finger from all sides, especially from the front. With the tenodesis effect of the MCP joint in different wrist positions, the finger naturally falls in the plane, which needs to be correct to function with the neighbor fingers.

13.8 Indication for Revision Surgery for Failed Finger Joint Fusion

The main reason to revise a finger joint arthrodesis is nonunion associated with pain and residual functional impairment. In rare occasion there is a fibrous pseudoarthrosis, which provides enough stability and thus no pain. Bone resorption at the osteotomy side and around the implants is often seen early in the postoperative course. If the biological surrounding of the joint is sound, prolonged immobilization might provide delayed healing. In cases of persistent pain after 6 months, reintervention needs to be evaluated.

13.9 Solutions for Failed Finger Joint Fusion

The only meaningful solution for a failed joint fusion is a rearthrodesis. In order to enhance the biological healing potential, the hardware must be removed completely and a comprehensive debridement of the bone is required. Biological healthy bone graft needs to be applied and a different bone fixation principle needs to be considered. Stern and Fulton[20] recommend a corticocancellous inlay graft with a longitudinal K-wire fixation. This is suitable for the DIP joint when there is enough bone length. In situations of significant bone defect an interposition graft is required and fixed according to the techniques described for revisions of failed implant arthroplasties.

Malunion, if functional problematic, requires corrective osteotomy. The principles for this procedure should follow the recommendations given in the chapter for PIP joint fusion after implant arthroplasty. It is crucial to control the correction in all three dimensions and in different positions of the finger.

13.10 Take-Home Message

Complications after surgery of finger arthritis are frequent. In order to find the correct revisions option, a meticulous analysis of the causes of failure is needed.

In PIP arthroplasty implant-related complications consist of loosening of the prosthesis, or in more complex joints, instability or joint luxation. Depending on the implant type and the soft tissue conditions, a revision includes either a soft tissue reconstruction with implant change or as salvage joint fusion. Unstable silicone implants can be replaced by more constrained two-component prosthesis. Since the implants leave often a significant bone defect and difficult biological conditions, a bone graft and a solid fixation is needed. For failed joint fusion with nonunion, a change in the fixation technique and biological healthy bone graft is needed.

References

[1] Ranney D. The hand as a concept: digital differences and their importance. Clin Anat. 1995; 8(4):281–287

[2] White WL. Why I hate the index finger. Hand (N Y). 2010; 5(4):461–465

[3] Sierakowski A, Zweifel C, Sirotakova M, Sauerland S, Elliot D. Joint replacement in 131 painful osteoarthritic and post-traumatic distal interphalangeal joints. J Hand Surg Eur Vol. 2012; 37(4):304–309

[4] Neukom L, Marks M, Hensler S, Kündig S, Herren DB, Schindele P. Silicone arthroplasty versus screw arthrodesis in distal interphalangeal joint osteoarthritis. J Hand Surg Eur Vol. 2020; 45(6):615–621

[5] Yamamoto M, Chung KC. Joint fusion and arthroplasty in the hand. Clin Plast Surg. 2019; 46(3):479–488

[6] Foliart DE. Swanson silicone finger joint implants: a review of the literature regarding long-term complications. J Hand Surg Am. 1995; 20(3):445–449

[7] Herren DB, Keuchel T, Marks M, Schindele S. Revision arthroplasty for failed silicone proximal interphalangeal joint arthroplasty: indications and 8-year results. J Hand Surg Am. 2014; 39(3):462–466

[8] Wagner ER, Luo TD, Houdek MT, Kor DJ, Moran SL, Rizzo M. Revision proximal interphalangeal arthroplasty: an outcome analysis of 75 consecutive cases. J Hand Surg Am. 2015; 40(10):1949–1955.e1

[9] Aversano FJ, Calfee RP. Salvaging a failed proximal interphalangeal joint implant. Hand Clin. 2018; 34(2):217–227

[10] Takigawa S, Meletiou S, Sauerbier M, Cooney WP. Long-term assessment of Swanson implant arthroplasty in the proximal interphalangeal joint of the hand. J Hand Surg Am. 2004; 29(5):785–795

[11] Herren DB, Schindele S, Goldhahn J, Simmen BR. Problematic bone fixation with pyrocarbon implants in proximal interphalangeal joint replacement: short-term results. J Hand Surg [Br]. 2006; 31(6):643–651

[12] Drake ML, Segalman KA. Complications of small joint arthroplasty. Hand Clin. 2010; 26(2):205–212

[13] Pugliese D, Bush D, Harrington T. Silicone synovitis: longer term outcome data and review of the literature. J Clin Rheumatol. 2009; 15(1):8–11

[14] Atkinson RE, Smith RJ. Silicone synovitis following silicone implant arthroplasty. Hand Clin. 1986; 2(2):291–299

[15] Herren DB. Current European practice in the treatment of proximal interphalangeal joint arthritis. Hand Clin. 2017; 33(3):489–500

[16] Swanson AB, de Groot Swanson G. Flexible implant resection arthroplasty of the proximal interphalangeal joint. Hand Clin. 1994; 10(2):261–266

[17] Tägil M, Geijer M, Abramo A, Kopylov P. Ten years' experience with a pyrocarbon prosthesis replacing the proximal interphalangeal joint. A prospective clinical and radiographic follow-up. J Hand Surg Eur Vol. 2014; 39(6):587–595

[18] Reissner L, Schindele S, Hensler S, Marks M, Herren DB. Ten year follow-up of pyrocarbon implants for proximal interphalangeal joint replacement. J Hand Surg Eur Vol. 2014; 39(6):582–586

[19] Murray PM, Linscheid RL, Cooney WP, III, Baker V, Heckman MG. Long-term outcomes of proximal interphalangeal joint surface replacement arthroplasty. J Bone Joint Surg Am. 2012; 94(12):1120–1128

[20] Stern PJ, Fulton DB. Distal interphalangeal joint arthrodesis: an analysis of complications. J Hand Surg Am. 1992; 17(6):1139–1145

[21] Vitale MA, Fruth KM, Rizzo M, Moran SL, Kakar S. Prosthetic arthroplasty versus arthrodesis for osteoarthritis and posttraumatic arthritis of the index finger proximal interphalangeal joint. J Hand Surg Am. 2015; 40(10):1937–1948

4

14 Management of Complications of Thumb CMC Surgery: Trapeziectomy, Arthrodesis, and Total Joint Arthroplasty

Filip Stockmans

Abstract

Thumb carpometacarpal joint surgery is the most commonly performed joint surgery in the hand. Clinically, the predominant complaint is pain. Once conservative treatment no longer controls the symptoms, surgery can offer a solution. Trapeziectomy with or without ligamentoplasty is by far the most common procedure. Reported complication rates are around 5% but it is not clear if this is the true complication rate. The main reason for revision surgery after trapeziectomy is ongoing or recurrent pain followed by functional impairment due to metacarpal instability and/or collapse. Removal of bony remnants of the trapezium, if present, and revision ligamentoplasty is the preferred treatment. In selected cases, fusion of the first and second metacarpal base can be considered as ultimate salvage procedure. Trapeziometacarpal fusion is mostly preferred for young, high demand patients. The main complications are nonunion and soft tissue irritation due to the dorsal hardware. Meticulous surgical technique is mandatory when performing this procedure with special attention to bone preparation, the use of bone grafts, and correct use of fixation material. Hardware removal after complete bony healing can be indicated in case of persistent soft tissue irritation. Total joint arthroplasty is not universally accepted. Current implants have 10-year joint survival rates around 90%. The majority of problems are related to the cup positioning and cup fixation. Cup revision can be performed but is not always feasible. Trapeziectomy combined with a ligamentoplasty is a good salvage option with good clinical outcome.

Keywords: CMC arthritis, trapeziometacarpal arthroplasty, trapeziometacarpal arthrodesis, trapeziectomy, revision surgery

14.1 Introduction

The thumb carpometacarpal (TMC) joint is the second most commonly affected joint by osteoarthritis. The clinical picture can often not be correlated with the radiographic findings. The most common complaints are pain, stiffness, decreased pinch strength, and overall disability. Conservative treatment is multimodal with splinting, physiotherapy, nonsteroidal anti-inflammatory drugs and steroid injections to control patient's symptoms. Once these treatments no longer control the symptoms, surgical treatment can be considered. Meanwhile many surgical options have been proposed: trapeziectomy with or without tendon interposition is probably the most com-

monly used surgical procedure to cure the patient's symptoms. Trapeziectomy has typically been associated with a good outcome regarding pain management but the major drawback is variable shortening of the thumb column which may lead to decreased grip strength and decreased mobility. Other surgical methods include arthrodesis, arthroscopic partial resection of the trapezium and/or metacarpal base, metacarpal extension osteotomy, and total joint arthroplasty using an implant. All these procedures have been shown to give favorable outcomes and all do have their specific indications and complications. No treatment option has been shown to be superior to another. In this chapter, we will focus on the complications of reconstructive surgery. Probably the most common complication is related to the surgical approach itself: injury to the dorsal sensory branch of the radial nerve. Next, specific complications related to trapeziectomy with and without ligamentoplasty and two types of trapezium sparing techniques: arthrodesis and total joint arthroplasty will be discussed. Carpometacarpal arthrodesis and carpometacarpal joint arthroplasty are usually chosen for so-called higher demand patients. In carpometacarpal arthrodesis, thumb column stability is the main theoretical advantage; in carpometacarpal joint arthroplasty, rapid recovery and more physiologic joint mobility are the main acclaimed advantages.

14.2 Injury to Sensory Nerve Branches

Branches of dorsal sensory radial nerve (DSRN) and lateral antebrachial cutaneous nerve (LACN) are at risk during surgical exposure of the TMC joint. The nerve branches are deep to the superficial venous system and should be visualized and protected during surgical approach. Injury can be caused by transection, excessive traction, or coagulation. This risk is even more important whenever revision surgery is undertaken on the TMC joint. The reported symptoms by the patient are variable from hypoesthesia over dysesthesia to hyperesthesia. Neuroma formation is probably the most feared complication. Initial treatment should be conservative with physiotherapy, pain management including neuromodulating medication, and desensitization. Referral to a pain specialist should be considered for these patients to optimize nonsurgical treatment. Surgical exploration is only considered if the symptoms persist for at least 6 months.[1] Surgery consists of neurolysis of the sensory branches from the surrounding scar. In case of neuroma formation, excision of the neuroma can be considered in combina-

4

tion with nerve grafting or nerve conduit. Many other treatment options are available.[2]

14.3 Trapeziectomy with and without Ligamentoplasty

Trapeziectomy was already proposed by Gervis in 1949[3] as a treatment option for osteoarthritis of the TMC joint. The ligamentoplasty has been added to the procedure since there was concern about the subsidence of the metacarpal into the empty space after resection of the trapezium. The reported failure rate of these procedures is under 5%[4,5]; it is not clear if this is the true failure rate since these data are retrieved from retrospective studies. Although the complication rate is low, one needs to realize that multiple revision surgeries are frequent within this group.[4] The main complications are incomplete trapeziectomy, symptomatic scaphotrapezoid arthritis, and problematic subsidence of the thumb metacarpal.

14.3.1 Incomplete Trapeziectomy

It is not uncommon to see residual shells of trapezium on postoperative radiographs after piecemeal resection of the trapezium. Although not all residual trapezium will be problematic, those located at the metacarpal base between the first and second metacarpal will be problematic. Often, they represent a remnant of the typical medial intermetacarpal osteophyte. Resection is recommended and is usually associated with suspension of the metacarpal.[1]

14.3.2 Scaphotrapezoid Arthritis

Unaddressed scaphotrapezoid arthritis has been recognized as a cause of residual pain after trapeziectomy.[6] Although systematic hemiresection of the proximal pole of the trapezoid is recommended by some authors, others question systematic resection.[7] One of the reasons to be cautious about systematic resection of the proximal trapezoid is related to midcarpal instability, as in resection of the distal pole of the scaphoid there is a theoretical concern regarding the stability of the proximal carpal row. A recent cadaver study demonstrated that up to 4-mm resection of proximal trapezoid has a negligible effect upon lunocapitate and scapholunate stability.[8] Most authors recommend interposition of a tendinous slip into the dead space after partial trapezoid resection.[9]

14.3.3 Problematic Subsidence of the Thumb Metacarpal

Some subsidence is expected after trapeziectomy.[10] Only when subsidence causes instability of the metacarpal base or impingement onto the distal pole of the scaphoid it becomes a reason for revision surgery. Whenever there

is a problem with the stability of the first metacarpal base after trapeziectomy, ligamentoplasty should be the first option. The preferred tendon is the flexor carpi radialis (FCR). Most authors prefer to use only half the FCR tendon since the FCR is considered to be an important secondary stabilizer of the scaphoid and the loop of the distally based tendon slip around the remaining FCR tendon adds a dynamic component to the ligamentoplasty during grip. In case the FCR tendon has been used, ruptured, or compromised during the previous surgery, a slip of the abductor pollicis longus or extensor carpi radialis longus or brevis can be used.[11] The surgical procedure remains similar to the conventional ligamentoplasty with a metacarpal bone tunnel, and the distally based tendon slip is looped around its remaining half to add the dynamic component to the reconstruction. More recently a suture button device has been introduced as a less invasive alternative for tendon harvesting.[12] Careful technique is mandatory when using these devices since poor technique can lead to overtightening of the suspension resulting in stiffness and painful contact between the base of the first and second metacarpal. Also fracturing of the second metacarpal has been reported and is related to multiple drilling of the bone tunnel or suboptimal positioning of the suture bottom device.[13] In case of major instability or failed revision soft tissue suspension arthroplasty, bony fusion between the base of the first and second metacarpal can be considered. The technique has been described for paralytic conditions but can be used as a last resort in these cases.[14] Patients need to be informed about the fixed abducted/opposed position of the intermetacarpal fusion which implies that the hand can't be flattened out anymore. The use of bone graft between the base of the first and second metacarpal is necessary and rigid fixation with locking plates is preferred.[15]

14.4 Trapeziometacarpal Arthrodesis

In the case of carpometacarpal arthrodesis, the most common problems encountered are nonunion, hardware irritation, malposition, and scapho-trapezio-trapezoidal (STT) arthritis.

14.4.1 Nonunion

In the case of carpometacarpal arthrodesis, the most common problem is related to achieving bony union with reported nonunion rates between 0 and 58%.[16,17] In an effort to achieve more stable fixation, different techniques were used. Currently dorsal locking plates are preferred. However, these plates are not always well tolerated and the dorsal approach is associated with irritation of the dorsal sensory branch of the radial nerve.[18]

Initial surgical technique used K-wires with or without tension banding. Since K-wires cannot reliably achieve

4

compression, tension banding was added to provide both compression and increased stability.[19,20] From biomechanical models, we know that the joint reaction forces are amplified throughout the thumb column. One kilogram of key pinch results in almost 10- to 20-kg joint reaction force in the CMC joint.[21] Even crossed K-wires combined with tension banding will be put to test under these particular conditions. Over time different fixation methods have been proposed, such as compression screws and various types of staples.[18] The most obvious solution would be the use of plate and screw fixation. Initially, mostly compression plates were used. Together with the development of dedicated plates for the hand, plate fixation was introduced. This had a positive influence on nonunion rates but new problems were identified related to hardware intolerance (see later).[22] The big advantage was the rigid fixation that could be achieved in combination with compression. Plates can be associated with the use of lag screws and/or K-wires. The next step was the introduction of the locking plates.[15] These made the constructs more rigid but this can come at the price of decreased compression when all screws are placed in locking mode. An advantage of locking plates is no need of purchasing the second cortex, preventing protruding screws which can lead to complications such as tendon rupturing.[17] An alternative method is the use of only compression screws to achieve stable fixation without the use of dorsal hardware. Dorsal hardware has been associated with irritation of the extensor tendons, hence making plate removal sometimes necessary. As in any arthrodesis method, not only nonunion can be a problem but also material malpositioning.

Whatever techniques are used, probably the most important step is the careful preparation of the bone surfaces. One should also keep in mind that these joints are affected by osteoarthritis with variable amounts of bone sclerosis and deformation. Adequate preparation of the bone surfaces is mandatory and can be challenging on the trapezium with its limited bone stock. The addition of bone grafts has a positive influence on healing rates regardless of the fixation technique used.[23]

14.4.2 Hardware-Related Problems

Although the introduction of plate and screw fixation was found to be positive for achieving better union rates, the complication rate remained relatively high.[22] Plate fixations are applied on the dorsal metacarpal surface which makes the dorsal sensory branch of the radial nerve susceptible for encasement in reactive scar tissue. Next the plate is in close contact with the extensor tendons of the thumb. Depending on the case, problems with the extensor tendons can lead to stiffness from adhesion as well as tendinitis through irritation of the tendon during its gliding over the hardware.[22] As plate designs evolved, initially there was a decrease in profile height

with improved hardware tolerance. However, the introduction of locking plates came at the price of a slightly higher plate profile.

In order to avoid dorsal hardware, a minimal invasive fixation technique was introduced using cannulated headless compression screws.[24] This technique even allows a complete arthroscopic technique without conventional arthrotomy. As in any minimally invasive technique, implant malposition can occur with screw penetration into the adjacent joints.[17]

14.4.3 Malpositioning and Reduced Mobility

Some patients will be unhappy with the loss of mobility in the carpometacarpal joint since the optimal position for fusion is with the first metacarpal in 30 to 45 degrees of palmar abduction and 30 to 45 degrees of pronation.[25] This results in the inability to lay the hand flat on the table since the thumb is in a fixed palmar abduction. As in any arthrodesis method, not only nonunion can be a problem but also malpositioning.

14.4.4 STT Arthritis

Fusion of the carpometacarpal joint will result in compensatory mobility in the adjacent proximal and distal joints. In the case of carpometacarpal arthrodesis, the more proximal scapho-trapezio-trapezoidal joint is of particular concern.[26] Secondary degeneration of this joint can be the source of recurrent pain problems for the patient. Different treatment options have been described to treat STT arthritis; STT fusion is no option after carpometacarpal fusion.[27] Two options can be considered to treat this condition. One option is to undo the arthrodesis, resect the trapezium, and perform a ligamentoplasty. The other option is resection of the STT joint.[28] This can be done with an open or arthroscopic procedure.[27] Distal scaphoid excision is contraindicated if there is either scapholunocapitate pathology or midcarpal instability.[29]

14.5 Thumb Carpometacarpal Joint Arthroplasty

Different types of implants have been designed to replace part or the total surface of the trapeziometacarpal joint. In this chapter the total joint arthroplasty and pyrocarbon interposition arthroplasty will be discussed.

14.5.1 Total Joint Arthroplasty

Total joint arthroplasty of the carpometacarpal thumb joint is still not universally accepted, although several studies report acceptable long-term outcomes and joint survival.[16] The complications are those of any joint arthroplasty with the exception of infection. The most common complications are related to the cup positioning in the trapezium. Cup malpositioning is not only associated with joint luxation but also with increased poly wear and cup loosening. Regarding cup loosening, one has to keep in mind that it is very hard to distinguish aseptic loosening from low-grade infection.[30]

Cup Positioning

There is no doubt that cup positioning is the single most important part of total joint replacement. Since the total joint arthroplasty is a ball-and-socket joint with just a single point of rotation, both location of this rotation point and cup orientation are important. Regarding cup positioning, one of the limiting factors is the relative small trapezium which forces cup positioning rather lateral, to avoid penetration of the trapeziotrapezoidal joint. In the dorsopalmar direction, a midposition is preferred for having maximal bone stock around the cup. Cup orientation is, in general, assessed with referral to the trapezioscaphoid joint surface. An orientation parallel to this joint is preferred. Although this is a fairly straightforward choice, the importance of cup orientation has to be seen on the ball-and-socket side where maximal coverage of the ball needs to be assured over the full range of thumb motion including motion during wrist flexion extension. Currently, it is unclear whether cup positioning with reference to the scaphotrapezial joint can/will solve all problems, it certainly will decrease luxation rates.[31] Meanwhile design innovations have also focused on improving luxation rates. These came from looking at hip arthroplasty where the introduction of dual mobility cups also decreased luxation rates.[32] Several dual mobility implants are being used now with encouraging short-term results but currently there are no long-term results available yet. In the long term the poly wear is a point of concern in a dual mobility design since poly thickness is around 2 mm at the articulating part.

Revision Surgery

Revision surgery after total joint arthroplasty needs to be divided in revisions, maintaining the total joint and conversion to a form of trapeziectomy. Cup revision is probably the most frequent type of joint-sparing revision surgery. Cup revision can be indicated in cases of recurrent luxation, cup loosening, or poly wear.[33] Cup revision is only feasible in the presence of sufficient bone stock in the trapezium. There is a substantial risk for trapezium fracture during revision surgery and patients should be informed. Whenever cup replacement is not feasible, an alternative treatment should be considered. Since these implants are modular, the metacarpal stem can be left in place. First the neck is separated from the stem and a complete trapeziectomy is performed. Since it is not feasi-

ble to drill a bone tunnel through the metacarpal base, a Weilby ligamentoplasty is preferred.[34] The results of these revision procedures are comparable to primary ligamentoplasty procedures.[35]

14.5.2 Pyrocarbon Interposition Arthroplasty

An alternative for total joint arthroplasty is the interposition of a spacer in the resected TMC joint space. Hemiresection arthroplasty was introduced as an alternative for TMC arthrodesis in higher demand patients.[36] Over time different materials have been used; resorbable synthetic implants can generate tissue reaction and hence have largely been abandoned.[37] Pyrocarbon is an inert ceramic material with excellent biocompatibility and favorable characteristics to interact with cartilage and bone.[38] The Pyrodisk, pyrocarbon, implant is designed to be used after distal hemitrapeziectomy for Eaton Glickel stage II or III CMC thumb joint arthritis.[39] The implant is a nonanatomic biarticular disc with convex surfaces and a central hole to allow movements along three axes. A strip of tendon (flexor carpi radialis or abductor pollicis longus) is used to align and stabilize the disc after resection of the joint by passing the tendon through the trapezium, the disc, and the base of the first metacarpal. The implant comes in various sizes (diameter and height) for optimal implant size selection to create a stable joint and to prevent impingement. A retrospective study by van Laarhoven et al has demonstrated clinical outcomes comparable to those of total joint arthroplasty with implant survival rates of 91%.[40] In their cohort of 164 thumbs, revision surgery had to be performed for disc dislocation (2%) or STT arthritis (4%). The revision surgery consisted of implant removal, completing the trapeziectomy combined with a ligamentoplasty, which resulted in comparable results to primary procedures.[40]

14.6 Arthroscopy

Arthroscopic debridement with or without soft tissue interposition is in essence a variant of the hemiresection arthroplasty.[36] This relative novel surgical technique for CMC arthritis is less invasive compared to the open technique and preserves all the ligaments and its proprioceptive nerve endings.[41] A recent systematic review found that there is a modest improvement after undergoing surgery of the CMC joint with arthroscopic-assisted techniques. Approximately 64 to 100% of patients were satisfied and the combined complication rate was low (4%).[42] In addition to the complications already mentioned above, specific complications related to the technique are portal-related nerve and tendon irritation and injury.[42] In case of insufficient pain relief, all open options for the treatment of TMC arthritis remain possible as salvage option.

14.7 Take-Home Message

As is true for most surgical treatments, the best strategy to avoid complications is careful patient selection, meticulous technique, and adequate follow-up of operated patients. No treatment for thumb CMC arthritis has been shown to be superior to the other. Surgeon's preference and experience will play an important role in patient and procedure selection. Every procedure has its own type of complications. In general, surgery of the trapeziometacarpal joint starts with careful joint exposure and adequate attention for the cutaneous sensory nerve branches. Most patients treated for basal thumb joint arthritis are satisfied. Trapeziectomy with or without ligamentoplasty has a low complication rate but those patients who need revision surgery represent a challenging subgroup who sometimes need multiple revision surgeries. Revision with resuspension using one of the remaining tendon slips is the recommended treatment. In selected cases, an arthrodesis between the base of the first and second metacarpal can be considered. Trapeziometacarpal arthrodesis is a fairly demanding procedure and nonunion is the most frequent complication. Revision arthrodesis with bone grafting is recommended. Total joint arthroplasty remains controversial and its complications are well documented. Most complications are related to the cup positioning and fixation. In selected cases, cup revision surgery is feasible; if not, trapeziectomy with Weilby ligamentoplasty is recommended.

References

[1] Hess DE, Drace P, Franco MJ, Chhabra AB. Failed thumb carpometacarpal arthroplasty: common etiologies and surgical options for revision. J Hand Surg Am. 2018; 43(9):844–852

[2] Watson J, Gonzalez M, Romero A, Kerns J. Neuromas of the hand and upper extremity. J Hand Surg Am. 2010; 35(3):499–510

[3] Gervis WH. Osteo-arthritis of the trapezio-metacarpal joint treated by excision of the trapezium. Proc R Soc Med. 1947; 40(9):492

[4] Mattila S, Waris E. Revision of trapeziometacarpal arthroplasty: risk factors, procedures and outcomes. Acta Orthop. 2019; 90(4):389–393

[5] Wilkens SC, Xue Z, Mellema JJ, Ring D, Chen N. Unplanned reoperation after trapeziometacarpal arthroplasty: rate, reasons, and risk factors. Hand (N Y). 2017; 12(5):446–452

[6] Irwin AS, Maffulli N, Chesney RB. Scapho-trapezoid arthritis. A cause of residual pain after arthroplasty of the trapezio-metacarpal joint. J Hand Surg [Br]. 1995; 20(3):346–352

[7] Hasselbacher K, Steffke M, Kalb K. Is chronic, untreated scapho-trapezoid arthrosis after resection arthroplasty of the carpometacarpal joint clinically relevant? Handchir Mikrochir Plast Chir. 2001; 33(6):418–423

[8] Alolabi N, Hooke AW, Kakar S. The biomechanical consequences of trapeziectomy and partial trapeziodectomy in the treatment of thumb carpometacarpal and scaphotrapeziotrapezoid arthritis. J Hand Surg Am. 2020; 45(3):257.e1–257.e7

[9] Moreno R, Bhandari L. FCR interposition arthroplasty for concomitant STT and CMC arthritis. Tech Hand Up Extrem Surg. 2019; 23(1):10–13

[10] Abdallah Z, Saab M, Amouyel T, Guerre E, Chantelot C, Sturbois-Nachef N. Total trapezectomy for osteoarthritis of the trapeziometacarpal joint: clinical and radiological outcomes in 21 cases with minimum 10-year follow-up. Orthop Traumatol Surg Res. 2020; 106(4):775–779

[11] Jones DB, Jr, Rhee PC, Shin AY, Kakar S. Salvage options for flexor carpi radialis tendon disruption during ligament reconstruction and tendon interposition or suspension arthroplasty of the trapeziometacarpal joint. J Hand Surg Am. 2013; 38(9):1806–1811

[12] Yao J, Zlotolow DA, Murdock R, Christian M. Suture button compared with K-wire fixation for maintenance of posttrapeziectomy space height in a cadaver model of lateral pinch. J Hand Surg Am. 2010; 35(12):2061–2065

[13] Khalid M, Jones ML. Index metacarpal fracture after tightrope suspension following trapeziectomy: case report. J Hand Surg Am. 2012; 37(3):418–422

[14] Shah A, Ellis RD. Thumb-index metacarpal arthrodesis for stabilization of the flail thumb. J Hand Surg Am. 1994; 19(3):453–454

[15] Bamberger HB, Stern PJ, Kiefhaber TR, McDonough JJ, Cantor RM. Trapeziometacarpal joint arthrodesis: a functional evaluation. J Hand Surg Am. 1992; 17(4):605–611

[16] Vermeulen GM, Slijper H, Feitz R, Hovius SE, Moojen TM, Selles RW. Surgical management of primary thumb carpometacarpal osteoarthritis: a systematic review. J Hand Surg Am. 2011; 36(1):157–169

[17] Satteson ES, Langford MA, Li Z. The management of complications of small joint arthrodesis and arthroplasty. Hand Clin. 2015; 31(2):243–266

[18] Chamay A, Piaget-Morerod F. Arthrodesis of the trapeziometacarpal joint. J Hand Surg [Br]. 1994; 19(4):489–497

[19] Alberts KA, Engkvist O. Arthrodesis of the first carpometacarpal joint: 33 cases of arthrosis. Acta Orthop Scand. 1989; 60(3):258–260

[20] Pardini AG, Lazaroni AP, Tavares KE. Compression arthrodesis of the carpometacarpal joint of the thumb. Hand. 1982; 14(3):291–294

[21] Cooney WP, III, Chao EY. Biomechanical analysis of static forces in the thumb during hand function. J Bone Joint Surg Am. 1977; 59(1):27–36

[22] Forseth MJ, Stern PJ. Complications of trapeziometacarpal arthrodesis using plate and screw fixation. J Hand Surg Am. 2003; 28(2):342–345

[23] Doyle JR. Sliding bone graft technique for arthrodesis of the trapeziometacarpal joint of the thumb. J Hand Surg Am. 1991; 16(2):363–365

[24] Faithfull DK, Herbert TJ. Small joint fusions of the hand using the Herbert Bone Screw. J Hand Surg [Br]. 1984; 9(2):167–168

[25] Mureau MA, Rademaker RP, Verhaar JA, Hovius SE. Tendon interposition arthroplasty versus arthrodesis for the treatment of trapeziometacarpal arthritis: a retrospective comparative follow-up study. J Hand Surg Am. 2001; 26(5):869–876

[26] Rizzo M, Moran SL, Shin AY. Long-term outcomes of trapeziometacarpal arthrodesis in the management of trapeziometacarpal arthritis. J Hand Surg Am. 2009; 34(1):20–26

[27] Catalano LW, III, Ryan DJ, Barron OA, Glickel SZ. Surgical management of scaphotrapeziotrapezoid arthritis. J Am Acad Orthop Surg. 2020; 28(6):221–228

[28] Garcia-Elias M, Lluch AL, Farreres A, Castillo F, Saffar P. Resection of the distal scaphoid for scaphotrapeziotrapezoid osteoarthritis. J Hand Surg [Br]. 1999; 24(4):448–452

[29] Deans VM, Naqui Z, Muir LT. Scaphotrapeziotrapezoidal joint osteoarthritis: a systematic review of surgical treatment. J Hand Surg Asian Pac Vol. 2017; 22(1):1–9

[30] Ganhewa AD, Wu R, Chae MP, et al. Failure rates of base of thumb arthritis surgery: a systematic review. J Hand Surg Am. 2019; 44(9):728–741.e10

[31] Caekebeke P, Duerinckx J. Can surgical guidelines minimize complications after Maïa® trapeziometacarpal joint arthroplasty with unconstrained cups? J Hand Surg Eur Vol. 2018; 43(4):420–425

[32] Terrier A, Latypova A, Guillemin M, Parvex V, Guyen O. Dual mobility cups provide biomechanical advantages in situations at risk for dislocation: a finite element analysis. Int Orthop. 2017; 41(3):551–556

[33] Cootjans K, Dreessen P, Vandenberghe D, Verhoeven N. Salvage revision arthroplasty after failed TMC joint prosthesis. Acta Orthop Belg. 2019; 85(3):325–329

[34] Weilby A. Tendon interposition arthroplasty of the first carpo-metacarpal joint. J Hand Surg [Br]. 1988; 13(4):421–425

[35] Lenoir H, Erbland A, Lumens D, Coulet B, Chammas M. Trapeziectomy and ligament reconstruction tendon interposition after failed trapeziometacarpal joint replacement. Hand Surg Rehabil. 2016; 35(1):21–26

[36] Eaton RG, Glickel SZ, Littler JW. Tendon interposition arthroplasty for degenerative arthritis of the trapeziometacarpal joint of the thumb. J Hand Surg Am. 1985; 10(5):645–654

[37] Lerebours A, Marin F, Bouvier S, Egles C, Rassineux A, Masquelet AC. Trends in trapeziometacarpal implant design: a systematic survey based on patents and administrative databases. J Hand Surg Am. 2020; 45(3):223–238

[38] Kawalec JS, Hetherington VJ, Melillo TC, Corbin N. Evaluation of fibrocartilage regeneration and bone response at full-thickness cartilage defects in articulation with pyrolytic carbon or cobalt-chromium alloy hemiarthroplasties. J Biomed Mater Res. 1998; 41(4):534–540

[39] Eaton RG, Glickel SZ. Trapeziometacarpal osteoarthritis: staging as a rationale for treatment. Hand Clin. 1987; 3(4):455–471

[40] van Laarhoven CMC, et al. Pyrolytic carbon disk interposition hemiarthroplasty as treatment for trapezial-metacarpal osteoarthritis: a long-term follow-up. J Hand Surg Am. 2020:published online

[41] Menon J. Arthroscopic management of trapeziometacarpal joint arthritis of the thumb. Arthroscopy. 1996; 12(5):581–587

[42] Wilkens SC, Bargon CA, Mohamadi A, Chen NC, Coert JH. A systematic review and meta-analysis of arthroscopic assisted techniques for thumb carpometacarpal joint osteoarthritis. J Hand Surg Eur Vol. 2018; 43(10):1098–1105

4

15 Treatment of Complications of Midcarpal Joints Arthritis

Eva-Maria Baur and Riccardo Luchetti

Abstract

Carpal procedures are various and delicate; therefore, the number of different complications is high. Especially nonunion, malunion, malalignment, and stiffness are well-known problems after these operations. Less frequent, but equally important are infection, complex regional pain syndrome (CRPS), nerve lesions, and hardware-associated problems. Some of them are related to the technique other generic. Their knowledge allows them to be prevented and recognized for early treatment. The prevention and the treatment are described in this chapter.

Keywords: midcarpal procedures, partial wrist fusion, proximal row carpectomy, wrist stiffness, complication of SNAC treatment, complication of SLAC treatment

15.1 Introduction

The most common indications for midcarpal procedures are advanced carpal collapse due to different pathologies such as scapholunate advanced collapse (SLAC) and scaphoid nonunion advanced collapse (SNAC) and scaphoid chondrocalcinosis advanced collapse (SCAC). Salvage procedures are also common for Kienböck disease—depending on stages, if revascularization or levelling operations are no more an option. Other less common indications, for instance, isolated midcarpal osteoarthritis (OA), are sometimes seen in systemic inflammatory diseases like rheumatoid arthritis (RA) or others. Radiolunate OA or dislocation is also common in RA.

Severe nonreducible instability could also be an indication for partial wrist fusion, if ligament repair or reconstruction fails to provide the required strength and stability.

Malunion and sequelae after distal radius fracture (DRF) could also be an indication for midcarpal procedures like partial wrist fusion, e.g., radioscapholunate (RSL) fusion, arthroplasty, or prosthesis.

Different procedures can be performed for the above-mentioned indications and diseases: Proximal row carpectomy (PRC), partial wrist fusions, denervation, resection arthroplasties, and prosthesis.

The least invasive procedure is denervation. Denervation was introduced in the 1990s in a partial or total manner for all kind of painful wrist disorders. The most common performed procedures are proximal row carpectomy and partial wrist fusions. The choice for one of these two techniques depends on the extent of arthrosis, preference of surgeon, and wishes of the patient. A prerequisite for performing a proximal row carpectomy is that the capitate cartilage is not damaged like in SLAC and SNAC stage 2. Partial wrist fusions can be performed for differ-

ent indications. Four-corner fusions (4CF) as well as two- or three-corner fusions can be used for SLAC/SNAC/SCAC stage 2 or 3.

Scaphocapitate or STT fusion is a salvage procedure in advanced Kienböck disease. STT fusion is an optional treatment for STT-OA or instability. RSL and RL fusion can be performed for arthrosis caused by DRF and RA, respectively. Resection arthroplasties without an interposition are rare in the wrist/midcarpal joint. Mostly, an interposition of a tendon or pyrocarbon or silicone implant is added.

Both total wrist prosthesis and partial prosthesis like a capitate head resection arthroplasty can be performed for midcarpal arthrosis. Naturally, no treatment is without complications and these will be discussed below.

15.2 Complications

Although not very invasive, denervation can lead to complications. A typical complication is a sensory nerve irritation. A lack of proprioception might occur after resection of the posterior interosseous nerve (PIN) but we only know this information for the healthy wrist.[1] Recurrence of pain or no release of pain at all can occur after denervation.

15.2.1 Infection

Infection can occur after every operation. Even though it is rare in elective hand surgery—at least less common than in foot surgery—probably one explanation is the better blood supply in the upper extremity as well as easier hygienic situation postoperatively. The first treatment is to clean the joint (several times) open or arthroscopic and give an antibiotic treatment. Arthroscopic procedures seem to have an advantage regarding number of operations and functional results.[2] If there has been a delay already, sometimes damage of the cartilage (and bone) is so high that only a (partial) or total wrist fusion is the option. Prosthesis after a severe joint infection has always the risk of recurrence of the infection, especially in proven osteitis.

15.2.2 Hardware-Associated Problems

These problems are common in every region of the body and can therefore occur in the midcarpal joint as well. As the carpal tunnel and the palmar portion of the carpal tunnel are convex, and mostly the hardware is placed from the dorsal aspect, the screws or wires can protrude in the carpal tunnel. Here is a risk of flexor tendon damage. Unfortunately, the carpal tunnel X-ray view is no more an option due to limited wrist extension after midcarpal fusion. So, in any case of suspicion make a postop computed tomography (CT) scan to be sure there is no risk of tendon rupture (▶ Fig. 15.1). Also in midcarpal partial wrist fusion, the protrusion of a wire in the PT (piso-triquetral) joint can occur. For preventing or detecting during the operation make a PT view (20 degrees of supination in lateral view) to ensure there is no screw or wire in the PT joint (▶ Fig. 15.2).

Extensor tendons are at risk in cases where plates or wires are placed on the dorsum of the wrist. Either you can bend the wires and bury them in between the metacarpal bones or leave them sticking out of the skin. I personally prefer to bury them. A risk of the wires could be "moving wires" down to the surface of the radius or get in conflict with the extensor tendons.

15.2.3 Malalignment

Malalignment is common after insufficient or "wrong" reduction. The functional range of motion (ROM) of the

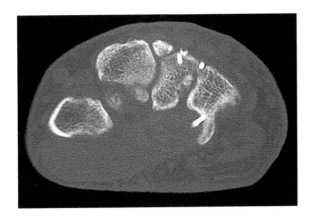

Fig. 15.1 Protruding screw in the carpal tunnel after 4CF (computed tomography [CT] scan).

wrist is 30-0-10 extension/flexion.[3] So, after midcarpal partial wrist fusion, this is what we want to get at least and what we can expect. A bit more can be expected after arthroscopic procedures than in open procedures due to less scarring postoperatively. For this purpose, reduction of the flexed lunate to a neutral position is needed—or even better—is a slightly extended position to get more wrist extension than flexion after partial fusion (Linscheid maneuver). A ROM of 40-0-20 extension/flexion is functional better than 20-0-40, because the powerful grip needs extension of the wrist. In SLAC (or SNAC) in combination with a misaligned DRF, the midcarpal reduction can be good, even though the total wrist ROM is worse, due to the malalignment of the DRF (▶ Fig. 15.3). Sometimes the reduction from the lunate in a correct or slightly overcorrected position is not easy—but very important for the postoperative result.

Regarding the ulnar translation of the lunate and triquetrum in SLAC we need to reduce it underneath the capitate in an anatomic position, depending on the shape of the lunate type 1 or 2. Here we do not recommend an overcorrection; otherwise, the wrist gets stiffer.

15.2.4 Nonunion

In partial wrist fusions, nonunion is a common problem. Percentages range from 5 to 40% as described in the literature. It also depends on the hardware material used for the arthrodesis. It seems that plates in partial wrist fusions have a more common nonunion rate (e.g., Mulford et al[4]: 4.9–13.6% K-wires vs. plates in their systematic review).

For the last 9 years, the author has been performing partial wrist fusion only with an arthroscopic-assisted approach with screws or K-wires. No differences are seen in our own series using screws or wires in the arthroscopic procedures.[5] We can see after a steep learning

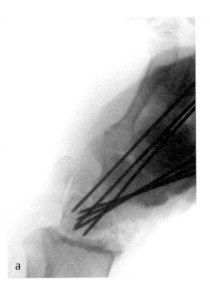
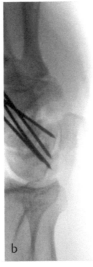

a
b

Fig. 15.2 (a, b) Intraoperative, two samples of PT view.

4

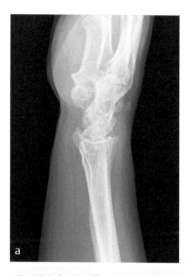
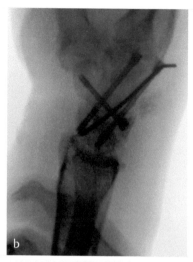
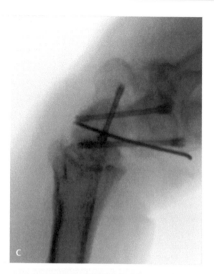

Fig. 15.3 (a–c) Different range of motion (ROM) in extension/flexion due to malaligned distal radius fracture (DRF), even with good reduction of the 4CF; Flex/Ext 0-0-80.

curve that the bony healing and postop ROM are better in arthroscopic than in open procedure. The ROM we get at the end of the operation in the OR, is what we can expect as final ROM—in contrast to open procedures, where a soft-tissue scarring decreases the ROM.

15.2.5 Secondary OA

Secondary OA is common in the long term after PRC, even though it's not always painful or need to be treated. If it is symptomatic, it can only be resolved by a total wrist fusion, prosthesis, or capitate head replacement. About 25 to 35% needs conversion to a total wrist fusion[6] or revision surgery in long-term follow-up.[7] An interposition arthroplasty with a tendon or artificial graft is an option, but there are no longstanding (good) results.

15.2.6 Prosthesis/Spacer

Well-known problems of prosthesis are either early or late loosening of prosthesis, as well as misplacement of the prosthesis. Early subclinical infection can lead to a loosening. The misplacement or misloading of the prosthesis leads more to a later loosening. Periprosthetic fractures of the bones can also be a problem. If the bony stock is very small to achieve bony healing, bone grafting can be used for resolution of the problem.

In case of spacers with no bony integration, the biggest problem is the dislocation besides the infection. This could be addressed with a stabilization procedure, like a ligamento-capsuloplasty. This does not always work. Sometimes the spacer has already molded a kind of a hole with stable walls, so just removal of the dislocated spacer can solve the problem.

15.2.7 Pain/CRPS

This can happen in every kind of operation. Anyway we need to check and exclude nerve, hardware, malreduction, etc., problems that we can solve and hence "heal" the CRPS. In a number of cases, we can figure out this and find an indication for revision surgery.[8] Plexus anesthesia and catheter insertion can be helpful in these cases to achieve as much less pain as possible after the secondary operation.

15.3 Stiffness

15.3.1 Causes of Stiffness

Stiffness can occur after a number of operations, although it seems to be more common in open than in arthroscopic procedures. Stiffness after carpal procedures (4CF or PRC) is determined by intra-articular, capsular, and/or extra-articular conditions. All of them can contribute to the stiffness, separately or in association. In the intercarpal fusion, all the procedures (2-3-4 bone fusion) that are used to fuse the midcarpal joint after scaphoid resection are to be considered as cause. Primary insult (chronic damage of the dorsal or palmar soft tissues) and prolonged immobilization had to be also considered. In 4CF and PRC, the intra-articular causes of rigidity are the fibrosis between the articular surface of the distal radius and the carpal bones (fibrotic tissue bands) and between the capsule and the carpal bones located mostly in the dorsal and less frequently in the volar part. In open surgery, the dorsal capsule contracture due to surgical approach is the main cause of wrist rigidity. It produces a loss of wrist flexion. This consequence is valid also for the

Table 15.1 Possible causes of secondary wrist rigidity (extra-articular or intra-articular)

- After trauma
  - Fracture
  - Fracture-dislocation
  - Dislocation
  - Ligament lesion
- After surgery
  - Dorsal wrist ganglia recurrence
  - Treatment of scaphoid fracture/nonunion
  - Intercarpal arthrodesis (four-bone fusion and so on)
  - Ligament reconstruction (SL ligament and so on)
  - Proximal row carpectomy
- Prolonged immobilization
- Erroneous wrist immobilization

Abbreviation: SL, scapholunate.

PRC when the traditional surgical way is used. However, loss of extension should be expected as palmar surgery is used, for example, in the PRC by the palmar approach.[9] The external causes of the wrist rigidity are the peritendinous and intertendinous adherence of extensor tendons as the dorsal approach is used (▶ Table 15.1). Postsurgery edema and complex regional pain syndrome (CRPS) are involved in the wrist stiffness with contemporary extension to the fingers.

Wrist stiffness is less present after arthroscopic surgery due to less soft tissues damage and exposition. The PRC and 4CF can be done by arthroscopy. However, skilled arthroscopists are needed to perform such a difficult surgery. Sometimes the arthroscopic procedure needs bigger portals or an accessory short open approach to complete the procedure. As these are used, the technique risks being closer to the open surgery with the same consequences. In addition, in the intercarpal bone fusion K-wires are frequently used as method of fixation instead of the screws or plate, as used in the open surgery, with less stability of intercarpal fusion. Therefore, if a prolonged protection through wrist immobilization is adopted in order to obtain healing of the intercarpal fusion, the consequences (wrist stiffness) are even more in open than in arthroscopic surgery.

All these causes of wrist rigidity should be considered as the clinician approaches to solve problems secondary to 4CF or PRC.

15.3.2 Treatment of Stiffness

As the wrist rigidity does not show any improvement after adequate rehabilitation, patients should be considered candidates for surgical intervention.

Surgical management of wrist stiffness consists of arthrolysis of the wrist. Preoperatively, X-ray, CT scan, and magnetic resonance imaging (MRI) of the wrist should be performed to confirm the consolidation of the arthrodesis and to exclude any carpal malunion or osteochondritis which needs a different surgical solution.

Arthrolysis can be performed by open or arthroscopic surgery.

Arthrolysis: Open Procedure

The open arthrolysis is much more indicated for the intercarpal fusion in open approach due to contemporary extensor tendon adherence that needs tenolysis procedure as well (▶ Fig. 15.4). Dorsal skin incision on the scar of previous surgery allows reaching directly the extensor tendons which are released by the adherence using scalpel or scissor. The extensor retinaculum is protected and the tendons are released passing under it using a dissector or periosteal elevator. Once the tendons are free, the procedure continues through a transversal capsular incision along the dorsal margin of the distal radius. This incision gets into the radio carpal joint. The first step is to remove the scar at the radial side at the cavity created after scaphoid resection. Then the adherences between the radius and the lunate and dorsally to the lunate are released. At the end of these two steps the wrist flexion is tested. As the flexion is sufficient, the procedure is stopped. If the wrist flexion is not sufficient, the release of the anterior part of the radiocarpal joint is required and it should be done using a curved dissector passed

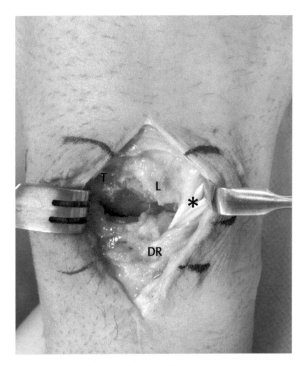

Fig. 15.4 Dorsal wrist arthrolysis using the same approach of the previous surgery (4CF). Dorsal capsule has been released exposing the radiocarpal joint (DR, distal radius; L, lunate; T, triquetrum).

radially to the lunate and under the lunate. The maneuver should be stopped as the ulnar margin of the radius is reached. Avoid, please, to release the ulnocarpal ligament to prevent an ulnar translation of the carpus.[10,11] The wrist motion is tested again in flexion and extension. The dorsal intercarpal plate should be removed if needed (malposition) or simply released from the adherence. If screws are used for intercarpal fixation, one has to pay attention to verify if any osteochondritis or screws subsidence is present. In case of subsidence, the screw should be removed.

Arthrolysis: Arthroscopic Procedure

Arthroscopic arthrolysis has been attempted in wrist stiffness due to intercarpal fusion but open conversion was always needed. 1–2 and 3–4 portals are used to scope the radial side of the wrist first. Arthroscopic arthrolysis of this part is feasible but as you try to enter into the radiolunate joint it is hard and difficult and the risk to damage the cartilage is very high. Therefore, the correct technical indication of arthrolysis for the intercarpal fusion is the open surgery.

Traditionally, the PRC is done by a dorsal approach. Palmar approach is rarely used but it is another approach to perform the same procedure with same or better results.[9] PRC has been demonstrated to be possible by arthroscopy, but it is time consuming and expertise in arthroscopy is a prerequisite. After removing the three proximal bones, a wider space in the RC joint is created with a new radiocapitate articulation. Despite of clinical expectation in terms of wrist ROM after PRC, stiffness rarely happens.

Management of this stiffness secondary to PRC passes through clinical examination and investigation by imaging. X-rays, CT scan, and MRI should be useful to understand the causes of the wrist stiffness. However, imaging investigations not always are clear and arthroscopy is needed for a direct evaluation and contemporaneous treatment (▶ Table 15.2). Arthroscopy is performed starting from the 1–2 and 3–4 portals distally to the radial styloid where the scaphoid was removed (▶ Fig. 15.5). Fibrotic scar is often present in the position of previous surgery (dorsal for the dorsal approach and palmar for the palmar approach). As the fibrotic bands and fibrosis are removed by using a shaver, the articular surface of the capitate is appreciated from the radial side. Its cartilage is evaluated and the lunate facet as well. Ulnarly to the capitate, the fibrosis should be removed using the 3–4 portal for the scope and 6 R for the shaver. In this RC joint space, fibrosis is found and removed, obtaining an improvement of the wrist motion. If necessary, the dorsal capsule and/or the palmar ligaments are released using scalpel, hook scalpel, shaver, or radiofrequency device. The resection of the palmar radiocarpal ligaments will improve the extension. The resection of the dorsal capsule will improve the wrist flexion. Radial styloidectomy might also be done when needed. Arthroscopic arthrolysis is an in-out procedure which has the advantage that the procedure can be stopped after the release of the fibrosis or the capsular resection if the fibrosis is absent. However, the external procedures, as for example the tenolysis, cannot be done.

Open arthrolysis should be also adopted with the same purpose, but it is an out-in procedure that doesn't stop until the internal joint is reached and released. It means that if the wrist stiffness is due to fibrotic bands or internal adherences, the capsule (dorsal or volar) has to be sectioned when you adopt an open procedure before removal of the internal fibrosis. For treatment of stiffness due to PRC performed by traditional dorsal approach, the surgical procedure is no longer different from that described for the intercarpal fusion. Simple elastic bandage is used at the end, promoting immediate wrist

Table 15.2 Arthroscopic wrist arthrolysis for suboptimal proximal row carpectomy (PRC) cases

Intra-articular findings	Procedure
Fibrosis/Fibrotic band	Remove
Capsular contracture	Release
Incorrect radiocapitate position	Relocation (palmar capsule resection)
Radial styloid impingement	Resection
Residual carpal bones	Remove
Radiocapitate articular degeneration	Debridement

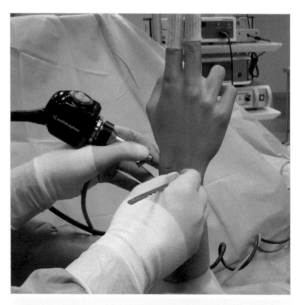

Fig. 15.5 Arthroscopic wrist arthrolysis. The scope is in 1–2 portal and hook blade in 6 R portal. The internal fibrosis and the capsule contracture are released.

motion. In wrist stiffness after PRC performed by palmar approach, the open arthrolysis is performed using a palmar access through the way of the previous surgery. The median nerve is released from the adherences and the flexor tendons as well. As the palmar capsule is reached, protecting the FPL and the median nerve in the radial side and the flexor tendons in the ulnar side, a transversal radiocarpal incision is done through the scar of the previous surgery. It corresponds to the volar border of the distal radius. The capitate is identified and its articular surface is evaluated and protected as that of the lunate facet of the distal radius. The radial side of the joint is released from the fibrotic tissue and the radial styloid is resected when needed. The ulnar side of the joint in respect to the capitate rarely needs to be treated. However, a dissector can enter into the joint space ulnarly to the capitate and the fibrotic bands can be released. The wrist flexion and extension is tested at the end. Rehabilitation starts immediately with two to three sessions per day but a palmar splint is used to maintain the wrist position at 30 degrees of extension between the sessions.

During the arthrolysis, both open and arthroscopically, the associated chondropathy or osteochondropathy must be well documented and taken into consideration (to compare for the patient symptoms and) for further management.

15.4 Take-Home Message

Specific and nonspecific complications (generic: like infection) are common in midcarpal procedures. CT scan as well as MRI is very useful for detection of problems like nonunion, hardware malpositioning, or soft tissue problems. Fortunately it is becoming easier to get these investigations to help us to detect the problems early so they can be treated. Don't hesitate to use these tools early and often enough. Some complications can be solved with a specific treatment, some not (infection, CRPS, secondary OA) and often lead to bad results.

References

[1] Hagert E, Persson JKE. Desensitizing the posterior interosseous nerve alters wrist proprioceptive reflexes. J Hand Surg Am. 2010; 35 (7):1059–1066

[2] Sammer DM, Shin AY. Comparison of arthroscopic and open treatment of septic arthritis of the wrist. J Bone Joint Surg Am. 2009; 91 (6):1387–1393

[3] Palmer AK, Werner FW, Murphy D, Glisson R. Functional wrist motion: a biomechanical study. J Hand Surg Am. 1985; 10(1):39–46

[4] Mulford JS, Ceulemans LJ, Nam D, Axelrod TS. Proximal row carpectomy vs four corner fusion for scapholunate (Slac) or scaphoid nonunion advanced collapse (Snac) wrists: a systematic review of outcomes. J Hand Surg Eur Vol. 2009; 34(2):256–263

[5] Baur EM. Arthroscopic-assisted partial wrist arthrodesis. Hand Clin. 2017; 33(4):735–753

[6] Chedal-Bornu B, Corcella D, Forli A, Moutet F, Bouyer M. Long-term outcomes of proximal row carpectomy: a series of 62 cases. Hand Surg Rehabil. 2017; 36(5):355–362

[7] Wall LB, Didonna ML, Kiefhaber TR, Stern PJ. Proximal row carpectomy: minimum 20-year follow-up. J Hand Surg Am. 2013; 38 (8):1498–1504

[8] Del Piñal F. Editorial. I have a dream … reflex sympathetic dystrophy (RSD or Complex Regional Pain Syndrome-CRPS I) does not exist. J Hand Surg Eur Vol. 2013; 38(6):595–597

[9] Luchetti R, Soragni O, Fairplay T. Proximal row carpectomy through a palmar approach. J Hand Surg [Br]. 1998; 23(3):406–409

[10] Viegas SF, Patterson RM, Ward K, Ward K. Extrinsic wrist ligaments in the pathomechanics of ulnar translation instability. J Hand Surg Am. 1995; 20(2):312–318

[11] Bain GI, Munt J, Turner PC. New advances in wrist arthroscopy. Arthroscopy. 2008; 24(3):355–367

4

16 Management of Complications after Salvage Procedures of the Radiocarpal and Distal Radioulnar Joint

Michel E. H. Boeckstyns, Peter Axelsson, Marion Burnier, Guillaume Herzberg, and Marjolaine Walle

Abstract

Partial wrist arthrodeses are relatively common motion-preserving procedures in both patients with rheumatoid arthritis (RA) and in nonrheumatoid patients. However, nonunion is a rather frequent complication. Union after total wrist (TW) arthrodesis is more reliable but obviously connected with an important functional disability, especially in nonrheumatoid patients and in RA patients with bilateral wrist destruction. Persistent pain is a frequent problem in nonrheumatoid patients.

TW replacement is another motion-preserving salvage procedure. Osteolysis and prosthetic loosening is then a concern. Contraindications are patients with poor bone stock and poor bone quality, young and physically very active patients, patients with pronounced joint laxity, patients with spontaneously ankylotic wrists, and noncompliant patients.

Symptomatic ulnar instability after Darrach's or Sauvé-Kapandji's procedures for distal radioulnar joint (DRUJ) problems is relatively frequent. Several soft tissue procedures to reduce the symptoms have been described. Prosthetic hemi- or total replacement of the DRUJ can also be used, but the technique and the learning curve may be challenging.

Keywords: arthrodesis, partial arthrodesis, total arthrodesis, joint replacement, radiocarpal joint, wrist, distal radioulnar joint

16.1 Radiocarpal and Total Wrist Arthrodesis

16.1.1 Definition of the Problem

Partial radiocarpal arthrodesis and total wrist (TW) arthrodesis are relatively common procedures that may be performed in two very distinct groups of patients, i.e., rheumatoid arthritis (RA) or nonrheumatoid patients. A specific analysis of their complications is seldom published. However, knowledge of these potential complications is interesting not only for scientific purposes but also because there are alternative treatments for both procedures. Therefore, potential complications of partial/total wrist arthrodesis should be discussed with each patient in a comprehensive informed consent manner, should surgery be chosen for this particular patient.

Complications after Radiolunate and Radioscapholunate Arthrodesis

Nonunion and secondary deterioration of the midcarpal joint are the most frequently reported complications.

Radiolunate (RL) Arthrodesis

In *rheumatoid patients*, RL arthrodesis is traditionally performed as open surgery,[1] although the use of arthroscopy has recently been advocated.[2,3] A distal ulna resection or Sauvé-Kapandji's (S-K) procedure is often combined with RL arthrodesis.[1] The indication to perform these procedures in a patient having a stable medical treatment is a painful wrist with caput ulnae syndrome, sometimes rupture(s) of the extensor tendons, and a radiographic carpal anterior and ulnar slide with severe involvement of radiocarpal joint space and a relative preservation of the midcarpal joint.

In *nonrheumatoid patients*, RL arthrodesis is traditionally performed as open surgery,[4] although some authors may also consider the use of arthroscopy.[2] A distal ulna resection or S-K procedure may be combined with RL arthrodesis, but the ulnar head should be preserved, if possible, in most of the nonrheumatoid patients.[2] The most frequent indications are painful articular distal radius malunion and chronic posttraumatic ulnar translation of the carpus, which usually is the consequence of a failed treatment or missed radiocarpal dislocation. In the following, the most common complications are reviewed and discussed.

Reduced Wrist Mobility

Some limitation of wrist motion should be expected after any partial wrist arthrodesis.[5] This should not be considered as a complication provided that 20 to 40 degrees of painless active wrist extension is preserved, which corresponds to a functional wrist.

Nonunion

Borisch and Haussmann[6] reported on 91 RL arthrodeses for rheumatoid patients at a mean follow-up of 5 years. No nonunion was reported. There are very few reports of RL arthrodesis in nonrheumatoid patients. Saffar[4] reported on a series of 11 RL arthrodeses performed mainly for symptomatic malunion after distal radial fractures. Only one nonunion was reported, salvaged by a bone grafting revision.

Secondary Deterioration of the Midcarpal Joint

In the series by Borisch and Haussmann,[6] there was a 6% revision rate to TW arthrodesis for secondary midcarpal arthrosis or arthritic destruction. Four percent displacements or malpositioning of the osteosynthesis material were reported. Trieb[1] reported secondary deterioration of the midcarpal joint in about 40% in a long-term follow-up study. He mentioned that this complication should not necessarily be considered as a failure of this procedure. We share this opinion since we observed in our series a constant but very slow secondary degeneration of the midcarpal joint that was most often well tolerated in RA patients. Overall, the complication rate after RL arthrodesis for RA wrist is low.[6,7,8,9] In the series by Safar,[4] secondary osteoarthritis (OA) in adjacent joints was not reported. The ulnar head was preserved in 72% of the cases. We have the same experience. It is our opinion that maintaining the height of the radiolunate original joint (with a massive corticocancellous bone graft if necessary) is of paramount importance if the secondary degeneration of the radioscaphoid joint is to be avoided.

Radioscapholunate (RSL) arthrodesis

In *rheumatoid patients*, RSL arthrodesis is traditionally performed as open surgery, often in conjunction with resection of the ulnar head. The indication is the same as for RL arthrodesis in a patient with a more severely destroyed radioscaphoid joint space. There are very few reports of RSL arthrodesis in RA patients since the RL arthrodesis usually provides satisfactory results.

Reduced Wrist Mobility

Garcia Elias emphasized the usefulness of combining RSL arthrodesis with distal scaphoid excision in terms of flexion and radial deviation.[10] This was confirmed in subsequent series.[11,12,13,14]

Nonunion

Ishikawa et al[7] and Honkaken et al[15] reported on small series of RSL in RA patients with a 100% union rate and very few complications.

In *nonrheumatoid patients*, RSL arthrodesis follows the same indication as for RL arthrodesis when there is also destruction of the radioscaphoid joint space. The surgical approach is usually dorsal but an anterior approach has recently been recommended.[11]

Mühldorfer-Fodor et al[14] reported on 47 cases of RSL arthrodesis for *posttraumatic OA* at a mean follow-up of 2 years (20 with distal scaphoidectomy). There was a 20% nonunion rate in the group where distal scaphoidectomy was not performed. Distal scaphoidectomy appeared to lessen the risk of nonunion and to improve radial devia-

tion. Degeorge et al[12] reviewed 75 cases of RSL for posttraumatic OA at a mean of up to 9 years. RSL was performed alone in 33, with distal scaphoid excision in 26, and distal scaphoid excision with triquetrum excision in 16. Fifty-six percent had combined distal scaphoid excision. The nonunion rate was 42% after RSL without distal scaphoid excision and only 9% with distal scaphoid excision. They concluded that after resection of the distal scaphoid, there might be less stress on the radioscaphoid arthrodesis, resulting in a better healing rate.

Secondary Deterioration of the Midcarpal Joint

In the series by Mühldorfer-Fodor et al,[14] there was a 20% of secondary arthrosis in adjacent joints in both groups. In the series by Degeorge et al,[12] the rate of secondary midcarpal OA was 44%. This rate was not influenced by distal scaphoid excision.

Complications after Total Wrist Arthrodesis

Persistent pain and hardware irritation is a frequent problem in nonrheumatoid patients.

In *rheumatoid patients*, TW arthrodesis is most often performed using a Mannerfelt pin technique.[16,17] The results in terms of pain relief are usually very good as well as the union rate.[1] The postoperative disability due to a nonmobile wrist is not a complication per se.

Malpositioned Arthrodesis

Poor arthrodesis position should be considered as a complication since not enough extension impairs prehension in patients with already weakened fingers. Barbier et al[18] reported on 18 cases, with 44% presenting at follow-up with a wrist position in either slight flexion or less than 10 degrees of extension. The average position of TW arthrodesis was 8 degrees of extension and 9 degrees of ulnar deviation. Three patients would have preferred a more functional position.

Nonunion and Hardware Problems

Recently, Dréano et al[16] reported on a series of 19 cases. There were 1 nonunion, 21% painful prominence of hardware, and 21% pin migration or breakage. Kluge et al[17] reported on 93 cases using a modified Clayton-Mannerfelt technique with 2% nonunion, 3% prominence of hardware, and 2% third metacarpal fracture.

Overall, nonunion is very rare after TW arthrodesis but hardware problems do exist and should be minimized. We sometimes use multiple k-wire fixation in order to provide a tailored extension-ulnar deviation position and to minimize hardware problems.

4

In *nonrheumatoid* patients, TW arthrodesis is most often performed using a dorsal plating technique, although some authors are using less invasive hardware.[19,20] Several authors have emphasized that there may be significant complication rates after this procedure. This knowledge is useful when discussing with a patient the choice of TW arthrodesis versus TW replacement. Sauerbier et al[21] reported on 60 cases at a mean of 3 years follow-up with AO plate fixation. Sixty-two percent underwent surgery before TW arthrodesis. He found 95% with persistent pain and 8% of reoperations. De Smet and Truyen[22] reported on 36 cases at a mean of 7 years follow-up and fixation with AO plate and bone graft. There were 83% with persistent pain at follow-up and 58% reoperations.

16.1.2 Treatment of Complications: Nonunion and Hardware Problems

Failure of SL and RSL arthrodesis due to nonunion can in selected cases be salvaged by a new attempt to obtain union by performing revision of all fibrous tissue in the interosseous spaces, filling these with cancellous bone graft, and performing a stable internal fixation. However, often the solution will be to convert a partial arthrodesis to a TW arthrodesis. An alternative solution is conversion to a TW replacement. Reoperation of a failed TW arthrodesis will usually be a new TW arthrodesis as described for the partial arthrodeses.

In the case of pain due to hardware problems (nerve and tendon irritation or subcutaneous prominence of the fixation material), the advice is to remove the hardware after consolidation of the arthrodesis.

16.1.3 Rehabilitation

As a general rule, the wrist is immobilized in a cast or splint until bony union of the arthrodesis is radiographically ascertained. However, in low-demand RA patients the casting period may be a few weeks only (mainly to relieve postoperative pain). If a rigid and solid fixation of the arthrodesis is performed (usually plate and screw fixation), immobilization can be omitted in all compliant patients. If the bone is very osteoporotic, locking screws are recommended.

16.1.4 Tips and Tricks

- RSL arthrodesis in RA patients has a higher risk of nonunion and severe stiffness when compared with RL arthrodesis. RL arthrodesis is usually sufficient to stabilize an RA wrist.
- Because of the strong association with caput ulnae syndrome, stabilized distal ulnar head resection or S-K procedure is often combined with RL arthrodesis in RA patients. Ulnar head replacement is rarely indicated.

- RL arthrodesis is a reliable motion-preserving procedure in case of chronic ulnar translation of the carpus in nonrheumatoid patients, provided that the height of the carpus is preserved or restored.
- The addition of a resection of the distal pole of the scaphoid in RSL arthrodesis in nonrheumatoid patients has a positive influence on both bone healing and residual postoperative motion.

A TW replacement option (see next) should be discussed, especially in bilateral wrist destruction. However, TW arthrodesis is preferred in heavy manual workers and noncompliant patients.

16.2 Total and Interpositional Wrist Replacement

16.2.1 Definition of the Problem

Prosthetic wrist replacement is an alternative option for the treatment of painful destroyed wrists, mainly in older, low-demand patients. First-generation implants—silicone spacers—gave promising early results in RA patients but the long-term results were discouraging due to a high incidence of failure, mainly breakage of the implant.[23] The procedure has been abandoned in the wrist. The next generations consisted of bulky multicomponent implants, requiring substantial bony resection. Long-term implant survival has been deceiving.[24] The fourth-generation of implants was introduced in the late 1990s.[25] In the following, the most important complications are analyzed.

Early Postoperative Complications: Periprosthetic Infection and Instability

The incidence of early deep infection is less than 2% with current implant techniques and the use of perioperative antibiotics.[26,27] Clinical signs of an acute infection after TW replacement are pain, erythema, edema, prolonged postoperative wound effusion, or dehiscence. Serial blood tests including C-reactive protein (CRP) and white blood cell count confirm the diagnosis.

Instability with dislocation was common with the first version of the Universal implant (Integra, Plainsboro, NJ, USA) but this problem has been solved with the modified versions, the Universal 2 (Integra, Plainsboro, NJ, USA) and the Freedom (Integra, Plainsboro, NJ, USA), and has not been a major problem with the Re-motion (Stryker, Kalamazoo, MI, USA), the Maestro (Biomet, Warsaw, IN, USA), or the Motec (Swemac, Linköping, Sweden). Nevertheless, patient selection is of paramount importance and the severely destroyed unstable wrist or other conditions causing general joint laxity are still relative contraindications. A rheumatoid wrist stage 3 according to the Simmen classification (▶ Fig. 16.1) is considered a contraindication by many surgeons not only because of instability but also due to lack of bone stock.

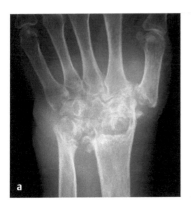 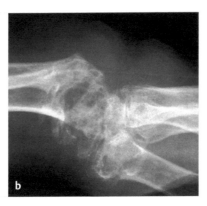

Fig. 16.1 (a, b) Severely unstable rheumatoid wrist (Simmen stage 3). Prosthetic replacement is generally considered contraindicated in this condition.

4

Rotational instability of the pyrocarbon interpositional replacement Amandys (Tornier SAS-Bioprofile Grenoble, France) has been reported.[28] When early postoperative dislocation occurs, it is usually caused by improper implant size or insufficient capsular reconstruction.

Late Complications: Osteolysis and Aseptic Prosthetic Loosening

Focal periprosthetic radiolucency after resurfacing replacement of the wrist, with or without frank loosening of the components, has repeatedly been reported.[29,30,31,32,33,34] Radiolucency is the radiographical sign of periprosthetic osteolysis. In most cases, it is confined to the part of the implant components located near the joint space and less than 2 mm in width. In some cases, the radiolucent area increases but this tends to stabilize after 1 to 3 years.[29] Implant loosening may be the result and it mainly affects the carpal component. Periprosthetic osteolysis without implant loosening is usually painless. The mechanism causing osteolysis is not clear but involves multiple factors, including micromotion, particulate debris-induced bone resorption, stress shielding, and increased intra-articular pressure. Implant survival rates vary considerably in the literature (▶ Table 16.1).

16.2.2 Treatment of Complications

Prosthetic Infection

Prosthetic infection requires resection of all infected tissue as soon as possible after diagnosis. The treatment should preferably be conducted by a team that is specialized in bone infections and will include removal of the implant and cement if this was used. Tissue samples for bacteriological investigation must be collected and antibiotic treatment initiated. Initially, broad-spectrum antimicrobial treatment is given and targeted therapy should follow as the causative agent is identified. An antibiotic spacer can be inserted if revision replacement is considered. However, implant survival after revision replacement is deceiving (see below). We recommend antibiotic

Table 16.1 Reported cumulative survival of latest generation implants

Publication	Implant survival	Type of implant	Rheumatoid disease (%)
Ferreres et al[35]	100% at 5 y	Universal 1	68
Sagerfors et al[36]	95% at 8 y	Maestro	81
	94% at 8 y	Remotion	78
	92% at 8 y	Universal 2	92
Boeckstyns et al[37]	90% at 9 y	Remotion	77
Chevrolier et al[38]	60% at 10 y	Remotion/ Universal 1	50
Ward et al[39]	40% at 10 y	Universal 1	100
Honecker et al[40]	69% at 10 y	Remotion	83
Pfanner et al[33]	64% at 12 y	Universal 2	100

treatment for at least 6 weeks and subsequent TW arthrodesis, provided there is no longer evidence of active infection. Antibiotic treatment is continued for a further 6 weeks after arthrodesis.

Instability

Dislocated TW replacement can usually be managed by closed reduction, but if there is an identifiable cause to the instability, such as wrong implant size or pronounced joint laxity, the risk of redislocation is high and surgical treatment is needed. Some cases can be solved by exchanging the polyethylene insert with a thicker one, and others by tightening or reconstructing the joint capsule. Instability of pyrocarbon interpositional replacement is often caused by a too large implant, and the problem can be solved by either changing to a smaller implant or deepening the carpal cavity. TW arthrodesis is the final solution for any recurrent instability. Conversely, preoperative ankylotic wrists tend to remain rather rigid after replacement.[37]

Osteolysis and Prosthetic Loosening

Narrow areas of radiolucency confined to the articulating extremity of the implant components should be no cause of concern. A broader but still limited radiolucency may look dramatic on radiographs and tempt the surgeon to revise and bone graft the osteolytic area, even if there is no pain (▶ Fig. 16.2). However, in the authors' experience, osteolysis will recur, and therefore it is recommended to follow asymptomatic patients carefully without taking action until implant loosening should occur. Painful osteolysis and loosened implant components require surgical action (▶ Fig. 16.3). In the situation of aseptic loosening of the carpal component alone, this component can be exchanged while preserving the radial component. When both components have loosened and an acceptable bone stock still is present, total prosthetic exchange can be an option. However, we must take into consideration that implant survival after revision is much less favorable than after primary replacement. TW arthrodesis as the alternative option must be discussed with the patient before a shared decision is made. In the case of metallosis, implant loosening must be considered to be due to a reaction to metallic debris. Seen in the light of the poor results after revision arthroplasty in general and of the favorable results after salvage arthrodesis, a new attempt to implant a prosthesis with metallic components seems not rational in this situation.

16.2.3 Rehabilitation

TW replacement is protected with a dorsal splint for 1 to 3 weeks with the wrist in 20 degrees of extension, after which unloaded mobilization of the wrist is initiated and

splinting continued intermittently. The elbow is immobilized when replacement is combined with any procedure on the distal radioulnar joint (DRUJ). After 6 weeks,

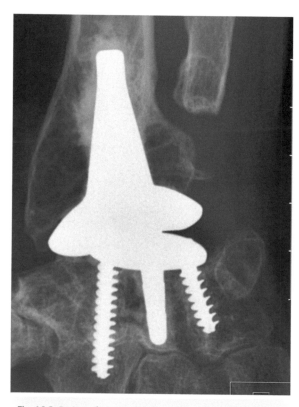

Fig. 16.2 Periprosthetic osteolysis. In this case, the condition was painless and the implant components had not subsided. The exact cause of osteolysis is not clearly known but is probably multifactorial. Surgical intervention is not indicated but close observation is recommended.

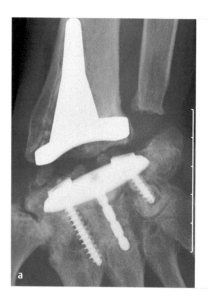
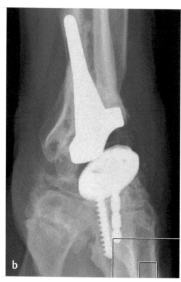

Fig. 16.3 (a, b) Subsidence of the implant components resulting in severe pain. A salvage procedure is needed: implant extraction and arthrodesis or revision arthroplasty.

osseointegration of the implants is expected to have taken place and splinting is discontinued.

16.2.4 Tips and Tricks

- As for any implant management, preoperative adminis- tration of antibiotics before joint replacement is impor- tant but the available evidence does not show added benefit of postoperative antibiotic prophylaxis or con- tinuation beyond 24 hours.[41]
- Owing to scarce and limited literature, there are major limitations to recommending the discontinuation of disease-modifying antirheumatic drugs. Methotrexate is by far the best studied conventional synthetic dis- ease-modifying antirheumatic drug and it seems rea- sonable to continue administering methotrexate during the perioperative period.[42] However, there is no con- sensus on this recommendation among rheumatolo- gists.
- In order to avoid postoperative instability, carefully test the tension and stability of the prosthetic wrist at the end of the operation and, if necessary, adjust it by inserting a thicker implant (if too loose) or by resecting more bone (if too tight).
- Select your patients thoughtfully. Contraindications are patients with poor bone stock and poor bone quality, young and physically very active patients, patients with pronounced joint laxity, patients with spontaneously ankylotic wrists, and patients that are not compliant.

16.3 The Distal Radioulnar Joint

16.3.1 Definition of the Problem

Ulnar Instability after Ulnar Head Resection (Darrach's Procedure) and Arthrodesis of the DRUJ Combined with Ulnar Metaphyseal Pseudarthrosis (Sauvé-Kapandji's Procedure)

Soft tissue stabilizers, including the triangular fibrocarti- lage complex (TFCC), the pronator quadratus muscle, the subsheath of the sixth compartment, and interosseous membrane, all contribute to the stability of the DRUJ while the bony geometry offers little support. Darrach's procedure is the most commonly performed operation for painful DRUJ degeneration, especially in rheumatoid patients, but it removes the ulnar bony support of the carpus, which eliminates the efficiency of all the stabiliz- ing soft tissues, leaving the ulnar stump unstable. As a result, convergence and impingement of the radius and the ulna occur during forearm loading and rotation (▶ Fig. 16.4). Instability is experienced by up to 60% of the patients.[43] In elderly, low-demand patients this usually is well tolerated but for younger, active people it may cause painful clicking. After the S-K procedure, the risk of ulnar

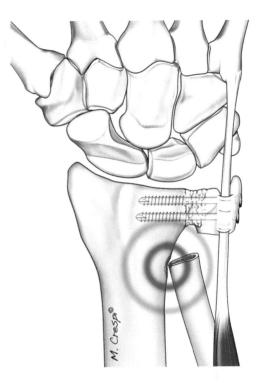

Fig. 16.4 Convergence and painful impingement of the radius and the ulna after the Sauvé-Kapandji's procedure.

translation of the carpus is reduced, but radioulnar impingement is still a problem. Although the S-K proce- dure is thought to be more appropriate for posttraumatic cases in younger, high-demand patients, the evidence for this assumption is weak.[44]

Instability after DRUJ Replacement

Prosthetic replacement of the DRUJ includes hemire- placement (partial- or total ulnar head replacement) and total joint replacement, which also replaces the articular surface of the sigmoid notch. DRUJ replacements were initially used as salvage procedures after failed ulnar head resections and S-K procedures but are now frequently used as primary procedures.

Total ulnar head replacement involves complete replacement of the ulnar head with a stemmed implant. Clinically relevant instability is rare[45,46] and can usually be avoided by careful patient selection and soft tissue handling. Malalignment after distal radius fractures, gross instability of the DRUJ after injury of the TFCC, and weak soft tissues after multiple procedures or inflammatory arthritis are relative contraindications.

Conversely, implant instability is not a concern when using a total DRUJ implant like the APTIS (Aptis medical, Louisville, KY, USA) as it is of a constrained design that also replaces the function of the soft tissue restraints.

4

Infection, Aseptic Loosening, and Implant Durability after DRUJ Replacement

The incidence of deep infection after DRUJ replacement is low and similar to that after TW replacement. According to reports and our experience, the rate of aseptic implant loosening using today's implants is low, if a properly sized implant stem is used.[45,46,47] Most series report an implant survival equal to or greater than 95% at 5 years for the implants currently available.[45] Likely, the reason is that the DRUJ is protected by the muscular dynamics during forearm loading. Furthermore, regarding the APTIS, the large degree of freedom of motion and the longer stem that widely transmits the load along the implant-bone interphase play a role.

16.3.2 Treatment of Complications

Distal Ulnar Instability after Resection and the Sauvé-Kapandji's Procedure

Several soft tissue procedures have been described to reduce ulnar instability, including extensor carpi ulnaris and/or flexor carpi ulnaris tenodesis (▶ Fig. 16.5), sometimes combined with soft tissue interposition, such as the pronator quadratus muscle. These stabilizing procedures can be used primarily or as an attempt to address radio-ulnar impingement as a salvage operation. If the problem persists, prosthetic replacement is to be considered.

Instability after Ulnar Head Replacement

Instability of the DRUJ may be asymptomatic but if painful, stability must be restored. Exchange to a larger head together with tightening and reinforcement of the joint capsule, with the extensor retinaculum, can be the solu-

tion. If the constraining soft tissues are insufficient, the brachioradialis wraparound technique or a revision to a total DRUJ implant is indicated (▶ Fig. 16.6).

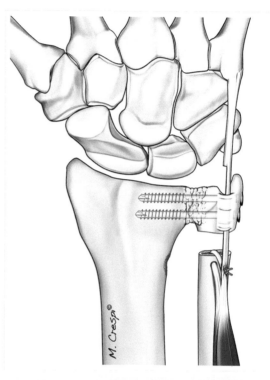

Fig. 16.5 Tenodesis for ulnar instability after the Sauvé-Kapandji's procedure. In this case, a dynamic proximal tenodesis is shown. When loading the forearm, the extensor carpi ulnaris muscle tends to pull the ulna away from the radius.

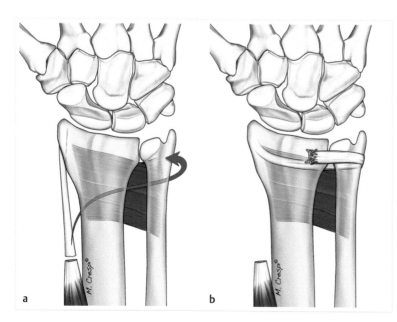

a   b

Fig. 16.6 (a, b) The brachioradialis wraparound procedure for stabilizing an ulnar head prosthesis.

Aseptic Loosening

If the ulnar stem of an ulnar head or total DRUJ prosthesis has loosened, revision of the stem, perhaps to a larger size, with bone grafting or bone cement must first be considered. If needed, revision of an ulnar head prosthesis to a total DRUJ implant can be performed.

However, if the radial component of a total DRUJ implant has loosened, there is little chance of successful immediate replacement of this component. In these cases, explantation of the prosthesis and ultimately proximal radioulnar arthrodesis creating a one-bone forearm may be the result.

Infection

Treatment of ulnar head implant infection is similar to the treatment of radiocarpal implant infection described above.

16.3.3 Tips and Tricks

- To avoid complications related to DRUJ replacement, meticulous adherence to technical recommendations is important, especially for the APTIS implant.

- When performing an ulnar head replacement, careful attention should be given to ulnar head sizing and tightening of the surrounding soft tissues. Oversizing should be avoided as a too big head might dislocate immediately or later after stretching of the soft tissues. A too small head can easily be changed if needed. If the sigmoid notch is deformed or flat, it can be contoured or deepened with a burr. If full stability is not achieved at the end of the procedure, we recommend to leave the implant in place and use a stricter rehabilitation program as even unstable implant might be asymptomatic.
- Take care not to place the ulnar head too distally in order to avoid impaction on the carpus.
- If only the radial component of a total DRUJ implant has loosened, simultaneous removal of the ulnar stem is a major undertaking (▶ Fig. 16.7). We recommend to leave it in place, since our experience is that this might be well tolerated. If necessary, it could be removed at a later time or possibly used for another attempt with a radial component.

16.4 Take-Home Message

The incidence of nonunion after partial wrist arthrodesis is relatively high. Persistent pain after TW arthrodesis is

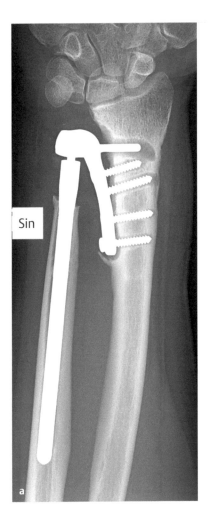
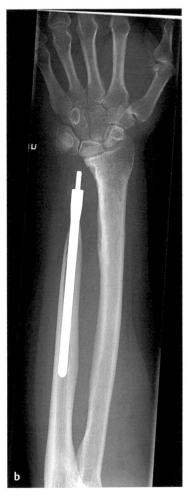

Fig. 16.7 (a, b) Loosening of the radial component of an Aptis prosthesis. The ulnar component is solidly osseointegrated. In this condition, removal of the radial component alone is recommended as a first attempt since the result will be well tolerated by many patients. Removal of an osseointegrated ulnar implant requires an extensive ulnar osteotomy.

4

frequent in nonrheumatoid patients. Young age, poor bone stock, high demands, and poor compliance contraindicate TW replacement due to the risk of aseptic prosthetic loosening. Distal ulnar instability is frequent after DRUJ resection arthroplasties. DRUJ replacements can solve this problem, but these techniques may be challenging to learn.

References

[1] Trieb K. Treatment of the wrist in rheumatoid arthritis. J Hand Surg Am. 2008; 33(1):113–123

[2] Ho PC. Arthroscopic partial wrist fusion. Tech Hand Up Extrem Surg. 2008; 12(4):242–265

[3] McGuire DT, Bain GI. Radioscapholunate fusions. J Wrist Surg. 2012; 1(2):135–140

[4] Saffar P. Radiolunate arthrodesis. In: Watson HK, Weinzweig J, eds. The wrist. Philadelphia: Lippincott, Williams & Wilkins; 2001:867–874

[5] Calfee RP, Leventhal EL, Wilkerson J, Moore DC, Akelman E, Crisco JJ. Simulated radioscapholunate fusion alters carpal kinematics while preserving dart-thrower's motion. J Hand Surg Am. 2008; 33(4):503–510

[6] Borisch N, Haussmann P. Radiolunate arthrodesis in the rheumatoid wrist: a retrospective clinical and radiological long-term follow-up. J Hand Surg Am. 2002; 27(1):61–72

[7] Ishikawa H, Murasawa A, Nakazono K. Long-term follow-up study of radiocarpal arthrodesis for the rheumatoid wrist. J Hand Surg Am. 2005; 30(4):658–666

[8] Motomiya M, Iwasaki N, Minami A, Matsui Y, Urita A, Funakoshi T. Clinical and radiological results of radiolunate arthrodesis for rheumatoid arthritis: 22 wrists followed for an average of 7 years. J Hand Surg Am. 2013; 38(8):1484–1491

[9] Raven EE, Ottink KD, Doets KC. Radiolunate and radioscapholunate arthrodeses as treatments for rheumatoid and psoriatic arthritis: long-term follow-up. J Hand Surg Am. 2012; 37(1):55–62

[10] Garcia-Elias M, Lluch A, Ferreres A, Papini-Zorli I, Rahimtoola ZO. Treatment of radiocarpal degenerative osteoarthritis by radioscapholunate arthrodesis and distal scaphoidectomy. J Hand Surg Am. 2005; 30(1):8–15

[11] Quadlbauer S, Leixnering M, Jurkowitsch J, Hausner T, Pezzei C. Volar radioscapholunate arthrodesis and distal scaphoidectomy after malunited distal radius fractures. J Hand Surg Am. 2017; 42(9):754.e1–754.e8

[12] Degeorge B, Montoya-Faivre D, Dap F, Dautel G, Coulet B, Chammas M. Radioscapholunate fusion for radiocarpal osteoarthritis: prognostic factors of clinical and radiographic outcomes. J Wrist Surg. 2019; 8(6):456–462

[13] Montoya-Faivre D, Pomares G, Calafat V, Dap F, Dautel G. Clinical and radiological outcomes following radioscapholunate fusion. Orthop Traumatol Surg Res. 2017; 103(7):1093–1098

[14] Mühldorfer-Fodor M, Ha HP, Hohendorff B, Löw S, Prommersberger KJ, van Schoonhoven J. Results after radioscapholunate arthrodesis with or without resection of the distal scaphoid pole. J Hand Surg Am. 2012; 37(11):2233–2239

[15] Honkanen PB, Mäkelä S, Konttinen YT, Lehto MU. Radiocarpal arthrodesis in the treatment of the rheumatoid wrist: a prospective midterm follow-up. J Hand Surg Eur Vol. 2007; 32(4):368–376

[16] Dréano T, Bouillis J, Ropars M. [Evaluation of a technical modification to Mannerfelt's total wrist fusion technique in a series of 19 rheumatoid wrists]. Chir Main. 2014; 33(5):344–349

[17] Kluge S, Schindele S, Henkel T, Herren D. The modified Clayton-Mannerfelt arthrodesis of the wrist in rheumatoid arthritis: operative technique and report on 93 cases. J Hand Surg Am. 2013; 38(5):999–1005

[18] Barbier O, Saels P, Rombouts JJ, Thonnard JL. Long-term functional results of wrist arthrodesis in rheumatoid arthritis. J Hand Surg [Br]. 1999; 24(1):27–31

[19] Orbay JL, Feliciano E, Orbay C. Locked intramedullary total wrist arthrodesis. J Wrist Surg. 2012; 1(2):179–184

[20] Rancy SK, Ek ET, Paul S, Hotchkiss RN, Wolfe SW. Nonspanning total wrist arthrodesis with a low-profile locking plate. J Wrist Surg. 2018; 7(2):127–132

[21] Sauerbier M, Kluge S, Bickert B, Germann G. Subjective and objective outcomes after total wrist arthrodesis in patients with radiocarpal arthrosis or Kienböck's disease. Chir Main. 2000; 19(4):223–231

[22] De Smet L, Truyen J. Arthrodesis of the wrist for osteoarthritis: outcome with a minimum follow-up of 4 years. J Hand Surg [Br]. 2003; 28(6):575–577

[23] Brase DW, Millender LH. Failure of silicone rubber wrist arthroplasty in rheumatoid arthritis. J Hand Surg Am. 1986; 11(2):175–183

[24] Cooney WP, III, Beckenbaugh RD, Linscheid RL. Total wrist arthroplasty: problems with implant failures. Clin Orthop Relat Res. 1984 (187):121–128

[25] Menon J. Universal total wrist implant: experience with a carpal component fixed with three screws. J Arthroplasty. 1998; 13(5):515–523

[26] Berber O, Garagnani L, Gidwani S. Systematic review of total wrist arthroplasty and arthrodesis in wrist arthritis. J Wrist Surg. 2018; 7(5):424–440

[27] Herzberg G, Boeckstyns M, Sorensen AI, et al. "Remotion" total wrist arthroplasty: preliminary results of a prospective international multicenter study of 215 cases. J Wrist Surg. 2012; 1(1):17–22

[28] Bellemère P, Maes-Clavier C, Loubersac T, Gaisne E, Kerjean Y. Amandys(®) implant: novel pyrocarbon arthroplasty for the wrist. Chir Main. 2012; 31(4):176–187

[29] Boeckstyns MEH, Herzberg G. Periprosthetic osteolysis after total wrist arthroplasty. J Wrist Surg. 2014; 3(2):101–106

[30] Cobb TK, Beckenbaugh RD. Biaxial total-wrist arthroplasty. J Hand Surg Am. 1996; 21(6):1011–1021

[31] Badge R, Kailash K, Dickson DR, et al. Medium-term outcomes of the Universal-2 total wrist arthroplasty in patients with rheumatoid arthritis. Bone Joint J. 2016; 98-B(12):1642–1647

[32] Kennedy JW, Ross A, Wright J, Martin DJ, Bransby-Zachary M, MacDonald DJ. Universal 2 total wrist arthroplasty: high satisfaction but high complication rates. J Hand Surg Eur Vol. 2018; 43(4):375–379

[33] Pfanner S, Munz G, Guidi G, Ceruso M. Universal 2 wrist arthroplasty in rheumatoid arthritis. J Wrist Surg. 2017; 6(3):206–215

[34] Reigstad O, Holm-Glad T, Bolstad B, Grimsgaard C, Thorkildsen R, Røkkum M. Five- to 10-year prospective follow-up of wrist arthroplasty in 56 nonrheumatoid patients. J Hand Surg Am. 2017; 42(10):788–796

[35] Ferreres A, Lluch A, Del Valle M. Universal total wrist arthroplasty: midterm follow-up study. J Hand Surg Am. 2011; 36(6):967–973

[36] Sagerfors M, Gupta A, Brus O, Pettersson K. Total wrist arthroplasty: a single-center study of 219 cases with 5-year follow-up. J Hand Surg Am. 2015; 40(12):2380–2387

[37] Boeckstyns ME, Herzberg G, Merser S. Favorable results after total wrist arthroplasty: 65 wrists in 60 patients followed for 5–9 years. Acta Orthop. 2013; 84(4):415–419

[38] Chevrollier J, Strugarek-Lecoanet C, Dap F, Dautel G. Results of a unicentric series of 15 wrist prosthesis implantations at a 5.2 year follow-up. Acta Orthop Belg. 2016; 82(1):31–42

[39] Ward CM, Kuhl T, Adams BD. Five to ten-year outcomes of the Universal total wrist arthroplasty in patients with rheumatoid arthritis. J Bone Joint Surg Am. 2011; 93(10):914–919

[40] Honecker S, Igeta Y, Al Hefzi A, Pizza C, Facca S, Liverneaux PA. Survival rate on a 10-year follow-up of total wrist replacement implants: a 23-patient case series. J Wrist Surg. 2019; 8(1):24–29

[41] Siddiqi A, Forte SA, Docter S, Bryant D, Sheth NP, Chen AF. Perioperative antibiotic prophylaxis in total joint arthroplasty: a systematic review and meta-analysis. J Bone Joint Surg Am. 2019; 101(9):828–842

[42] Fleury G, Mania S, Hannouche D, Gabay C. The perioperative use of synthetic and biological disease-modifying antirheumatic drugs in patients with rheumatoid arthritis. Swiss Med Wkly. 2017; 147: w14563

[43] Minami A, Iwasaki N, Ishikawa J, Suenaga N, Yasuda K, Kato H. Treatments of osteoarthritis of the distal radioulnar joint: long-term results of three procedures. Hand Surg. 2005; 10(2–3):243–248

[44] Verhiel SHWL, Özkan S, Ritt MJPF, Chen NC, Eberlin KR. A comparative study between Darrach and Sauvé-Kapandji procedures for post-traumatic distal radioulnar joint dysfunction. Hand (N Y). 2019; •••:1558944719855447

[45] Moulton LS, Giddins GEB. Distal radio-ulnar implant arthroplasty: a systematic review. J Hand Surg Eur Vol. 2017; 42(8):827–838

[46] Calcagni M, Giesen T. Distal radioulnar joint arthroplasty with implants: a systematic review. EFORT Open Rev. 2017; 1(5):191–196

[47] Axelsson P, Sollerman C, Kärrholm J. Ulnar head replacement: 21 cases; mean follow-up, 7.5 years. J Hand Surg Am. 2015; 40(9):1731–1738

4

Section 5

Ligament Surgery

17 Management of Complications of Ligament Repair of Thumb and Finger Joints

Mike Ruettermann

Abstract

The complications of surgical treatment of the most common and functionally critical ligamentous injuries of the thumb and fingers are described in chronological order (short-, mid-, and long-term complications). Conservative and operative management options of these complications are explained. The ulnar collateral ligament (UCL) of the thumb is the most affected ligament. The radial collateral ligament (RCL) of the thumb and the volar plate of the proximal interphalangeal (PIP) joints of the fingers are injured less often.

Iatrogenic nerve injury, wound healing problems, and wound infections, including osteomyelitis, can occur in the short term after operative treatment. Mid-term complications comprise nerve compression due to scarring, stiffness, and persistent instability of the joint. Long-term recurrence of instability after months or years of intensive use after a successful primary repair is a possible complication and does resemble chronic gamekeeper's thumb. Chronic pain is mostly caused by cartilage damage.

An easily reproducible pull-out tendon graft technique for secondary RCL as well as UCL reconstruction for the metacarpophalangeal (MCP) joint of the thumb is presented. With slight modifications regarding the soft tissue dissection, this pull-out tendon graft technique can also be used for severe instabilities of PIP joints.

The most common complications of volar plate injuries and their conservative and surgical treatments are stiffness and instability, leading to subluxation and in the long run secondary arthritis.

Diagnostic pearls are presented as well as technical tips. Foreign body materials, like bone anchors, interference, or locking screws, are discussed regarding their value in secondary cases. Finally, differential indications for secondary surgery with regard to specific joints are detailed.

Keywords: complications, radial/ulnar collateral ligament repair, stiffness/instability MCP/PIP/DIP joint, subluxation thumb/finger joint

17.1 Introduction

The primary treatment of injuries of ligament lesions of the small joints of the thumb and fingers, such as metacarpophalangeal (MCP), proximal, and distal interphalangeal (PIP and DIP) joints, is in most cases nonoperative, especially when there is no extensive instability: less than 30 degrees of laxity or less than 20 degrees more laxity compared to the contralateral side with a discrete end point to

the joint opening. Also, volar plate injury is mostly treated nonoperatively, unless there is gross instability.

The nonoperative treatment is generally done by splinting or buddy taping, ideally without immobilizing other joints that are not affected. For volar plate injuries, a dorsal extension block is added in cases of dorsal subluxation. For the ulnar collateral ligament (UCL) lesion of the MCP joint of the thumb, a Stener lesion[1] has to be ruled out because the retracted part cannot heal. Stability of the UCL should be tested in 40 degrees of flexion, as, otherwise, the volar plate will stabilize the joint such that a relevant lesion of the collateral ligament could be missed clinically.[2] A Stener lesion is possible in case of complete UCL injuries of the MCP joint of the thumb, without a clinical end point on valgus stress. It needs to be ruled out by ultrasound or magnetic resonance imaging (MRI) if one does not operate anyway. Nonoperative treatment will not lead to sufficient healing and stability if the distally avulsed ligament is retracted behind the adductor aponeurosis like in a Stener lesion. The distally avulsed ligament cannot get into contact with its insertion at the base of the proximal phalanx without surgical readaptation.

17.2 Indications for Surgery

If nonoperative treatment does not lead to sufficient stability or there is extensive instability including (sub) luxation in the first place, surgery is indicated. Other indications for primary surgical repairs are an open injury or the Stener lesion as mentioned above. Bony ligament avulsions, which include a relevant part of the joint surface and lead to instability of the joint, should be treated as fractures. Reposition and fixation of a significant bony fragment will correct the joint instability.

Surgical repair of the ligamentous injury is either done by suturing of the ligaments in cases of intrasubstance injuries, which are rare, or by reattachment of the ligament with or without a bony fragment at the side of the bony fracture. This is the distal attachment at the base of the proximal phalanx in the majority of cases.

In volar plate injuries of the PIP joints, there is mostly no need to fix a bony fragment, unless it is a relevant part of the joint surface and would be classified as a fracture rather than a volar plate lesion.[3] In cases of severe luxation with significant instability or patient incompliance with regard to postoperative immobilization, temporary fixation of the joint with a K-wire may be indicated.

This chapter deals with the management of complications of surgical ligament repair of thumb and finger joints. Fractures, as well as dislocations caused by a fracture, are beyond the scope of this chapter and are discussed in Chapter 7.

Most injuries happen to the stable hinge joints, like the PIP joints, in the form of dislocations caused by hyperextension due to a ball striking a fingertip. These dislocations can be dorsal, lateral, or volar, and most of them can be treated nonoperatively. UCL lesions of the thumb are ten times more common than radial collateral ligament (RCL) injuries.[4]

Notwithstanding which ligament of which joint has to be treated, complications can be classified according to when they appear postoperatively as short-, medium-, and long-term complications.

17.2.1 Short-Term Complications and Their Treatment

These can affect tissues in the anatomical area of the procedure and resemble general hand surgery complications.

Intraoperative complications like iatrogenic *nerve injury* of the branch of the dorsal radial superficial nerve on the dorsoulnar side of the thumb, for example, should ideally be noticed immediately and microsurgically repaired directly. This is also important in cases of injuries of palmar finger nerves during repairs of ligaments or volar plates.

Postoperative *hematomas* or *wound healing problems* should be treated accordingly if they have a relevant extend.

Wound infections can be overcome by rest and topical antiseptic treatment if detected early. In advanced infection, debridement and antibiotic treatment may be necessary. Special care must be taken when K-wires have been used for temporary fixation of the joint. If there is any risk of *osteomyelitis*, the hardware needs to be removed and the osteomyelitis treated. If this complication is not taken seriously and treated accordingly, the joint will get infected, leading to long-term complications with joint damage resulting in pain, stiffness, etc.

Nerve compression due to scarring can occur in the course of wound healing, especially after wound healing problems, hematomas, or wound infections. In most cases, conservative scar treatment with massage and silicone application solves the problem. In persistent cases, corticosteroid injections into the scarred area might help; otherwise, surgical neurolysis is indicated.

Missed *sharp nerve injuries* require microsurgical repair or proximal resection and translocation in muscle or bone. If direct repair is feasible after resection of the neuroma, it should be done. In case of defect with a distance, the approach should be based on the anatomical location and the patient's wishes. A detailed discussion of the options with the patient and informed consent are mandatory in these cases.

The approach with the best cost-benefit ratio for the patient should be chosen.

If, for example, direct repair of the distal dorsoulnar branch of the thumb, which comes of the superficial radial nerve, is not feasible, it should be denervated proximally. For an injury of the palmar ulnar digital nerve of the thumb, microsurgical interposition of a nerve graft is indicated if the thumb is otherwise functional.

17.2.2 Mid-Term Complications and Their Treatment

After healing of the ligament repair in a cast or splint, there is frequently *stiffness*, which generally can be improved by exercises and hand therapy. Additionally, dynamic splints may lead to further improvement of the range of motion.

If these measures do not lead to a sufficient function, and there is no further progress, surgical revision may be indicated if the patient is motivated.

Depending on the primary injury, especially on which other structures, such as flexor or extensor tendons, have been affected, there needs to be a precise evaluation of the problem.

In cases of a passively mobile joint with limited active flexion or extension, tenolysis of the extensor or flexor tendon, respectively, could be the next step. This should be done after complete maturation of the scar tissues. Beforehand a corticosteroid injection could be given if the area of the scarring can clinically be identified.

A surgical revision in wide-awake local anesthesia without tourniquet (WALANT) is helpful, as the results can be actively verified during the procedure.

If the tendons are gliding, but the joint itself is contracted despite consequent hand therapy and dynamic splinting, a surgical approach with stepwise arthrolysis is an option. The long-term results of arthrolysis, especially of the PIP joints, are less predictable than those of tenolysis.

The most important mid-term complication is *persistent instability of the joint* due to insufficient primary repair/healing. This can be caused not only by short-term complications, like infection, but also by inadequate quality of the remnants of the ligament in cases of direct suturing of intrasubstance lesions.

Insufficient healing to the periosteum in cases of a distal avulsion can also cause this problem, which happens if a Stener lesion is treated conservatively.

Another reason may be the formation of a pseudarthrosis when a small bony fragment fixed at the repair site is not healed. This might happen if the bone part is fixed in malposition; it is rotated in a way that the cortical bone or the joint surface is in contact with the cancellous bone at the fracture site. Secondary fixation can be considered, but this is a technically demanding procedure as the bony fragment is often small, but needs to be debrided, repositioned, and fixed adequately. Since that is not feasible in many cases, excision of the small bone fragment and reinsertion or reconstruction of the ligament are advisable.

In most cases of failed primary surgical repair of a collateral ligament, there are not sufficient remnants of the ligament in a secondary procedure. Often a reconstruction with an augmentation or replacement graft is necessary.

An exception to this is an insufficient distal repair, in which no bone anchor has been used so far. This permits the use of a bone anchor with attached sutures to fix the remnant of the ligament with a reasonable chance of success.

However, in most cases a reconstruction with a graft is necessary. The reference standard graft is the palmaris longus tendon if this is available. Another option is a graft taken from the flexor carpi radialis tendon, mostly as a partial lengthwise split. Other tendons can be used, too, but this has to be weighed up against the downsides of the specific donor-site morbidity. Alternatively, a piece of extensor retinaculum can be used as a graft for augmentation of the ligament's remnants but is not easy to harvest or handle as a pull-out graft. Other options are artificial grafts that are available as ligament augmentation. Their use has to be weighed against the extra costs and possible reaction to foreign body material.

An example of a secondary collateral ligament reconstruction with a palmaris longus tendon graft for the UCL of the MCP joint of the thumb is described in detail below.

Complications of Volar Plate Injuries

Most volar plate injuries of the MCP and PIP joints are treated conservatively in the first place. If closed reposition is not feasible, open reposition is performed. The most common complications of conservative and surgical treatment are *stiffness and instability*, leading to *subluxation* which subsequently could lead to *osteoarthritis*.

Stiffness is treated with hand therapy and dynamic splinting. If there is a remaining functional flexion contracture without arthritic changes in the joint, an arthrolysis is indicated in a motivated patient. This is ideally done via mid-axial incisions. A stepwise approach with a release of the collateral ligaments, the checkrein ligaments, and the proximal part of the volar plate is the method of choice. The joint should be straight at the end of the procedure without a tendency to spontaneous flexion. Otherwise, more extensive dissection of remaining adhesions is needed. Instability is hardly ever seen; recurrent flexion contracture is more likely.

Consequent exercises and splinting are mandatory after arthrolysis.

Instability with dorsal luxation can be treated by reinsertion of the volar plate, for which one or two suture-bone anchors can be used. With these, the proximal part of the volar plate can be fixed to the head of the proximal phalanx in most cases. An additional K-wire for temporary fixation of the joint protects the repair. It can be removed after about 4 weeks. Dorsal splinting to prevent reluxation should be continued until the volar plate has healed, at least 8 weeks in cases of complete instability.

17.2.3 Long-Term Complications and Their Treatment

A *recurrence of instability* after months or years with intensive use after a successful primary repair does resemble chronic gamekeeper's thumb. It can be treated like persistent instability of the joint.

If *chronic pain* develops over time, this is mostly caused by cartilage damage. Pain progresses faster in cases where the ligament repair is not stable enough and leads to laxity and subluxation of the joint with consequent accelerated cartilage damage. Treatment is the same as for any other form of posttraumatic osteoarthritis.

If conservative treatment does not provide sufficient relief, surgery is indicated.

If the pain due to cartilage damage is not yet severe and persistent, a ligament reconstruction could be performed. Arthrodesis is the most promising option regarding pain relief, as arthroplasty in joints with already injured collateral ligaments results in more complications.[5] Depending on the affected joint, arthrodesis can be performed with K-wires, cerclages, screws, or plates. But not all patients are happy with an arthrodesis of, for example, their thumb MCP joint as this can lead to difficulties with one or more specific activities, especially in young, more demanding patients. Adequate preoperative information and realistic expectations are essential.[6]

In joints that are less prone to strain, like the PIP joints of the ring- and little finger, arthroplasty is an alternative. (Especially new generation) Silicone spacers do have some intrinsic stability and can be used, but the results in posttraumatic cases with ligament injuries are less rewarding and lasting than those in primary arthritis.

17.3 Operative Technique

17.3.1 Preferred Method of Secondary Ligament Reconstruction of the Radial/Ulnar Collateral Ligament of the Thumb MCP Joint

Multiple methods of repair of the collateral ligaments of the MCP of the thumb have been described, but none has been shown to be superior.[7] The original method described by Littler's group[8] is technically demanding. It makes it difficult to precisely place the distal tunnel, which is important with regard to joint movement.[9]

An alternative method is a pull-through tendon graft with two oblique transverse tunnels: one in the distal first metacarpal and one in the base of the proximal phalanx of the thumb (▶ Fig. 17.1).

The old scar can mostly be used as incision. If needed, this can be extended proximally or distally. Special care is taken to carefully dissect and protect the branch of the

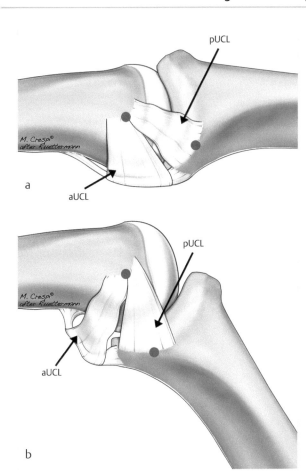

Fig. 17.1 Normal ulnar collateral ligament complex (view of the thumb metacarpophalangeal joint from the ulnar side): **(a)** in extension, **(b)** in flexion. pUCL = proper ulnar collateral ligament (tight in flexion with a maximum around 40 degrees) and aUCL = accessory ulnar collateral ligament (tight in extension). *Red dots*: the ideal position of the bone tunnels for the pull-out tendon graft.

superficial radial nerve. The extensor hood has to be dissected, and its components identified, which mostly is cumbersome as there is scarring from the previous procedure. For UCL reconstruction, the adductor tendon in the extensor hood has to be opened longitudinally and the capsule of the MCP joint opened, with the preference to use the same access as the previous operation, if this can be identified. In an RCL repair, there is of course no adductor tendon.

Structurally stable tissue components should be kept to be readapted as an augmentation to the tendon graft, but soft scar tissue has to be debrided. If nonabsorbable sutures have been used before, these should be removed. A bone anchor may stay in place, as long as it does not interfere with drilling the tunnels. An interference screw is often an obstacle for the ideal position of the tunnels and needs to be removed.

Identifying the proximal and distal stumps of the collateral ligament as well as the accessory collateral ligament is frequently difficult. Viable tissue should be kept to be fixed to the tendon graft, ideally in its original fiber direction, which avoids tensioning of the capsule–ligament complex in the wrong direction.

The joint surface is inspected to verify that there is no relevant cartilage damage. The joint is irrigated and mobility, as well as stability and subluxation, need to be assessed. If there is any stiffness, this should be taken care of by further dissection by opening the recessus of the MCP joint capsule with a blunt instrument.

Then a tunnel is drilled from ulnar to radial at the midpoint of the origin of the UCL complex at the head of the first metacarpal. A second one is drilled at the insertion of the proper UCL at the base of the proximal phalanx of the thumb. The tunnels are converging to increase the stability of the tendon graft. Special care is taken to place the tunnel away from the concavity of the joint surface of the proximal phalanx base to avoid cartilage damage (▶ Fig. 17.2).

A palmaris longus tendon graft is harvested through a transverse incision in the distal carpal line with the help of a tendon stripper. Care must be taken to protect the median nerve. If the surgeon is not experienced in this technique or encounters any difficulty, it is advisable to harvest the graft via multiple transverse incisions instead of one.

The length of the graft is adapted so that it has the optimal length for passing through both bone tunnels from drill hole to drill hole. This can be simulated by placing the graft on top of the thumb. The graft is made a little bit shorter because it needs to be tensioned. If the graft is thin, it can be folded in half so that two times the thickness of the graft is used; mostly the length is sufficient to do so. Then the tendon graft is armed with, for example, 3–0 slow resorbable sutures on a straight needle in a Bunnell fashion on both ends, grasping at least one centimeter of each tendon end. With these sutures, the graft is pulled through the drill holes and brought out through the skin on the other side, dorsal to the line of the midlateral approach to the thumb to avoid nerve injury. If no straight needle is available, this maneuver can be carried out by using a cannula through which the sutures are passed. After that, the graft is pulled into the tunnels and tensioned by pulling the sutures through the skin on the opposite side.

Adequate tensioning can be tested clinically by holding the sutures under tension while testing the stability of the MCP joint. The sutures are passed through a piece of a soft silicone tube with a length that corresponds to the distance between both tunnels. Then the sutures are tied on the outside of this silicone tube, which prevents skin necrosis (▶ Fig. 17.2). Adequate tension can be verified under direct vision in the surgical field, as well as tested manually. Then the joint is reconstructed by fixing the remnants of the proper and accessory collateral ligament to each other and the graft in the original anatomic

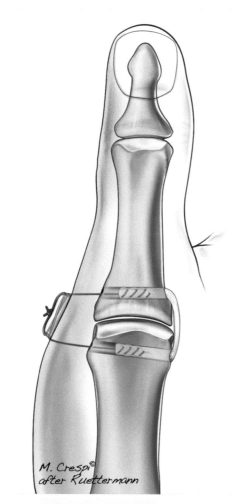

M. Crespi©
after Ruettermann

Fig. 17.2 Dorsal view of the metacarpopharangeal (MCP) joint of a right thumb: ulnar collateral ligament (UCL) reconstruction with a pull-out tendon graft. Proximal and distal bone tunnel and the pull-out suture tied over a silicone tube on the skin on the contralateral side.

direction of their fibers and closing the capsule, which is important for the stability of the joint.[10]

The transverse fibers of the extensor hood and the insertion of the adductor (UCL) or abductor (RCL) pollicis are readapted.

If there is any doubt regarding the stability of the reconstruction or the patient's compliance as to wearing his cast or splint, a K-wire can be placed as temporary fixation of the MCP joint of the thumb. The skin is closed taking special care not to injure the branch of the superficial radial nerve.

A dressing is applied, and a cast or splint is made including the proximal phalanx of the thumb for 4 weeks. Interphalangeal joint movement should be possible.

After that, a small splint that prevents radial deviation but allows flexion and extension of the MCP joint of the

thumb is worn for another 4 weeks (a K-wire has to be removed at this time).

Depending on the ligament repaired radially or ulnarly, directed stress on the tip of the thumb is to be avoided for 12 weeks.

This technique is easy to reproduce. The tunnels are easier to drill in the correct position than those in the original Littler technique. If no anchors or interference screws had been used in the previous, failed repair, the graft can also be fixed in a groove created at the site of the tunnel entrance point and fixed with a bone anchor.

The technique can be applied for RCL as well as UCL repair for the MCP joint of the thumb. With slight modifications regarding the soft tissue dissection, this pull-out tendon graft technique can also be used for severe instabilities of PIP joints.

17.4 Foreign Body Material

Foreign body material is frequently used in primary repairs these days, but this does only lead to a satisfactory result if the anatomy is restored. I have seen many patients that had a short period of initial stability, until they started load bearing. Then the artificial material ruptured as it had been used as sole reconstruction, without debridement and suturing the remaining ligament and capsular tissues. Several patients I saw had had a repair of UCL with a proximal and a distal bone anchor that had been placed and tied extracapsular, which did not and cannot lead to sufficient stability.

In secondary revisions of failed surgical repairs, there has already been a problem with healing. Anchors, nonresorbable sutures, or interference screws in the area of the revision surgery can be an obstacle to adapt the remaining healthy tissues or drill any bone tunnels at the optimal position. Especially larger interference or locking screws can pose a severe problem as there is a risk of intra-articular fracture by drilling necessary additional tunnels. If foreign body material is used in a secondary surgical revision, it needs to have an added value that has to be weighed against disadvantages like infection, foreign body reaction, and additional costs.

17.5 Joint Specific Issues

Repair of an unstable UCL of the MCP joint of the thumb is always indicated, as its stability is necessary for pinch grip. RCL lesions of this joint are less common, they occur only in 29%, mostly distally,[11,12] and surgical repair is indicated if the patient has functional complaints.

RCL or UCL lesions of the MCP joints of the fingers are less common due to their less exposed anatomic situation and more stabilization through the intrinsic muscles. These provide more stability as there is no opposition like in the thumb through which the protective effect of the intrinsic muscles varies depending on the angle of opposition and supination.[13] However, if there are functional complaints, the collateral ligaments of these MCP joints of the finger can be repaired with bone anchors[14] or using tendon strips from the extensor hood, as has been described for rheumatic hands.[15]

Collateral ligament lesions of PIP joints often heal well with conservative treatment, so that a primary surgical repair is not done very often. If this has been performed with an insufficient result, a secondary reconstruction with a tendon graft is feasible. Depending on the quality of the remnants of the original ligament, a bone anchor can aid in refixation, an augmentation graft can be sutured to the remnants, or longer grafts can be used with a pull-through technique, along the lines of the above-described method for collateral ligament reconstruction of the MCP joint of the thumb. This is mostly indicated in the PIP joint of the index finger as insufficiency of the RCL of the index PIP joint becomes symptomatic during pinch grip.

Ligamentous lesions of the DIP joints are mostly treated conservatively, and primary surgical repair is done rarely if at all. Persisting symptomatic problems due to insufficient collateral ligaments or subluxation are treated mainly by arthrodesis due to the limited functional restriction and predictable results.

17.6 Take-Home Message

As in all cases of complications, the best way to treat them is to avoid/prevent them. Therefore, some details should be taken into account when dealing with ligamentous injuries of small joints of the thumb and fingers in the first place. In MCP collateral ligament injuries, a missed Stener lesion leads to instability when treated conservatively. If there is doubt and a Stener lesion cannot be ruled out by clinical testing, additional ultrasound, MRI, or better surgical exploration should be performed. If there is clearly no end point at all, surgery is indicated.

In volar plate injuries, the most common complication is stiffness. Thus, early active motion should be recommended if there is no recurrent subluxation.

17.7 Diagnostic Pearls

- A radiograph should be taken at first to prevent further dislocation of a bony fragment by clinical testing.
- Clinical testing should be done under local anesthesia and joint stability should be compared to the contralateral side.

17.8 Technical Tips

- Use grafts if tissue quality is insufficient in primary repairs.

- Local grafts, like tendon strips, cause more problems with stiffness than free tendon grafts (palmaris longus, partial flexor carpi radialis, or parts of the extensor retinaculum). On the other hand, infections due to free tendon grafts have rarely been reported.
- If a bone anchor is used in the primary repair, there is in general sufficient stability, and an additional K-wire is not necessary.
- In an attempt of secondary reconstruction of a collateral ligament, symptomatic osteoarthritis of the joint has to be ruled out; if needed, obtain a computed tomography (CT) scan.

References

[1] Stener B. Displacement of the ruptured ulnar collateral ligament of the metacarpo-phalangeal joint of the thumb. J Bone Joint Surg Br. 1962; 44-B:869–879

[2] Harley BJ, Werner FW, Green JK. A biomechanical modeling of injury, repair, and rehabilitation of ulnar collateral ligament injuries of the thumb. J Hand Surg Am. 2004; 29(5):915–920

[3] Jespersen B, Nielsen NS, Bonnevie BE, Boeckstyns ME. Hyperextension injury to the PIP joint or to the MP joint of the thumb: a clinical study. Scand J Plast Reconstr Surg Hand Surg. 1998; 32(3):317–321

[4] Moberg E, Stener B. Injuries to the ligaments of the thumb and fingers; diagnosis, treatment and prognosis. Acta Chir Scand. 1953; 106 (2–3):166–186

[5] Wagner ER, Robinson WA, Houdek MT, Moran SL, Rizzo M. Proximal interphalangeal joint arthroplasty in young patients. J Am Acad Orthop Surg. 2019; 27(12):444–450

[6] Rigó IZ, Røkkum M. Not all non-rheumatoid patients are satisfied with thumb metacarpophalangeal joint arthrodesis. J Plast Surg Hand Surg. 2013; 47(2):144–146

[7] Daley D, Geary M, Gaston RG. Thumb metacarpophalangeal ulnar and radial collateral ligament injuries. Clin Sports Med. 2020; 39(2):443–455

[8] Glickel SZ, Malerich M, Pearce SM, Littler JW. Ligament replacement for chronic instability of the ulnar collateral ligament of the metacarpophalangeal joint of the thumb. J Hand Surg Am. 1993; 18(5):930–941

[9] Bean CH, Tencer AF, Trumble TE. The effect of thumb metacarpophalangeal ulnar collateral ligament attachment site on joint range of motion: an in vitro study. J Hand Surg Am. 1999; 24(2):283–287

[10] Kim BS, Doermann A, McGarry M, Akeda M, Ihn H, Lee TQ. Dorsoradial instability of the thumb metacarpophalangeal joint: a biomechanical investigation. J Hand Surg Am. 2017; 42(12):1029.e1–1029.e8

[11] Coyle MP, Jr. Grade III radial collateral ligament injuries of the thumb metacarpophalangeal joint: treatment by soft tissue advancement and bony reattachment. J Hand Surg Am. 2003; 28(1):14–20

[12] Schroeder NS, Goldfarb CA. Thumb ulnar collateral and radial collateral ligament injuries. Clin Sports Med. 2015; 34(1):117–126

[13] Jakubietz RG, Erguen S, Bernuth S, Meffert RH, Gilbert F, Jakubietz M. An anatomical study on the Stener-type lesion of the radial collateral ligament of the metacarpophalangeal joint of the thumb. J Hand Surg Eur Vol. 2020; 45(2):131–135

[14] Waxweiler C, Cuylits N, Lumens D, et al. Surgical fixation of metacarpophalangeal collateral ligament rupture of the fingers. Plast Reconstr Surg. 2019; 143(5):1421–1428

[15] Wood VE, Ichtertz DR, Yahiku H. Soft tissue metacarpophalangeal reconstruction for treatment of rheumatoid hand deformity. J Hand Surg Am. 1989; 14(2 Pt 1):163–174

5

18 Treatment of Complications after Scapholunate Ligament Repair

Marc Garcia-Elias, Mireia Esplugas, and Alex Lluch

Abstract

Systematic analysis of complications after ligament reconstruction for carpal instabilities is difficult, due to inconsistent reporting of the great number of surgical techniques used. Mistaken indications should not be considered as complications. Loss of scaphoid or lunate correction, loss of scapholunate joint reduction, dorsolateral scaphoid subluxation, wrist stiffness, and problems affecting the bones, tendons, and nerves are some of the complications that may happen after scapholunate ligament reconstruction and will be discussed in this chapter.

Keywords: scapholunate ligament, scapholunate complication, scapholunate gap, scapholunate ligament reconstruction, carpal collapse, wrist stiffness, tendon complication, nerve complication

18.1 Complication versus Mistake

A mistake is defined as an act or judgment that is misguided or wrong. On the contrary, a complication is an extra problem that appears and makes a situation more difficult than it previously was.

There seems to be a good agreement in literature to when a ligament reconstruction is indicated in an unstable scapholunate (SL) joint and when it is not. If problems arise after a tendon reconstruction performed while misalignment is not easily reducible, there is a combined instability, or, even worse, there is damaged cartilage or carpal collapse, these situations should not be considered complications but mistaken indications. Poor results are not always the consequence of a complication after a ligament reconstruction; sometimes they result from a wrong interpretation of what is unstable and what is not.[1]

Complications after scapholunate ligament (SLL) repair procedures are frequent.[2,3] SL dysfunction represents a broad spectrum of injuries, from a partial stable lesion to arthropathy. Depending on the stage of SL instability, different techniques may be indicated. Considering this, and also the trend to minimally invasive procedures, we will focus on the prevention and treatment of the complications found after the following four procedures:

- Open three-ligament tenodesis procedure (3LT).[4,5]
- Open antipronation spiral SLL tenodesis using extensor carpi radialis longus (ECRL) slip.[6]
- Arthroscopic dorsal-SLL tenodesis with flexor carpi radialis (FCR) or ECRL.[7]
- SL screw fixation to maintain reduction of SL interval after SLL reconstruction.[8] Each technique may have its own specific complications. The complications most often seen are discussed in this chapter and are shown in ▸ Table 18.1.

18.2 Treatment of Complications after Scapholunate Ligament Repair

18.2.1 Loss of Scapholunate Reduction

Scapholunate Gap Tyranny

- Problem: Maintenance of SL joint intraoperative reduction in the frontal plane is usually not achieved, despite the use of SL or scaphocapitate Kirschner wires (KW), or even with tendon fixation with biotenodesis screws (▸ Fig. 18.1).
- Treatment: Postoperative SL gap recurrence is common, but frequently this radiological finding is clinically asymptomatic and doesn't need to be treated. Only cases associated with dorsoradial translation of the scaphoid, sometimes with a positive Watson test, require surgical treatment as will be explained later.
- Rehabilitation: Strengthening of distal row supinator muscles (APL in neutral forearm rotation and ECRL/ECRB in forearm pronation), as in all SLL reconstructive procedures.[9]

Table 18.1 Complications after SLL reconstruction

1. Loss of SL reduction:
   SL gap widening
   Dorsal scaphoid translation
   Scaphoid flexion
   Lunate flexion
2. Loss of carpal reduction: Ulnar carpal translation
3. Stiffness:
   Extracapsular origin
   Intracapsular origin: Carpal collapse, chondrolysis
4. Tendons:
   Flexor tendons: FCR tendonitis, FDP adhesions
   Extensor tendons: Rupture, adhesions
5. Bone:
   Fracture: Scaphoid, Lunate, radius
   Avascular necrosis
   Osteolysis
6. Nerve: Radial, median, ulnar
7. Infection

Abbreviations: FCR, flexor carpi radialis; FDP, flexor digitorum profundus; SL, scapholunate; SLL, scapholunate ligament.

• Tips and Tricks: Ligament augmentation with internal brace devices may, theoretically, decrease recurrence of the SL gap. A systematic review for anterior cruciate ligament repair in the knee with some form of internal bracing concludes that it increases the success rate.[10]

This aspect has not yet been demonstrated in the wrist. Avoid ligament reconstruction procedures in static SL dysfunction.

Dorsal Scaphoid Translation

• Problem: Dorsoradial scaphoid translation is directly related to persistent pain and weakness. Scaphoid remains flexed, which is associated with a limited wrist extension. Secondary degenerative radioscaphoid cartilage changes will certainly develop in the future (▶ Fig. 18.2a–c).

• Treatment: When symptomatic, proximal carpal row (PCR) resection or radioscapholunate (RSL) fusion may relieve patient's symptoms and maintain functional mobility. In both cases, cartilage of the head of the capitate needs to be preserved. If the lunocapitate joint is affected but radiolunate cartilage remains in good condition, scaphoid resection and midcarpal (MC) fusion (lunocapitate, lunocapitohamate, or four corner) are indicated.

Dorsal scaphoid translation increases when a dorsal distal radius malunion is associated. In such cases, prior correction of the dorsally tilted distal radius can limit dorsoradial scaphoid translation and facilitate symptomatic improvement. For the same reason, any SLL reconstruction performed in a wrist with a distal radius dorsal malunion has a higher failure rate (▶ Fig. 18.3).

• Rehabilitation: MC mobility around dart throwing motion axis in RSL fusion. Radiocarpal (RC) mobility in MC fusion.

• Tips and Tricks: Arthroscopic PCR, RSL, or MC fusion preserves extra-articular vascularization and, so,

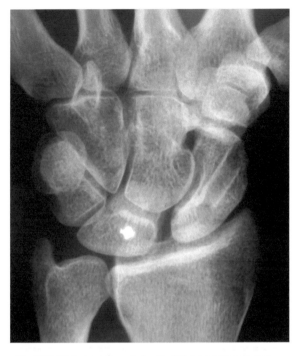

Fig. 18.1 Widening of scapholunate (SL) joint intraoperative reduction 3 years after a three-ligament tenodesis (3LT) procedure. Despite the moderate gap, the scaphoid is no longer flexed or pronated and the patient is asymptomatic.

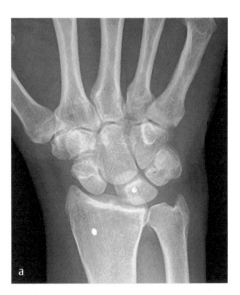
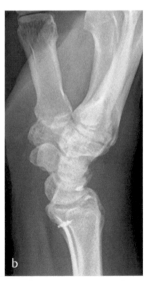
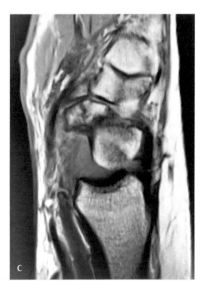

Fig. 18.2 (a–c) Recurrence of scapholunate (SL) malalignment after an antipronation spiral tenodesis **(a,b)**. Scaphoid flexion and dorsal translation induce high loading in a small joint area of the scaphoid fossa that will end in chondral damage **(c)**.

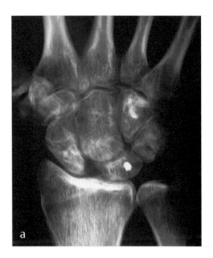
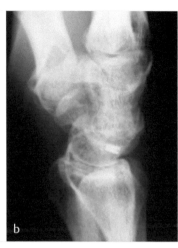

Fig. 18.3 (a,b) Early symptomatic malalignment recurrence after a three-ligament tenodesis (3LT) procedure performed in a wrist with a distal radius dorsal malunion. (Courtesy of Dr. P. Forcada.)

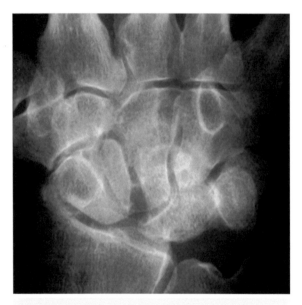

Fig. 18.4 Static flexion deformity of the lunate (volar intercalated segment instability [VISI]) in a lunotriquetral (LT) dysfunction may create confusion as the scapholunate (SL) space seems to be wider in the anteroposterior (AP) view. Look at the altered Gilula lines in the ulnar side of the wrist.

facilitates bone fusion. Correct lunate extension deformity to allow proper range of motion. Avoid overcorrection at the lunocapitate fusion in the frontal plane. MC joint stabilization with KW avoids RC joint screw protrusion if some degree of collapse occurs before MC fusion is achieved.

Scaphoid Flexion Persistence

• Problem: Postoperative scaphoid flexion persistence can be either associated or not associated to a dorsoradial scaphoid translation. When scaphoid flexion is associated with a scaphoid dorsoradial translation, both should be faced as described previously.
  Isolated scaphoid flexion is associated with a carpal height loss. This condition may evolve to an MC misalignment. Whether this misalignment will lead to an MC clinical instability or not is uncertain.
• Treatment: No preventive surgical treatment of isolated scaphoid flexion persistence should be planned while the patient is free of symptoms.
• Rehabilitation: Strengthening of distal row supinator muscles.[9]
• Tips and Tricks: Using ECRL as a donor tendon for SLL reconstruction induces greater scaphoid extension and supination than FCR.[5]

Volar Intercalated Segment Instability (VISI) of the Lunate

• Problem: Permanent malalignment in flexion of the lunate after SLL surgery or development of a progressive flexion deformity. A fixed VISI deformity in a static lunotriquetral (LT) dysfunction may be confused with an SL joint gap, and may explain a permanent lunate flexion malalignment even after an SLL reconstruction. This describes a wrong indication rather than a complication (▶ Fig. 18.4). Overcorrection of lunate position during SL ligamentoplasty followed by several weeks of pinning would also explain a lunate flexion deformity (▶ Fig. 18.5).
• Treatment: Any soft tissue procedure aimed to correct a static VISI deformity has high chances of failure. PCR or MC fusion will probably be needed.
• Rehabilitation: Strengthening of distal row pronator muscle (ECU) with the forearm in supination after LT ligament repair or pinning.[11]
• Tips and Tricks: In arthroscopic SLL ligamentoplasty,[5] the lunate intraosseous tunnel must be parallel to the distal lunate surface to avoid lunate overcorrection in

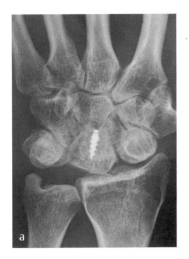 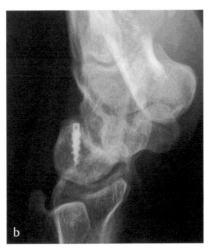

Fig. 18.5 (a,b) Static flexion deformity of the lunate 6 months after a three-ligament tenodesis (3LT) procedure secondary to overcorrection. No lunotriquetral (LT) dysfunction was found at the time of scapholunate (SL) ligament reconstruction.

VISI; a temporary radiolunate KW may help to stabilize a floating lunate during drilling. Check for an LT origin in cases of an apparent SL space widening plus a flexed lunate.

- Extension of the whole proximal carpal row, as it happens in a dorsal nondissociative instability, may be wrongly considered as secondary to an SLL dysfunction. Performing an SLL reconstruction in such cases has also to be considered a mistake and not a complication.

18.2.2 Loss of Carpal Reduction

Ulnar Carpal Translation

- Problem: Previously unidentified radiocarpal instability associated with SLL dysfunction secondary to RC ligaments insufficiency.
  Elongated long and short radiolunate, and dorsal radiocarpal ligaments do not prevent ulnar translation of the carpus. Any reconstruction focused just in the SLL complex will not solve both problems.
- Treatment: Procedures that add a reinforcement of radiocarpal ligaments, as the antipronation spiral tenodesis, will theoretically avoid ulnar translation of the carpus under loading. Radiolunate arthrodesis will also prevent ulnar carpal translation, but the procedure alone will not solve SL instability.
- Rehabilitation: Protected RC and MC joint mobility for 3 weeks. Strengthening of distal row supinator muscles.[9]
- Tips and Tricks: ECRL allows to obtain a tendon graft long enough to reconstruct the spiral ligament architecture. Arthroscopic-assisted spiral tenodesis avoids extended dorsal and volar approaches. Using interferential screws and augmentation with internal bracing add stability and may prevent the use of KW.

18.2.3 Stiffness

Extra-articular Origen

- Problem: Loss of RC and/or MC mobility. Secondary to excessive scarring, wrist or finger extensor tendons adhesions, complex regional pain syndrome 1 or 2.
- Treatment: Conservative first. Persistent symptoms may need arthrolysis, tendolysis, neuroma management, PCR, partial/total fusion.
- Rehabilitation: Neuropathic pain-specific programs; wrist or finger stiffness-specific programs.
- Tips and Tricks: Avoid KW through MC joint. Protect tendons and sensory branches from irritation. Early finger and wrist active motion.

Intra-articular Origen

Chondrolysis

- Problem: Damaged cartilage due to heating or intra-articular protrusion when pinning is used. This may end in RC or MC secondary stiffness.
- Treatment: Steroid injection. Selective joint denervation. Fusion.
- Rehabilitation: Orthosis to protect the affected joint.
- Tips and Tricks: Low velocity when pinning. Avoid reintroduction of a previously inserted KW. Detect articular KW protrusion.

Carpal Collapse

- Problem: The misaligned carpus becomes progressively stiff, and no longer reducible. In such a situation, the wrist is not unstable but collapsed. A previously collapsed wrist may be wrongly treated with a ligament reconstruction, which is a mistake, or a failed tendon

5

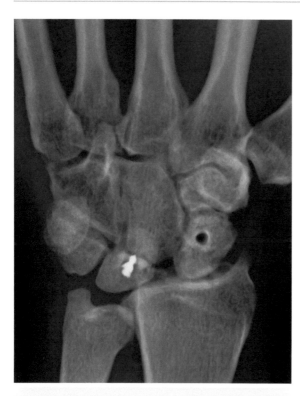

Fig. 18.6 Stiff collapsed carpus after a failed scapholunate ligament (SLL) reconstruction (three-ligament tenodesis [3LT]) due to a wrong indication (static deformity and carpal ulnar translation preoperatively).

reconstruction may end as a collapsed stiff carpus (▶ Fig. 18.6).

- Treatment: PRC or partial fusion if there is any preserved joint surface and reasonable wrist motion. Total fusion or arthroplasty if completely stiff or extensive chondral lesion.
- Rehabilitation: Strengthening of distal row supinator muscles.[9]
- Tips and Tricks: Recognize collapse before planning ligament reconstruction. Follow intra- and postoperative recommended steps in any ligament reconstruction procedure.

18.2.4 Tendon Complications

Flexor Tendons

FCR Tendonitis

- Problem: Painful FCR at the entrance of the tunnel located in the distal scaphoid, especially when the patient supports his flattened hand on a hard surface. Occurs when FCR is the donor tendon for reconstruction, or when an antegrade biotenodesis screw gets loose in the distal scaphoid.

- Treatment: Ultrasound-guided steroid injection. Resection of the remaining FCR. Removal of protruding biotenodesis screw.
- Rehabilitation: Local anti-inflammatory treatment.
- Tips and Tricks: Release of the FCR distal tunnel when harvesting the tendon slip. Check for biotenodesis screw protrusion with ultrasound.

Adhesions

- Problem: Loss of function of the flexor digitorum profundus (FDP) tendon secondary to adhesions. Volar central portal and volar extracapsular tendon plasty need FDP manipulation. Volar SL ligament reconstruction associates a volar RC capsulodesis with nonabsorbable suture knots. FDP adhesions may induce volar wrist pain and contribute to stiffness.
- Treatment and rehabilitation: Promote FDP gliding.
- Tips and Tricks: Careful FDP management. Short volar capsulodesis suture knots.

Extensor Tendons

Rupture

- Problem: Loss of function of extensor digitorum comunis (EDC) or extensor digiti minimi (EDM) tendons secondary to rupture.
  EDM is at risk in the radiocarpal 4/5 portal establishment, in the dorsal approach to the triquetrum in arthroscopic spiral SLL reconstruction, and when creating and closing the ulnar part of a Berger dorsal capsular approach. EDC tendons are at risk in the extracapsular tendon passing and in the dorsal central portal establishment in arthroscopic SLL repair, or when leaving extracapsular knots with cutting edges in capsulodesis (▶ Fig. 18.7a, b). EDC and EDM lesions may induce dorsal wrist pain and contribute to stiffness.
- Treatment: Tendon release and repair. Usually using grafts or tendon transfer. Performing the repair under wide-awake local anesthesia no tourniquet (WALANT) can be beneficial.
- Rehabilitation: Specific protocol for every repair procedure.
- Tips and Tricks: In arthroscopic SLL repair: avoid finger trap at the small finger to check EDM normal tension; skin incision and dissection parallel to tendons; distal part of the extensor retinaculum incision facilitates EDC manipulation and protection. In open procedures, extend dorsal capsulotomy beyond the EDM tendon to protect it.

Adhesions

- Problem: Finger and wrist stiffness secondary to EDC and extensor indicis propius (EIP) adhesions in the dorsum of the wrist. Dorsal wrist central arthroscopic

5

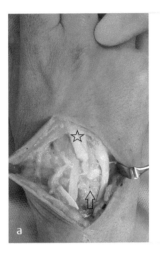 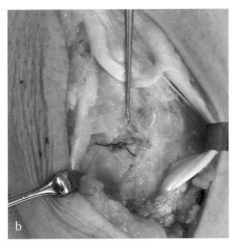

Fig. 18.7 (a,b) Extensor indicis propius (EIP) and extensor digitorum comunis (EDC) for the index finger rupture caused by a protruding rigid knot in the dorsal capsule. Ruptured tendons marked with a star, protruding suture with an arrow **(a)**. Better view of the suture after scar tissue and a slice of the capsule removal **(b)**.

5

portal needs EDC manipulation that may create adhesions.

Wrist stiffness or radial wrist pain secondary to adhesions between ECRL and ECRB when the first is the donor tendon. Arthroscopic techniques use distal mini-open ECRL harvesting that do not allow second compartment synovectomy or tendon release, and may favor secondary problems.

- Treatment: Tendon release, preferably with WALANT.
- Rehabilitation: Specific protocol for every tendon release procedure.
- Tips and Tricks: Perform wrist extensors release when harvesting. Protect properly EDC and EIP during surgery and promote early finger motion.

18.2.5 Bony Problems

Fractures

Scaphoid Fracture

- Problem: Fracture due to a weakened scaphoid after a tunnel is created following its axis. It can happen intra-operatively when the tunnel is done, when fixing the tendon with interferential screws, or when pinning the scaphoid if large KWs are used. Or it can be a consequence of a wrist trauma that happens after surgery (▶ Fig. 18.8a, b).
- Treatment: If a partial or stable scaphoid fracture is created intraoperatively, the tendon plasty is still contained within the tunnel, and a correct carpal alignment is achieved, a longer immobilization period until healing may be enough. If only interferential screws were planned as stabilizers, adding Kirschner pinning can be an option.

  Treatment of scaphoid fractures that occur after surgery will depend on the stability of the fracture itself. Non-displaced stable fractures can be treated conservatively. Unstable fractures will need stabilization. In case that

fixation is possible, consider using KW or plating, as screw fixation may be difficult due to the tunnel positioning. When the fracture compromises the tendon plasty SL joint stabilizing effect, PRC or partial fusions are indicated.

- Rehabilitation: Bone-healing promotion techniques (magnetotherapy) combined with early isometric strengthening of intracarpal supinator muscles into the cast.
- Tips and Tricks: As the shape of the scaphoid is extremely variable, check preoperatively with a computed tomography (CT) to identify those cases in which the scaphoid waist is narrow and twisted. Do not drill the tunnel too close to the limits of the scaphoid. Always use cannulated drills, and adapt the tendon slip to the tunnel size and not the opposite. Use tendon passers and try to pass the tendon smoothly. When using a biotenodesis screw, be sure that it follows the direction of the tunnel using fluoroscopy. Avoid transmitting too much strength on the KWs used as joysticks. Avoid too large KWs and too many attempts when pinning, and try not to place KWs entry point too close in the scaphoid.

Lunate Fracture

- Problem: Fracture that occurs in those techniques in which a bony tunnel is created in the lunate. As only a few procedures use lunate tunnels, lunate fractures are less frequent than scaphoid fractures.
- Treatment: Treatment depends on the stability of the fracture itself and in its repercussion on the tendon-plasty stability. PRC or partial fusions may be indicated.
- Rehabilitation: Same as in scaphoid fractures.
- Tips and Tricks: Do not drill the tunnel too close to the distal lunate surface, and keep parallel to the lunocapitate joint surface. Use KW as a joystick with caution, and avoid placing them in bony bridges that may break. When using a temporary SL screw fixation combined to

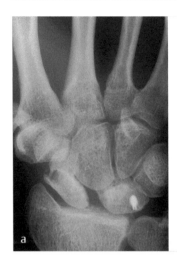 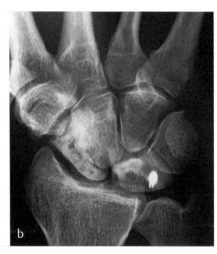

Fig. 18.8 (a,b) Scaphoid fracture after a scapholunate ligament (SLL) ligament reconstruction (a). This case ended with a proximal pole avascular necrosis (AVN) several months later (b).

an SLL reconstruction, correct positioning of the screw avoiding the bony tunnels is not easy. The screw should theoretically be placed in the SL axis of rotation. As this axis is slightly dorsal, ending in a too dorsal screw position may debilitate the bone. Incorrect orientation of the screw or insertion through a misaligned SL joint secondary to a dorsal scaphoid translation can also be a source of problems (▶ Fig. 18.9).

Radius Fracture

- Problem: Fracture that occurs in those techniques in which a bony tunnel is created in the radius (▶ Fig. 18.10).
- Treatment: Usually stable fractures that will heal conservatively.
- Rehabilitation: Same as scaphoid fractures.
- Tips and Tricks: Avoid placing the bony tunnel too close to the distal and radial corners of the radius.

Avascular Necrosis (AVN)

- Problem: Drilling a tunnel across the proximal scaphoid and extensive dissection in open procedures may interfere with the poor blood supply of this part of the bone[12] (▶ Fig. 18.8b).
- Treatment: PRC or scaphoidectomy and MC fusion.
- Tips and Tricks: Avoid extensive dissection of the scaphoid in open procedures. The need for that may indicate a static SL dysfunction, closer to collapse than to instability. Use a smaller drill or do a more vertical tunnel in small scaphoids.

Osteolysis

- Problem: Loosening of interferential/transarticular screws or KW associated with mechanical pain and bone resorption (▶ Fig. 18.11).

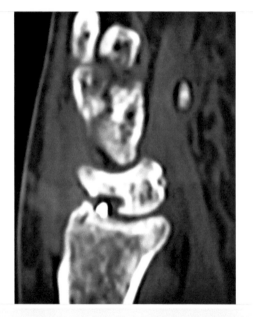

Fig. 18.9 Dorsal lunate fracture and loosening 5 months after screw temporary scapholunate (SL) fixation, due to incorrect positioning of the screw in the lunate (too dorsal).

- Treatment: Material removal before bone osteolysis.
- Rehabilitation: Orthosis for specific area immobilization and local magnetotherapy.
- Tips and Tricks: Avoid material overheating during its insertion. The trans-scaphoid screw insertion must exactly follow the joint rotation axis.

18.2.6 Nerve Complications

Radial Nerve

- Problem: Injury to the dorsal sensory branches of the radial nerve (DSBRN), which are at risk in either open

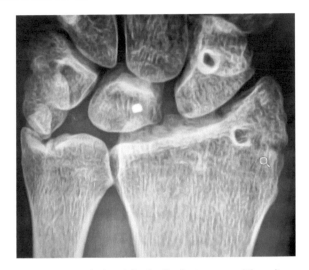

Fig. 18.10 Nondisplaced distal radius fracture around the radius tunnel 2 years after an antipronation spiral tenodesis.

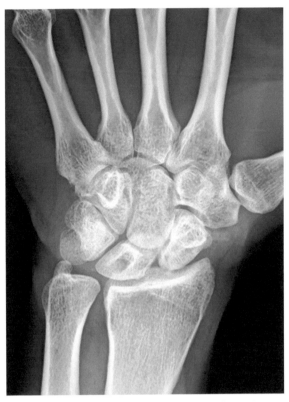

Fig. 18.11 Osteolysis around a biotenodesis screw in the lunate tunnel in a dorsal scapholunate ligament (SLL) arthroscopic reconstruction. Despite loss of reduction and osteolysis, this patient remains asymptomatic.

and arthroscopic techniques. Open approach to the radial part of the wrist, harvesting the slip of ECRL, passing it through the STT, establishing 1/2 RC portal, or pinning with KW are risky surgical steps.

- Treatment: Paresthesia is usually transient and is secondary to manipulation or contusion. Iatrogenic partial or total nerve injury will need repair or neuroma displacement.
- Rehabilitation: Neuropathic pain-specific programs.
- Tips and Tricks: Maintain DSBRN attached to the subcutaneous tissue and try not to individualize them in open approaches. Intracapsular ECRL passage from dorsal to volar. Protect KW entrance when pinning.

Ulnar Nerve

- Problem: Injury to the dorsal sensory branches of the ulnar nerve (DSBUN), at risk in ulnar-sided part of the surgical approach.
  Injury to the ulnar nerve in Guyon's canal in those reconstructions that create a dorsovolar tunnel in the triquetrum or reach the volar LT space, or when establishing the volar central arthroscopic portal.
- Treatment: Same as DSBRN for sensory branches. Surgical revision when low ulnar palsy does not recover.
- Rehabilitation: Neuropathic pain-specific programs.
- Tips and Tricks: Maintain DSBUN attached to the subcutaneous tissue in open approaches. Protect the ulnar neurovascular bundle toward the ulnar side when creating triquetrum tunnel. Always use KW and drill with the nerve and artery under direct control.

Median Nerve

- Problem: Injury to the thenar cutaneous branch when harvesting FCR, when creating the scaphoid tunnel, or when manipulating the volar part of it.

- Treatment and Rehabilitation: Same as the other sensory branches.
- Tips and Tricks: Stay in the radial side of FCR. Avoid blind dissection or cutting distal to the wrist flexion creases.

18.2.7 Infection

KW superficial intolerance/infection is not unusual when they are left out of the skin. Uncommonly, this superficial infection can deepen and carry a secondary chondrolysis or septic arthritis.

18.3 Take-Home Message

The complication rate after SL ligament reconstruction procedures is high, even in those cases with a correct indication. Maintenance of the correction seems to be related to perform the procedures in proper selected patients. Bone, nerve, and tendon complications can be lowered with an accurate surgical technique. Less invasive procedures, such as arthroscopically supported tendon reconstruction, can decrease extracapsular causes of stiffness.

References

[1] Garcia-Elias M, Ortega DM. Tendon reconstruction of the unstable scapholunate dissociation. A systematic review. In: Giddins G, Leblebicioğlu G, eds. Evidence based data in hand surgery and therapy. Budapest: Iris Publications; 355–68

[2] Naqui Z, Khor WS, Mishra A, Lees V, Muir L. The management of chronic non-arthritic scapholunate dissociation: a systematic review. J Hand Surg Eur Vol. 2018; 43(4):394–401

[3] Athlani L, Pauchard N, Detammaecker R, et al. Treatment of chronic scapholunate dissociation with tenodesis: a systematic review. Hand Surg Rehab. 2018; 37(2):65–76

[4] Garcia-Elias M, Lluch AL, Stanley JK. Three-ligament tenodesis for the treatment of scapholunate dissociation: indications and surgical technique. J Hand Surg Am. 2006; 31(1):125–134

[5] Kakar S, Greene RM, Garcia-Elias M. Carpal realignment using a strip of extensor carpi radialis longus tendon. J Hand Surg Am. 2017; 42 (8):667.e1–667.e8

[6] Chee KG, Chin AYH, Chew EM, Garcia-Elias M. Antipronation spiral tenodesis: a surgical technique for the treatment of perilunate instability. J Hand Surg Am. 2012; 37(12):2611–2618

[7] Corella F, Del Cerro M, Larrainzar-Garijo R, Vázquez T. Arthroscopic ligamentoplasty (bone-tendon-tenodesis): a new surgical technique for scapholunate instability: preliminary cadaver study. J Hand Surg Eur Vol. 2011; 36(8):682–689

[8] Fok MWM, Fernandez DL. Chronic scapholunate instability treated with temporary screw fixation. J Hand Surg Am. 2015; 40(4):752–758

[9] Esplugas M, Garcia-Elias M, Lluch A, Llusá Pérez M. Role of muscles in the stabilization of ligament-deficient wrists. J Hand Ther. 2016; 29 (2):166–174

[10] Van Eck CF, et al. Is there a role for internal bracing and repair of the anterior cruciate ligament? A systematic literature review. Am J Sports Med. 2017; 20:1–8

[11] Hagert E, Lluch A, Rein S. The role of proprioception and neuromuscular stability in carpal instabilities. J Hand Surg Eur Vol. 2016; 41 (1):94–101

[12] De Smet L, Sciot R, Degreef I. Avascular necrosis of the scaphoid after three-ligament tenodesis for scapholunate dissociation: case report. J Hand Surg Am. 2011; 36(4):587–590

19 Management of Complications Following Surgery to the Triangular Fibrocartilage Complex

Simon MacLean, Greg Bain, and Andrea Atzei

Abstract

Preventing complications in triangular fibrocartilage complex (TFCC) repair begins with a systematic approach. Patient history and clinical examination determines tear chronicity, stability, and the patient's functional demands. Basic and advanced imaging modalities define the anatomy of the tear, and the etiology of symptoms—whether it be primarily osseous, soft tissue, or a combination of both. Surgical treatment can then be directed appropriately. Arthroscopy plays a crucial role in both diagnosis and treatment. Complex procedures or salvage options may be warranted in advanced cases.

In this chapter we outline the complications of TFCC repair and our approach to this challenging injury. We present specific examples of challenging TFCC cases, and our TFCC tear management algorithm to help direct appropriate treatment for the wrist surgeon when treating these injuries.

Keywords: TFCC tear, TFCC reconstruction, algorithm, complications, salvage procedures

19.1 Introduction

Triangular fibrocartilage complex (TFCC) repairs are indicated in cases of persistent pain or instability of the distal radioulnar joint (DRUJ) following TFCC injury. Traumatic TFCC injuries are caused by axial loading, ulnar deviation and forced extremes of wrist rotation. Early diagnosis of an isolated TFCC tear is a challenge. In the absence of clear radiographic signs, the diagnosis is often missed at initial presentation. Other TFCC injuries occur in the setting of forearm or distal radius fractures and are often missed at the time of osteosynthesis.[1] Many TFCC injuries settle with nonoperative treatment. As a result, many TFCC tears remain undiagnosed, although a cohort will present later with ulnar-sided wrist pain or mechanical symptoms. Difficulty in initial diagnosis and delay in presentation presents a significant challenge to the wrist surgeon; chronic tears may have a poor capacity to heal following repair.

In the international literature, numerous papers report different surgical techniques of repair and reconstruction of the peripheral TFCC, using either traditional open or arthroscopic approach. Being mostly technical reports, these studies often lack adequate information regarding the type and incidence of complications. Even data from the few systematic reviews are lacking regarding the complications of these procedures: only limited reference can be found on persistence of pain and recurrence of DRUJ instability.[2,3,4,5] For both open and arthroscopic techniques, the incidence for postoperative pain is reported as high as 41%, and for DRUJ instability an incidence up to 16% is also reported. Furthermore, a detailed account of the causes for these complications is poorly reported.

Several challenges exist for the treating surgeon. A clear history is fundamental. Careful interpretation of clinical findings is required—particular coexisting injuries to the other ulnar-sided structures, and assessment of DRUJ instability. In addition, a careful review of radiological findings is required—including previous fractures, malunions, degenerative change, ulnar variance, and each individual TFCC component to assess for the anatomy of the tear. These parameters, as well as other patient and surgical factors, help direct repair strategy. As a result of this complex interplay of factors, surgical outcomes may be suboptimal and complications can occur.

19.1.1 Definition and Causes of Complications Following TFCC Repair and Reconstruction

For the purpose of this chapter, a complication is defined as an unfavorable event that arises during or in addition to a surgical procedure of TFCC repair and reconstruction, and is directly or indirectly linked to the surgical technique, either open or arthroscopic. For the evaluation of the possible causes of complications and failures of a surgical procedure, four phases were considered during the entire process: (1) preoperative diagnostic phase; (2) operative surgical phases, further divided in: (2A) perioperative and (2B) intraoperative; and finally (3) the rehabilitation phase.[6] Due to the number of technical advancements recently introduced to improve accuracy and facilitate surgery of TFCC repair and reconstruction, some complications have been recognized to be specifically related to the surgical procedures of TFCC repair and reconstruction. Accordingly, this chapter will focus on complications arising in the intraoperative phase. Undoubtedly, poor diagnostic work-up as well as wrong indications may doom surgery to failure. Even though peripheral TFCC tears represent the most common cause of ulnar-sided wrist pain and loss of function, it is also important to understand that, besides TFCC injury, there are other three main groups of pathologies that should be assessed: bone deformity, cartilage damage, and muscle/tendon disorders. Failure to recognize these disorders in the diagnostic approach may lead to complications and eventually failure of the surgical treatment. Thus, following the principles suggested by the "Four-Leaf Clover Algorithm" will facilitate decisions on treatment of DRUJ disorders.[7] Complications of arthroscopic surgery may occur in the perioperative phase of setup, but they may be strongly prevented with use of nonischemic finger traps and a traction force not exceeding 4 to 5 kg.[8] More accurately, these conditions relate to the learning curve and are absolutely rare in the operating room of an experienced surgeon. Intraoperative complications following TFCC repair and reconstruction may cause clinical complaints which are divided into two broad groups, as related to persistence or recurrence of (1) pain and (2) DRUJ instability.

19.2 Clinical Assessment

19.2.1 History and Examination

A number of TFCC tears following repair present with persistent instability of the DRUJ. In some cases, the surgeon performs a peripheral repair to the capsule and ECU subsheath but fails to appreciate or repair the foveal attachment onto the ulnar head. In other cases, a foveal repair is performed, which fails to heal, or a suboptimal technique is used. Patient factors—including comorbidities, hyperlaxity, or compliance with splinting or therapy —may also contribute to repair failure.

DRUJ instability is a spectrum and therefore clinical assessment can be challenging. In extreme cases, asymmetry and dorsal prominence of the ulnar are present on initial inspection. Previous scars from TFCC surgery may indicate the nature of previous surgery. Persistent foveal tenderness with a positive "foveal sign" is a sensitive and specific test for a persistent TFCC tear.[9] The press test and piano-key test may be positive. All instability tests should be performed on the contralateral wrist—appreciating that DRUJ laxity may be normal for the patient. An overall assessment of laxity, with the "Beighton Score" should be performed.[10] Other important tests include an ulnocarpal stress test and tests for DRUJ arthritis including the Grind test.

Other causes of ulnar-sided wrist pain should be considered, particularly ECU instability, lunotriquetral instability, or pisotriquetral osteoarthritis.

19.2.2 Investigations

Radiographic assessment includes inspection for previous fractures, particularly distal radius malunion at the DRUJ. A basal ulnar styloid fracture may affect the insertion of the TFCC foveal fibers. Nonunions in this region are not uncommon, which may in themselves produce pain, and associated persistent instability. Previous drill holes and anchors on radiographs may affect planned reconstruction techniques. Ulnocarpal abutment is not *always* associated with positive ulnar variance on static imaging, as it is a dynamic phenomenon. Abutment can occur with loading (clenched-fist view) and rotation (pronated view) (▶ Fig. 19.1). Degenerative changes at the DRUJ or

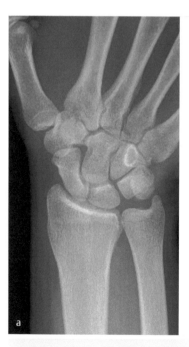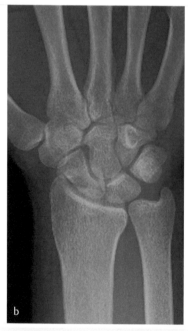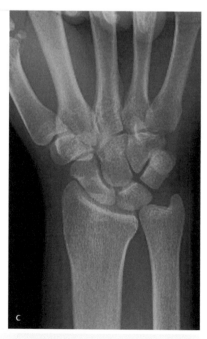

Fig. 19.1 Ulnocarpal abutment is usually associated with positive ulnar variance but this is not always the case such as in this patient. **(a)** Plain radiograph in the midpronated position. **(b)** Pronated view showing positive ulnar variance. **(c)** Clenched fist view showing further increase in ulnar variance.

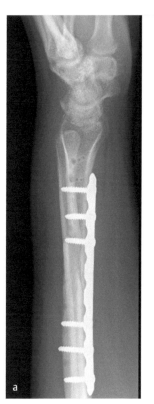
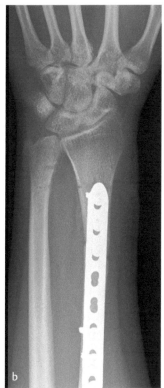
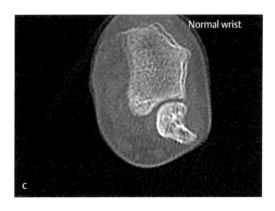
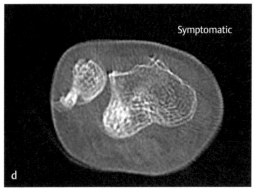

Fig. 19.2 A 20-year-old male with ulnar wrist pain following open reduction and internal fixation of his radial shaft. Plain lateral radiographs **(a)** showing full overlap of the radius and ulna at the forearm with only partial overlap at the wrist. Anteroposterior (AP) view **(b)** showing no gapping at the distal radioulnar joint (DRUJ). 4D-CT (computed tomography) scans of the normal **(c)** and symptomatic **(d)** wrist showing DRUJ incongruence, dynamic instability, and notching at the ulnar head due to bony impingement.

radiocarpal joint can occur and may warrant a salvage procedure.

3-Dimensional imaging includes computed tomography (CT) scanning of *both* wrists. Axial slices allow assessment of the morphology of the sigmoid notch, and review of the contralateral side allows comparison to a *normal* template, which is particularly useful if osteotomy ("notchplasty") is indicated.[11] Some patients will have dysplasia of both wrists and this will affect options for reconstruction.

Dynamic 4D CT scanning allows dynamic assessment of prosupination.[12] Cine images can be reformatted from different aspects depending on the surgeon's preference. Dynamic 2D axial sequences define the extent of DRUJ instability at different degrees of forearm rotation (► Fig. 19.2). The distal ulna is not tightly constrained in the sigmoid notch and a degree of dorsal and volar translation will occur in a normal wrist. This proportion is not well defined in the literature, but comparison to the asymptomatic side will assist the surgeon in cases of mild DRUJ instability. 4D scanning allows diagnosis of ulnar styloid triquetral impingement (► Fig. 19.3) and ulnocarpal abutment. 4D scanning also allows dynamic assess-

ment of the failed distal ulnar salvage procedure that presents with instability.

Magnetic resonance imaging (MRI) allows assessment of fixation failure. Metal suppression sequences can be helpful in cases where metallic anchors or other hardware has been used. Cystic change in the proximal ulnar lunate, triquetrum, or ulnar head can occur with ulnocarpal abutment. Ulnocarpal abutment may be seen directly on the 4D scan. On PD (proton density) views, the overall status of articular cartilage can be evaluated.

19.2.3 Arthroscopy

Arthroscopy may be both diagnostic and therapeutic. For arthroscopic assessment of the TFCC, we utilize a 3–4 portal with a 6-radial (6R) working portal on the radiocarpal joint, and DRUJ portal with the direct foveal portal for DRUJ exploration. Dry arthroscopy has several benefits. It allows accurate assessment of synovitis—as fluid insufflation tends to force blood out of synovial capillaries, it allows accurate assessment of tissue tension, and reduces postoperative edema and pain. The TFCC should be inspected for tissue quality and tear configuration.

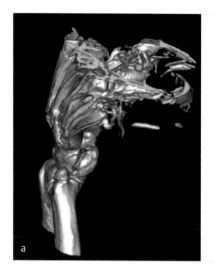
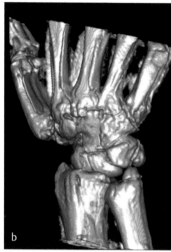

Fig. 19.3 (a,b) Ulnar styloid-triquetral impingement on 4D-CT (computed tomography) scanning. 3D reformats.

Previous sutures (broken or intact) may be present and may necessitate removal. A normal intact TFCC is naturally under tension and will "rebound" on trampoline testing. A positive trampoline test occurs when a probe ballots the surface and no rebound occurs, suggesting a tear of the peripheral attachments, as the TFCC loses its usual tautness.[6] A hook test is used to pull the ulnar insertion of the TFCC radial-wards to check for the integrity of the underlying foveal attachments.[13] The "reverse-hook" test checks the integrity of the radial attachments. Ballottement should occur with the wrist in neutral, pronation, and supination, which will selectively tension different volar and dorsal components of the TFCC.

19.3 General Overview of Complications Following TFCC Repair and Reconstruction

TFCC repairs are indicated in cases of posttraumatic pain or DRUJ instability, which persist after conservative treatment. Early clinical diagnosis of TFCC tears is a challenge to the wrist surgeon. Tears of the superficial component are amenable to simple capsular sutures. If there is significant involvement of the foveal insertions and chronic instability, the TFCC needs to be repaired to the ulnar fovea. Arthroscopy may also reveal chronic tears with poor healing capacity: for those tears, a reconstructive procedure is indicated. In the current clinical practice, arthroscopy is considered a mandatory completion to the diagnostic staging of TFCC tear. Based on the arthroscopic findings, indications can be established safely according to the different classes of Palmer 1B-type tears described in the treatment-oriented classification proposed by Atzei.[14,15] A systematic presentation of the complications occurring following the surgical treatment of the peripheral TFCC tears will be presented accordingly, along with

the recommendations for a strategy of prevention and treatment, as summarized in ▶ Table 19.1.

19.3.1 Complications Following Repair of Superficial Tears

Diagnosis of Class 1 distal peripheral tear is made exclusively by arthroscopy. Thus, the arthroscopic technique is also mandatory to perform the repair of the TFC proper to the dorsal capsule, in order to avoid the obvious drawbacks related to the soft tissue damage following the open approach to the tear. Since the first description of the different outside-in[16] and inside-out[17] techniques, the intolerance to the knot in the subcutaneous tissues has been a main issue, often requiring a second operation for knot removal, even when a resorbable suture is used.[18] Del Piñal et al recently described a technique for all-inside suturing that should be preferred for the treatment of Class 1 TFCC tear to circumvent the problem of knot intolerance.[19] Otherwise, it is recommended to refer the patient to the physiotherapist for skin desensitization. If physical therapy (PT) is not effective, surgery to remove the suture can be planned at least after 3 months postoperatively, to allow for proper healing of the repair. Another problem with the suture is related to the use of resorbable material, as it may cause a painful inflammatory synovitis due to the intra-articular suture resorption process. Use of high-strength nonabsorbable suture (such as FiberWire) is preferred. Furthermore, high-strength sutures offer the advantage of greater strength with smaller diameters, thus being preferable to use in small joint surgery. PT local anti-inflammatory treatment is recommended. Rare cases may require arthroscopic debridement if patient's complaints persist after 3 months postoperatively. The percutaneous suturing showed a significant risk of entangling the dorsal sensory branch of the ulnar nerve (DSBUN) or the tendons of

Table 19.1 Complications following peripheral TFCC tears repair and reconstruction presented according to the different classes of Palmer 1B-type tears described by Atzei: recommendations for prevention and treatment are also presented

Technique of Repair	Complications	Prevention strategy	Treatment
Repair of superficial tears (Type 1B–Class 1)			
Arthroscopic repair	Suture • Subcutaneous knot intolerance • Inflammatory synovitis during suture resorption	Prefer all-inside suture technique Prefer high-strength nonabsorbable suture	Desensitization therapy Physical therapy Suture removal at 3 months post-op
	Tendon entrapment • *ECU/EDQ* Nerve damage • *DSBUN/TAB of DSBUN*	Respect of anatomical landmarks and careful surgical technique. Blunt dissection of arthroscopic portals. Use dry arthroscopy.	Suture removal at 3 months post-op Tenolysis Desensitization therapy/neurolysis/neuroma revision and protection
Repair of deep tears (foveal repair) (Type 1B–Class 2-3)			
Open repair Arthroscopic repair	Generalities on fixation issues • *Eccentric setting causing anchor loosening/tunnel broadening and abrasion of the sutures* • *Early recurrence of pain and DRUJ instability* • *Small grasp of suture tearing TFCC edges*	Locate the foveal area by direct visualization (DRUJ exposure/ arthroscopy) Ensure proper positioning of anchor/tunnel at the fovea Debride foveal area and refresh tear's edges Be sure sutures grasp enough tissue of the TFCC	• The TFCC still has good quality: A) fixation using screw or small tunnels: new attempt of fixation B) fixation using large tunnel(s): allow for new bone formation and check with CT scan after 3 months • The TFCC has poor quality: Tendon graft reconstruction
	Screw fixation • *Poor strength of fixation* • *Poor bone quality* • *Screw eyelet to cut sutures during knot-tying*	Choose appropriate screw thread design according to bone characteristics/quality Avoid surgery on osteopenic bone. Prefer screws with smooth eyelet and high-strength suture	
	Partial repair • *Dorsal only repair causing residual palmar instability*	Accurate placement of the sutures Prefer ligament specific repair using 2 sutures	Complete the repair using a palmar (open) approach
	Knotting • *Soft tissues may be entangled with the suture* • *Over-tightening causes increased pressure on joint surfaces leading to arthritis*	Master suture management and sliding-knot technique Use dry arthroscopy Preserve physiological anteroposterior translation prior to secure the repair	Limit rehabilitation program Remove suture at 3 months post-op DRUJ arthroplasty/ulnar head prostesis
	Tendon entrapment/instability • *ECU/EDQ* Nerve damage • *DSBUN/TAB of DSBUN*	Respect of anatomical landmarks and careful surgical technique. Careful repair of the extensor retinaculum/ECU tendon sheath. Blunt dissection of arthroscopic portals. Use dry arthroscopy.	Suture removal at 3 months post-op. Tenolysis/reconstruction of extensor retinaculum/tendon sheath. Desensitization therapy/neurolysis/nerve stump revision and protection.

(Continued)

either the extensor carpi ulnaris (ECU) or extensor digiti quinti (EDQ).[20] Commonly, Class 1 tears are located close to the 6 R portal, whose area is often crossed by the transverse accessory branch of dorsal sensory branch of ulnar nerve (TAB of DSBUN), which is at risk of being caught and severed by the knot (► Fig. 19.4). Respect of anatomical landmarks and careful surgical technique, also to prepare a mini-open approach, may minimize this risk. Blunt dissection of the soft tissues around the arthroscopic portals and the use of dry arthroscopy, as popularized by del

Table 19.1 *(Continued)* Complications following peripheral TFCC tears repair and reconstruction presented according to the different classes of Palmer 1B-type tears described by Atzei: recommendations for prevention and treatment are also presented

Technique of Repair	Complications	Prevention strategy	Treatment
Reconstruction of nonrepairable tears (Type 1B–Class 4)			
Open repair Arthroscopic repair	Tendon graft • *Absent Palmaris Longus* • *Inadequate graft: Short/Thin*		Alternative donors may be used: (split) Ring FDS, strip of ECRL/FCR/BR
	Graft deployment and fixation • *Difficult graft insertion/passage* • *Difficult graft fixation*	Precise matching of graft/tunnel sizes Precise whipstitching of graft extremities Take advantage of dedicated tendon shuttling devices Graft Trimming or tunnel broadening according to specific anatomic conditions Use dry arthroscopy	
	Osseous tunnels • *Eccentric positioning* • *Fracture of the Ulnar Head*	Locate the foveal area by direct visualization (DRUJ exposure/arthroscopy) Use interference screw of appropriate size Avoid over stuffing of the tunnel	Above-elbow cast immobilization with for 5 weeks, then postpone rehabilitation for further 2 weeks
	Graft over-tightening • *Increased pressure on joint surfaces leading to arthritis*	Preserve physiological anteroposterior translation before completing the reconstruction	Limit rehabilitation program Remove graft DRUJ arthroplasty/ulnar head prostesis
	Tendon entrapment • *ECU/EDC/EDQ/FDP/FDS* Neurovascular damage • Ulnar neurovascular bundle	Respect of anatomical landmarks and careful surgical technique Blunt dissection of arthroscopic portals Dry arthroscopy	Suture removal at 3 months post-op Tenolysis/neurolysis Nerve/artery resection + tension-free anastomosis or grafting

Abbreviations: BR, brachioradialis; DSBUN, dorsal sensory branch of ulnar nerve; DRUJ, distal radioulnar joint; ECRL, extensor carpi radialis longus; ECU, extensor carpi ulnaris; EDC, extensor digitorum comunis; EDQ, extensor digiti quinti; FCR, flexor carpi radialis; FDP, flexor digitorum profundus; FDS, flexor digitorum superficialis; TAB of DSBUN, transverse accessory branch of dorsal sensory branch of ulnar nerve; TFCC, triangular fibrocartilage complex.

Piñal et al is recommended in order to reduce soft tissues infiltration and facilitate the smooth passage of the suture and grasper in and out of the joint, and prevent entanglement of the sutures along the path.[21] In case of tendon entrapment, tenolysis after suture removal is recommended, usually after 3 months postoperatively. In case of entrapment of the DSBUN or the TAB of DSBUN, desensitization therapy is recommended as a first choice of treatment. However, often the nerve may be damaged so severely, or even actually severed, that even neurolysis may not suffice and neuroma revision and protection may be necessary.

19.3.2 Complications Following Repair of Foveal Fibers

An increasing number of arthroscopic options for foveal repairs are becoming gradually more popular. However, most foveal repairs are still performed by open surgery. Regardless of the type of surgery, the techniques of foveal repair are performed by means of a suture anchor/screw or transosseous tunnels. Both types of surgery and fixation methods share some common issues.

As the foveal area is considered the isometric area of rotation of the DRUJ,[22] the suture anchor/screw or the transosseous tunnels must be accurately located within this area. Failure to reach proper positioning (eccentric setting) may cause displacing forces during forearm rotation. These forces may cause loosening of the anchor/screw or broadening of the tunnel, due to suture attrition over the tunnel's edges, hence leading to anchor/screw pull-out or suture rupture due to abrasion at the anchor/screw eyelet or over the tunnel's edges. Consequently, the repair may ultimately fail. In order to prevent this complication, it is recommended to ensure proper positioning of the anchor/screw or of tunnel within the fovea area by

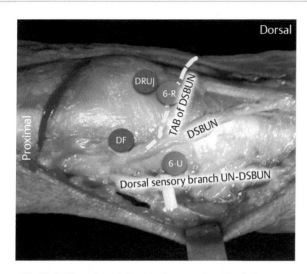

Fig. 19.4 Bifurcation of the dorsal sensory branch of ulnar nerve (DSBUN) and the transverse accessory branch of the dorsal sensory branch of ulnar nerve (TAB of DSBUN) crossing the ulnar side of the wrist tears in close relationship with the arthroscopic portals. Abbreviations: DF, direct foveal portal; DRUJ, distal radioulnar joint portal; 6 R, 6-radial portal; 6 U, 6-ulnar portal.

direct visualization of the foveal area: it requires appropriate surgical exposure of the ulnar head or use of DRUJ arthroscopy. Early recurrence of pain and DRUJ instability have been reported especially in patients with chronic injuries treated with transosseous fixation using small tunnels, either open or arthroscopic.[23,24] We believe that early failure of these cases may be related to the poor debridement of the foveal area and tear's edges, which were not included in the original techniques. Improved outcomes have been achieved with a similar technique by Iwasaki and Minami, who described an arthroscopically assisted technique using a 2.9-mm osseous tunnel at the foveal area.[25] They showed that bone bleeding from the transosseous tunnel could enhance adhesion of the avulsed TFCC to the foveal area. Therefore, careful debridement of foveal area and refreshment of tear's edges to a bleeding surface is strongly recommended, especially when a suture anchor/screw is used. For this purpose, wide exposure of the DRUJ and use of loupe magnification are recommended in open surgery. Due to the difficulties related to the exploration of such a narrow joint as the DRUJ, arthroscopy may represent an advantage for the surgeon, as it allows a magnified view and direct visualization of the TFCC tear site, with a very limited damage of surrounding tissues.

Specific complications are related to the use of a suture anchor/screw, whose strength of fixation may be reduced in case of poor bone quality. Currently, these devices are available with different thread configuration according to bone characteristics so that specific threads are used on cancellous bone, and other ones on cortical bone. How-

ever, as a general rule, use of a suture anchor/screw on the osteopenic ulnar head must be avoided. In cases where treatment cannot be postponed to allow for the improvement of bone quality, transosseous sutures should be preferred, as they rely on the strength of the metaphyseal cortex, which is always preserved.

Another unfortunate anchor/screw-related complication is associated with poor features of the eyelet of the anchor/screw, especially when it loads standard sutures (not high-strength sutures). If the eyelet is not smooth enough to allow free suture gliding, forceful knotting, especially using a sliding knot technique, may cause suture breakage by attrition on the eyelet edges. Treatment of this complication may be difficult as the presence within the foveal area of a properly located anchor/screw hinders positioning of a new anchor/screw or drilling of the ulnar tunnel for transosseous suture or, ultimately, for tendon graft reconstruction.

A specific complication more frequently related to the open dorsal approach to the DRUJ consists of the dorsal-only partial repair of the TFCC, in which just the dorsal DRUJ ligament is included in the repair. Often, in these cases, patients still complain about persistence of a residual palmar instability. Proper exposure and use of loupe magnification are recommended for use of either anchor/screw or transosseous fixation to prevent failure to include the palmar aspect of the TFCC into the stitch. The arthroscopic technique is less likely to develop this complication, as magnified visualization through the scope ensures accurate location of the stitch either at the convergence of both DRUJ ligaments or on each DRUJ ligament individually, in a ligament-specific technique.[26] This complication may be treated by repeating the foveal repair using the palmar approach, as suggested by Moritomo.[27]

Using arthroscopic knotting techniques, a specific complication may develop related to the risk that some nerve branch or tendon may be entangled with the sutures. A dedicated learning curve is required for managing the suture threads mainly with the use of the arthroscopic crochet hook or suture grasper, so as to help retrieve out of the joint, through the same portal, both suture extremities. Use of dry arthroscopy is crucial in order to preserve the quality of the soft tissues around the path for suture retrieval and knot sliding and tightening into the joint.

A general issue for any techniques of foveal repair is related to proper tensioning of the repair, especially in chronic lesions, when some scar tissue needs to be resected to prepare good quality tear's edges. Thus, the overtightening required to close the resulting gap may result in an increased tension across the DRUJ, eventually leading to early DRUJ arthritis. Likewise, in open repairs with dorsal approach, an increased pressure across the DRUJ is generated after a "pant-over-vest" overlapping repair of the extensor retinaculum, which is also often associated with restricted forearm pronation. As a rule of thumb, it is a good practice to ensure that the physiological

5

anteroposterior translation of the ulnar head is maintained before the repair is secured. Unfortunately, even if the typical disabling DRUJ pain, worsening during forearm rotation, presents since the early rehabilitation phase, the actual problem is recognized rather lately, when the chondral damage is already irreversible and joint arthroplasty/prosthesis remains the only treatment advisable.

19.4 Addressing Bony Morphology

19.4.1 Acute- on Chronic- with Positive Ulnar Variance

Two groups of TFCC tears are recognized—the acute traumatic and the chronic attritional type. The attritional type is often associated with positive ulnar variance, with characteristic findings on MRI scan, and a central tear of the TFCC. Chondral fissuring, ulcers, and flaps can affect the proximal, ulnar aspect of the lunate. These two types can coexist as a dual lesion (▶ Fig. 19.5). Failure of peripheral TFCC repair and persistent symptoms can occur if both wrist morphology (ulnar variance) and the TFCC repair are not addressed concurrently.

In these cases, we recommend initial arthroscopic evaluation of the wrist and TFCC, including debridement of the central tear back to stable margins. We then proceed with an open ulnar shortening osteotomy. Only after

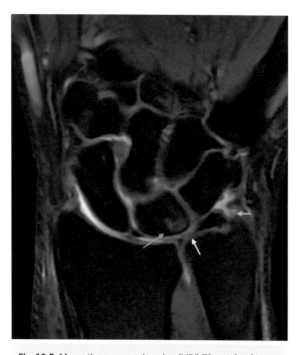

Fig. 19.5 Magnetic resonance imaging (MRI) T2-weighted image showing a dual lesion: a central degenerate and acute peripheral triangular fibrocartilage complex (TFCC) tear in a 30-year-old male. *White arrow*: central tear; *blue arrow*: peripheral tear; *orange arrow*; proximal ulnar-sided high signal in the lunate.

osteotomy can the correct repair tension be determined. Next, we perform an arthroscopic peripheral repair with mattress sutures.

19.5 Avoiding Problems with TFCC Tears: Challenging Scenarios

19.5.1 Missed TFCC Tear with Distal Radius Fixation

The incidence of TFCC tears with distal radius fracture is significant. With adequate alignment of the distal radius, most TFCC tears heal or become asymptomatic. Malunion can be subtle unless comparison is made to the contralateral side. Coronal malalignment has been shown to detension the secondary stabilizer effect of the distal oblique band of the interosseous membrane.[7] This can cause profound DRUJ instability (▶ Fig. 19.6). Careful evaluation with a CT is essential, and contralateral radiographs are needed to create a normal template for preoperative planning.

The distal radius is approached on the volar aspect with a distal flexor carpi radialis (FCR) approach. Previous hardware may require removal, or if the distal locking screws are appropriately positioned, only the shaft screws may require removal. The osteotomy is performed as per preoperative planning. Length, tilt, and radial inclination are restored. Coronal correction can be easily performed with a laminar spreader between the ulna and the proximal radius fragment. The proximal plate holes are redrilled and osteotomy stabilized. The DRUJ should then be clinically assessed at different degrees of rotation. It is important to determine DRUJ translation on the contralateral side prior to starting the procedure. Assessment of the bony morphology will often stabilize the wrist. Arthroscopic-assisted foveal repair is then commenced.

19.5.2 The Chronic TFCC Tear with DRUJ Instability

Transulnar Styloid TFCC Reconstruction

Indications for this procedure is DRUJ instability with a chronic foveal TFCC tear, 6 to 12 months after injury, or following failed repair with persistent instability.[28] MRI is required to evaluate that the TFCC is still attached to the distal radius and carpus. TFCC tears that involve the radial attachments are a contraindication for this procedure and can be identified with the "reverse-hook" test. In this setting, a reconstruction of both the origin and insertion of the volar and dorsal radioulnar ligaments is indicated.

Arthroscopy is performed as described previously. If the DRUJ is unstable, on probe testing, the translation can be seen to be much greater and extend beyond the rim of the sigmoid notch. A volar incision is made to harvest the PL tendon or half of FCR if the palmaris is absent; a mini-

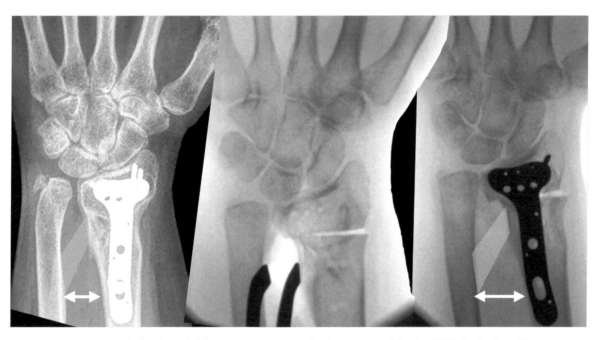

Fig. 19.6 Anteroposterior (AP) radiograph following previous open reduction and internal fixation (ORIF) distal radius with subsequent repair of triangular fibrocartilage complex (TFCC). The patient has significant distal radioulnar joint (DRUJ) instability. The plate is removed and a transverse osteotomy is performed. A laminar spreader is used to correct the coronal translation, retension the distal oblique band of the interosseous membrane, and the plate is replaced. An arthroscopic-assisted foveal repair was then performed.

mum length of 6 cm is required. Grasping sutures are placed in each end of the harvested tendon.

A 4-cm longitudinal incision is made directly over the ulnar styloid. The dorsal branch of the ulnar nerve is protected. The deep fascia is incised just volar to the sixth extensor compartment. The ulnar styloid is excised with sharp dissection to expose the ulnar fovea. Excision of the ulnar styloid can be challenging. Insertion of a suture (#2 Fiberwire, Arthrex, Naples, FL) into the ulnar styloid allows the styloid to be mobilized and then excised with sharp dissection (▸ Fig. 19.7).

The soft tissues are elevated off the volar DRUJ and volar capsule. The TFCC is elevated off the ulnar head. The 6R portal is opened to 1 cm to allow passage of the tendon graft. The foveal footprint is debrided.

Anchor preparation is performed with a 5.5-mm drill bit and tap, made into the ulnar fovea to a depth of 25 mm (▸ Fig. 19.8). The suture ends of the harvested PL tendon, and subsequently the tendon itself, are advanced from the 6R portal, through the TFCC. This is performed arthroscopically by passing the free ends of a looped suture through the TFCC with a 19-gauge hypodermic needle. The sutured ends of the PL graft are passed through the looped suture. Those suture ends are retrieved ulnarly, through the ulnar styloid approach, from the volar ulnar aspect of the wrist, taking care to protect the ulnar nerve. If too technically demanding to

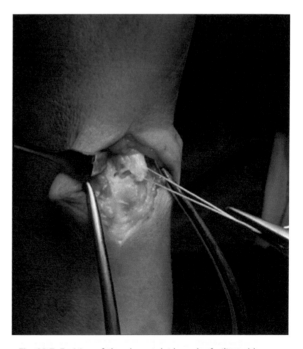

Fig. 19.7 Excision of the ulnar styloid can be facilitated by placing a suture into the ulnar styloid, to allow it to be mobilized and then excised with sharp dissection. (Copyright Dr. Gregory Bain, with permission.)

5

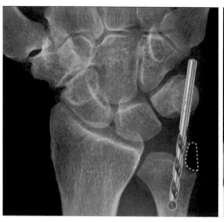

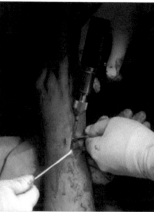

Fig. 19.8 Ulnar styloid excision and foveal suture anchor preparation. (Copyright Dr. Gregory Bain, with permission.)

perform arthroscopically, this technique can be replicated through a dorsal open approach. Both ends of the PL graft/suture complex are secured into the proximal ulnar with the 5.5-mm PEEK SwiveLock anchor (▶ Fig. 19.9).

Once secured, the DRUJ stability is assessed. Sutures arising from the anchor are used with an eyed needle to repair the extensor carpi ulnaris subsheath, as it is a secondary stabilizer. Layered closure is carried out with dissolvable sutures.

Patient is placed in an above-elbow backslab at 60 degrees of supination for 1 week. Thereafter, a Muenster splint is applied for a further 5 weeks. Afterward, a hand therapist supervises gentle range of motion exercises. At 10 weeks, the splint is discarded. The patient is advised not to perform any heavy lifting for 6 months.

The anatomic outcome of this procedure is a reconstruction and stabilization of the TFCC footprint to the fovea, increasing stability of the DRUJ and decreasing pain at the wrist.[29] Near full range of forearm rotation can be expected at 6 months.

19.5.3 The Chronic TFCC Tear with DRUJ Arthritis

Matched Distal Hemiresection Arthroplasty

For patients with chronic TFCC tears and arthritis involving the DRUJ, with an unstable and deformed distal ulna, the authors' preferred technique is the matched hemiresection developed by the late Dr. Jim Roth.[30]

The extensor retinaculum is divided over the fifth extensor compartment. The dorsal radioulnar joint capsule and the adherent infratendinous portion of the extensor retinaculum are divided 1 mm from their attachment to the sigmoid notch. No attempt is made to separate the dorsal capsule from the retinaculum, and the ECU is not removed from the retinacular flap.

An oblique osteotomy of the distal ulna is performed and the distal ulna shaped to match the contour of the distal radius throughout forearm rotation. Care is taken to

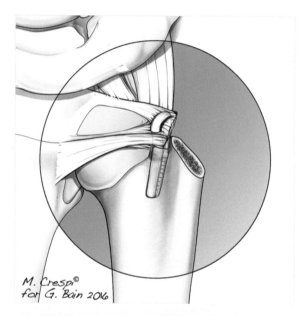

Fig. 19.9 Illustration of the tendon graft stabilization with an anchor. (Copyright Dr. Gregory Bain and Max Crespi, with permission.)

ensure that there is adequate resection and no impingement between the ulna and radius and the ulnar styloid and carpus. The joint is also examined with intraoperative fluoroscopy throughout supination and pronation.

The ulnar-based retinacular flap is undermined from the adjacent ulna and tendons, allowing it to be mobilized and used as an interposition graft. The technique helps to stabilize the distal ulna, as the ECU tendon is stabilized over the top of the distal ulnar stump. The ulnar-based retinacular flap is sutured to the 1-mm stump. The supratendinous portion of the retinaculum is repaired distally to prevent bowstringing of the extensor digiti minimi tendon (▶ Fig. 19.10).

19.6 Algorithm

We believe the best way to avoid complications when performing TFCC surgery is to perform a detailed clinical

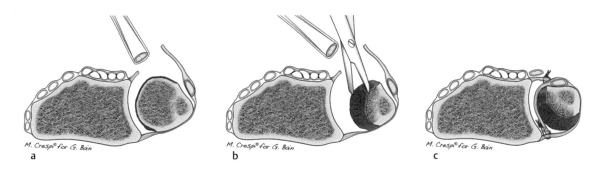

Fig. 19.10 **(a)** Cross-section at the level of the distal radioulnar joint showing the relationship of the extensor digiti minimi and the extensor carpi ulnaris. **(b)** The fifth extensor compartment is divided, the extensor digiti minimi is retracted, and the dorsal capsule and the infratendinous portion of the extensor retinaculum divided 1mm from their radial insertion. A matched resection of the distal ulna is then performed. **(c)** The ulnar-based retinacular flap is mobilized and then sutured to the 1-mm flap. This transfers the extensor carpi ulnaris to the dorsal aspect of the distal ulna. (Copyright Dr. Gregory Bain, Dr. Simon MacLean, and Max Crespi, with permission.)

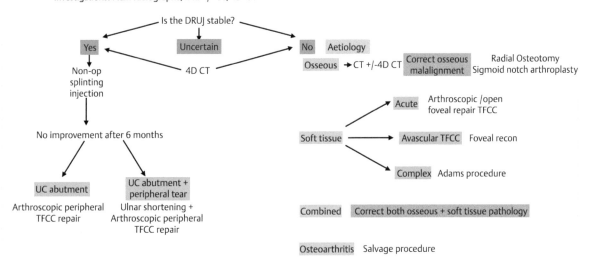

Fig. 19.11 Triangular fibrocartilage complex (TFCC) tear algorithm. (Copyright Dr. Simon MacLean and Dr. Gregory Bain, with permission.)

assessment, with a focused history, clinical examination, and investigations. Treatment will depend on a number of factors. We have introduced an algorithm for the painful TFCC tear. The algorithm is a framework for the wrist surgeon and highlights the key concepts when treating these injuries (▸ Fig. 19.11).

19.7 Take-Home Message

Effective treatment of TFCC tears and avoidance of complications depend upon a number of patient-related and surgical factors. A thorough history, clinical examination, and review of imaging should be performed. Arthroscopic assessment is fundamental to assess tear anatomy, acuity, and stability and helps direct surgical treatment. An algorithm-based approach can be used to avoid complications from TFCC repair.

Acknowledgments

Riccardo Luchetti (Rimini Hand Surgery and Rehabilitation Center, Rimini, Italy).

Lucian Lior Marcovici (Hand & Microsurgery Unit, Jewish Hospital of Rome, Rome, Italy).

References

[1] Richards RS, Bennett JD, Roth JH, Milne K, Jr. Arthroscopic diagnosis of intra-articular soft tissue injuries associated with distal radial fractures. J Hand Surg Am. 1997; 22(5):772–776

[2] Andersson JK, Åhlén M, Andernord D. Open versus arthroscopic repair of the triangular fibrocartilage complex: a systematic review. J Exp Orthop. 2018; 5(1):6

[3] Demino C, Morales-Restrepo A, Fowler J. Surgical management of triangular fibrocartilage complex lesions: a review of outcomes. J Hand Surg Am. 2019; 1(1):32–38

[4] Robba V, Fowler A, Karantana A, Grindlay D, Lindau T. Open versus arthroscopic repair of 1B ulnar-sided triangular fibrocartilage complex tears: a systematic review. Hand (N Y). 2020; 15(4):456–464

[5] McNamara CT, Colakoglu S, Iorio ML. A systematic review and analysis of palmer type I triangular fibrocartilage complex injuries: Outcomes of Treatment. J Hand Microsurg. 2020; 12(2):116–122

[6] Luchetti R, Atzei A, Rocchi L. [Incidence and causes of failures in wrist arthroscopic techniques]. Chir Main. 2006; 25(1):48–53

[7] Kakar S, Garcia-Elias M. The "four-leaf clover" treatment algorithm: a practical approach to manage disorders of the distal radioulnar joint. J Hand Surg Am. 2016; 41(4):551–564

[8] Leclercq C, Mathoulin C, Members of EWAS. Complications of wrist arthroscopy: a multicenter study based on 10,107 arthroscopies. J Wrist Surg. 2016; 5(4):320–326

[9] Tay SC, Tomita K, Berger RA. The "ulnar fovea sign" for defining ulnar wrist pain: an analysis of sensitivity and specificity. J Hand Surg Am. 2007; 32(4):438–444

[10] Beighton P, Solomon L, Soskolne CL. Articular mobility in an African population. Ann Rheum Dis. 1973; 32(5):413–418

[11] Wallwork NA, Bain GI. Sigmoid notch osteoplasty for chronic volar instability of the distal radioulnar joint: a case report. J Hand Surg Am. 2001; 26(3):454–459

[12] Carr R, MacLean S, Slavotinek J, Bain GI. Four-dimensional computed tomography scanning for dynamic wrist disorders: prospective analysis and recommendations for clinical utility. J Wrist Surg. 2019; 8(2):161–167

[13] Hermansdorfer JD, Kleinman WB. Management of chronic peripheral tears of the triangular fibrocartilage complex. J Hand Surg Am. 1991; 16(2):340–346

[14] Atzei A. New trends in arthroscopic management of type 1-B TFCC injuries with DRUJ instability. J Hand Surg Eur Vol. 2009; 34(5):582–591

[15] Atzei A, Luchetti R, Garagnani L. Classification of ulnar triangular fibrocartilage complex tears. A treatment algorithm for Palmer type IB tears. J Hand Surg Eur Vol. 2017; 42(4):405–414

[16] Bednar JM, Osterman AL. The role of arthroscopy in the treatment of traumatic triangular fibrocartilage injuries. Hand Clin. 1994; 10(4):605–614

[17] de Araujo W, Poehling GG, Kuzma GR. New Tuohy needle technique for triangular fibrocartilage complex repair: preliminary studies. Arthroscopy. 1996; 12(6):699–703

[18] Pederzini LA, Tosi M, Prandini M, Botticella C. All-inside suture technique for Palmer class 1B triangular fibrocartilage repair. Arthroscopy. 2007; 23(10):1130.e1–1130.e4

[19] del Piñal F, García-Bernal FJ, Cagigal L, Studer A, Regalado J, Thams C. A technique for arthroscopic all-inside suturing in the wrist. J Hand Surg Eur Vol. 2010; 35(6):475–479

[20] Estrella EP, Hung LK, Ho PC, Tse WL. Arthroscopic repair of triangular fibrocartilage complex tears. Arthroscopy. 2007; 23(7):729–737, 737.e1

[21] del Piñal F, García-Bernal FJ, Pisani D, Regalado J, Ayala H, Studer A. Dry arthroscopy of the wrist: surgical technique. J Hand Surg Am. 2007; 32(1):119–123

[22] Haugstvedt JR, Berger RA, Nakamura T, Neale P, Berglund L, An KN. Relative contributions of the ulnar attachments of the triangular fibrocartilage complex to the dynamic stability of the distal radioulnar joint. J Hand Surg Am. 2006; 31(3):445–451

[23] Nakamura T, Sato K, Okazaki M, Toyama Y, Ikegami H. Repair of foveal detachment of the triangular fibrocartilage complex: open and arthroscopic transosseous techniques. Hand Clin. 2011; 27(3):281–290

[24] Iwasaki N, Nishida K, Motomiya M, Funakoshi T, Minami A. Arthroscopic-assisted repair of avulsed triangular fibrocartilage complex to the fovea of the ulnar head: a 2- to 4-year follow-up study. Arthroscopy. 2011; 27(10):1371–1378

[25] Iwasaki N, Minami A. Arthroscopically assisted reattachment of avulsed triangular fibrocartilage complex to the fovea of the ulnar head. J Hand Surg Am. 2009; 34(7):1323–1326

[26] Atzei A, Rizzo A, Luchetti R, Fairplay T. Arthroscopic foveal repair of triangular fibrocartilage complex peripheral lesion with distal radioulnar joint instability. Tech Hand Up Extrem Surg. 2008; 12(4):226–235

[27] Moritomo H. Open repair of the triangular fibrocartilage complex from palmar aspect. J Wrist Surg. 2015; 4(1):2–8

[28] Ross M, Di Mascio L, Peters S, Cockfield A, Taylor F, Couzens G. Defining residual radial translation of distal radius fractures: a potential cause of distal radioulnar joint instability. J Wrist Surg. 2014; 3(1):22–29

[29] Bain GI, Tu CG. Transulnar styloid foveal TFC reconstruction: with a palmaris longus tendon graft. Tech Hand Up Extrem Surg. 2020; 25(1):10–13

[30] Bain GI, Pugh DMW, MacDermid JC, Roth JH. Matched hemiresection interposition arthroplasty of the distal radioulnar joint. J Hand Surg Am. 1995; 20(6):944–950

Section 6

Soft-Tissue Surgery

20 Complications Following Treatment of Dupuytren's Disease and Their Management

Paul M.N. Werker and Ilse Degreef

Abstract

There is a variety of surgical and nonsurgical options for the treatment of Dupuytren's disease. Understandably, they all have their advantages and disadvantages. Important disadvantages include complications. The purpose of this chapter is to list the most relevant treatment options and their complications and management. Ultimately, prevention is prime priority, but if complications occur, proper treatment and open communication with the patient are paramount. Prior to treatment it is important to allow for information-based decision making after sufficient explanation followed by properly reporting of the decision.

Keywords: Dupuytren's disease, complications, fasciectomy, fasciotomy, collagenase, radiotherapy, steroids, systemic treatment

20.1 Introduction

Dupuytren's disease (DD) is a very common benign hand infliction. It is a disease of all ages, but is most prevalent in people of over 60 years. Prevalence investigations in our countries has shown that more than 20% of the population of over 50 years of age has signs of the disease and 4% of these people have actual contractures.[1] Histopathologically, DD is a fibromatosis that develops and spreads along the palmar fascia of the hand. First, nodules form that harbor conglomerates of myofibroblasts that deposit superfluous extracellular matrix. This process may progress into the formation of cords, which ultimately may contract, causing extension deficits foremost of the ulnar fingers. Similar diseases occur in the soles of the feet (M. Ledderhose) and in the tunica albuginea of the penis (M. Peyronie) and pads may form on the dorsum of the proximal interphalangeal (PIP) knuckles (Garrod's pads). Pain is often a sign of early disease, which usually subsides when the disease advances. Functional problems in most people only occur after substantial contractures have formed, turning the affected fingers into hooks that catch on handles and crockery, and make the use of gloves cumbersome. Many tasks of daily living that require straight fingers also become more difficult (washing, shaking hands, caressing, etc.).

The disease has a genetic basis and runs in families: using Genome Wide Association Studies (GWAS), over 25 loci in the genome have been associated with it.[2] Its emergence is possibly triggered by direct repetitive microtrauma and even more remote trauma to the extremity, for instance, following distal radial fractures seem to influence the disease. Exposure to vibration, diabetes mellitus, liver disease, antiepileptic drug use, alcohol abuse, and smoking have also been indicated as being influential.[3,4] Both hands may be affected, but usually in a different phase and the disease in general starts in the little and ring fingers, although all fingers may be affected.

As clinicians we only see the more advanced stages of the disease, and relatively little is known about the natural course of the disease. Recent research has shown that, in general, DD progresses at a constant pace, but it may also be stable for a considerable time and in some cases even regress.[5]

The disease is chronic and at present cannot be cured. When an affected hand can no longer be put flat on the table (table top test), a patient should be referred to a specialist to discuss treatment. Flexion contractures of the metacarpophalangeal joints (MCPJ) usually can be redressed during treatment. Those of the proximal interphalangeal joints (PIPJ) are more difficult to correct, especially once they are over 60 degrees of flexion, possibly because the joint capsule also becomes involved and the central slip of the extensor tendon attenuates. Treatment for the last 200 years has been symptomatic and surgical, although some local treatments (steroid injections, local radiotherapy, and TNF-alfa blockers) aim at stabilizing the disease or even inducing regression of early disease.[6] During surgery, which still is the mainstay of treatment, cords causing contractures can be transected or excised, with or without replacement of the overlying skin. Besides, in recent decades, collagenase has been introduced into the market for the treatment of flexion contractures. It has now become clear that it is just as effective in the short and long run as percutaneous needle fasciotomy (PNF) and has recently been taken off the market in Europe.

Every treatment has its advantages and disadvantages (including complications) and every surgeon involved in the treatment of DD should develop a treatment algorithm that is adapted to the population one sees, and apply treatments that are effective in the short term with a limited risk of complications and with an acceptable durability of the results. Most less invasive treatments such as PNF and collagenase have a very low chance at causing complications, but pay a price of a more limited durability. However, these treatments often can be repeated more than once and as such postpone more aggressive treatments.

Each patient should be involved in the choice for the best fitting treatment at the most appropriate time. Recurrences after the more extensive surgical interventions should be treated by specialists, since there is a much higher likelihood of complications and any further recurrence should be prevented at any cost.[7]

The prime subject of this chapter is to provide an overview of potential complications, a way to prevent and a way to deal with them. There have been a number of excellent papers dedicated to this topic and the aim of this chapter is to summarize these and add our personal experience which we have collected over the past decades as specialists in the treatment of this disease in Belgium (ID) and The Netherlands (PW).[8,9,10] The discussion will be treatment-based and therefore some overlap is unavoidable. For young less experienced colleagues an important message at this stage is: apply shared decision-making, explain the most common possible complications to the patient before you embark on any treatment. Make sure the patient understands the choices and risks. Please try to avoid complications during surgery. Don't get depressed when they occur, because they will, and if they do, treat them as best as you can and explain everything in detail to the patient, and—last but not least—report them appropriately in your operating notes, so that for subsequent surgeries they are well documented, informing the next surgeon about the situation so he/she can take them into account when confronted with yet another recurrence.

20.2 General Overview of Complications of Fasciectomy

Fasciectomy can be performed segmentally, limited to the areas of pathology, or radically. In any case, it entails incision of the skin and the elevation of skin flaps.

Wound-healing disturbances including skin sloughing (22.9%, range 0–86) and incisional scar pain (17.4%) were the most frequently found complications in the review of Denkler in 2010.[8] The authors have experienced this problem more often following Bruner's incisions than following Z-plasties. Skin slough should be treated depending on its extent: small areas can be left alone, larger areas (complete flap loss) should be surgically debrided and primarily or secondarily skin grafted.

Neuropraxia of one or both digital nerves is very common after fasciectomy and may occur in up to 50% of cases.[9] It is due to the fact that the nerves are manipulated on one hand (neuropraxia), and vascularly segmentally supplied on the other. In the more extensive procedures, these tiny vessels are easily damaged (devascularization), especially when the neurovascular (nv-) bundle is completely encased by pathology. This neuropraxia can be a complete conduction block and by definition temporary and usually recovers in 2 to 3 months. However, if the sensation only recovers partially and the digital nerve was macroscopically intact, it must have suffered more internal damage due to ischemia which may have caused some axonotmesis, while visually intact. Not much can be done in such a situation, although sensory re-education may

improve the quality of the sensibility to some extent. Besides all this, it is good to realize that in the areas of fasciectomy the sensibility in the elevated skin flaps usually diminishes to the level that is normally achieved following skin grafting. This is only seldom reported in the literature, but good to bring across to our patients. The same goes for the incidence of cold intolerance, which has been found to be as high as 44% following fasciectomy.[11]

The incidence of iatrogenic division of the digital nerves in primary cases is about 2% and may increase to up to 20% in recurrent cases.[8] The high numbers of nv-bundle injuries in recurrent cases is caused by the presence of scar tissue, making it sometimes impossible to distinguish the digital nerve from the pathology. The patient should be warned beforehand for this situation.

Similar figures apply for digital artery injuries, although the reported incidence may be lower than factual. The reason for this is that this injury may be simply overlooked, especially on the ulnar side of the little finger and the radial side of the thumb and index, where the smallest nondominant digital arteries are situated. These are often tiny, in the long fingers especially distal to PIPJ and when operating using a tourniquet and after exsanguination of the extremity. We therefore plea strongly against the latter maneuver: elevating the arm while disinfecting or after draping is in general enough to evacuate the blood to such an extent that it leaves a bloodless field, without emptying the blood vessels completely. Operating using wide-awake local anesthesia no tourniquet (WLANT) may be an alternative, with which we have no experience.

A sharp digital nerve transection that occurs during surgery should always be repaired microsurgically. The result of such a repair is often quite good and the sensibility may return to the same level as that of a digital nerve that has been completely freed from its surroundings but left anatomically in continuity for the reasons mentioned earlier. A transected nerve that is not repaired will form a neuroma. Eight percent of these neuromas may cause neuropathic pain.[12] Repair of the nondominant digital artery is a questionable act in our view if very small (<0.5 mm), because the other digital artery will be able to feed the whole finger. Injury to the dominant artery (usually situated at the side closest to the middle finger) should always be repaired with microsurgical techniques. Most often, insufficient pinking up of a treated finger immediately after tourniquet release following fasciectomy is caused by vasospasm rather than arterial transection. A wait-and-see policy usually may suffice. In addition, the digit can be warmed, or treated with antispasm agents such as papaverine or lidocaine, and/or placed in slight flexion to relieve undue tension on the vessel. Within 10 minutes, the digit will usually pink up. If not, amputation of part of the finger may be unavoidable, but may also be postponed for a few days. The level of amputation usually is transarticular at the PIPJ and closure can usually be achieved using a dorsal flap. This level of amputation does leave an unsightly hand and some patients prefer ray amputation or transposition if indicated at the risk of painful neuroma formation.

20.2.1 Specific Complications of Limited Fasciectomy (LF)

Limited fasciectomy (LF) is still the most commonly performed treatment modality for DD. It entails the preoperative identification of the pathology that needs to be removed, the elevation of the skin off the pathology and its excision, taking care to protect the neurovascular (nv-) bundles.

A plethora of incisions are described for getting access to the finger, These incisions can be grouped into the straight-line incision that is closed after the incorporation of Z-plasties, the Bruner Zig-Zag incision that can be closed using Y-V-plasties, or the McCash transverse incisions at the level of the transverse ligament of the palmar aponeurosis that crease more distally. The transpositions serve two purposes: recruitment of extra skin from the side to increase the length and in case of the straight-line incision the prevention of skin contractures. Remaining skin defects in the McCash technique can be left to heal by secondary intention. An additional benefit of this technique is that there is hardly any risk for a hematoma collection after surgery. Downsides are the more limited surgical exposure and the longer healing time of the wounds, for which the patient should be warned. A longitudinal incision with Z-plasties offers—especially once the Z-plasties are cut—a better access to the whole finger than the McCash technique. A longitudinal incision with Z-plasties carries less risk for skin slough, since the flaps usually are of more even thickness, or at least the thinnest at their apex and not halfway as is often the case with zig-zag incisions. Downside of the Z-plasties may be the development of a transverse contracture where the flaps of the Z-plasty meet, which may hamper flexion in the early phases of the rehabilitation. An extra word of caution is needed for mirroring zig-zag incisions of joining fingers that meet too distal in the webspace. They may cause a web space contracture that is not only unsightly, but also cumbersome for the patient, since it limits abduction of the fingers. Iatrogenic longitudinal skin contractures should be prevented (by performing Z-plasties before skin closure) or treated as soon as the wounds have healed and the hand function has recovered substantially, since they may hinder further functional recovery. Another word of caution about Z-plasties: there is usually ample surplus to be recruited from the sides at the level of the proximal phalanx half way the palm-finger and the PIP-creases, but there is very little skin to be recruited from the sides in the distal palm. As a consequence, the Z-plasty at the level of the proximal phalanx can be big and include most of the skin between the ear-

lier named creased, whereas a Z-plasty in the distal palm of especially the ring and middle finger can only have limbs of 0.75 cm.

Elevation of the skin off the pathology and its excision can be a challenge, since the nv-bundles can be displaced. A classical place of displacement is just proximal to natatory ligament, where the nv-bundle can be displaced toward the middle of the ray and lie superficial to a spiral cord, which originates from McGrouther's layer 2 of the pretendinous cord. Pathognomonic of this is the presence of fat in between the skin and the cord in the distal palm (Short-Watson sign). More distally, the pathology may develop in the palmodigital spiraling system, the lateral digital sheet fibers, and in Grayson's and Cleland's ligaments and since they are all interconnected and originally run in different planes, they can also cause spiraling of the nv-bundles at various places in the finger as described by Hettiaratchy and Tonkin in 2010.[13,14] In primary cases, the nv-bundles are usually easily identifiable just distal to the transverse ligament of the palmar aponeurosis and can be traced distally, or can be identified distal of the pathology and traced proximally. In recurrent cases, the plain between the pathology and the nv-bundles may be less clear and there may even be pathology between digital artery and nerve, placing either of them extra at risk for injury.

Reduced sensibility at physical examination in a previously operated finger is a warning sign for earlier damage to the corresponding nerve and artery. In such cases, an extra warning to the patient that the finger may lose its sensation completely on that side of the finger, or worse, even become ischemic and may ultimately turn into gangrene.

In 2% of cases a hematoma may form after LF; in theory, more often it may form if skin closure and bandaging is performed before tourniquet release. If not evacuated, this may cause skin flap problems and often is the beginning of an early recurrence. For this reason, we see every patient after LF back on the day after surgery, inspect the wound, and act if necessary.

A rare complication of fasciectomy is infection and should be treated as any other infection: with antibiotics if superficial, and by incision, drainage, and wash out if deep.

Cold sensitivity is almost inevitable after any (surgical) trauma to the hand or a finger and especially people who work in the cold should be warned against it, since it occurs in 44% of cases. In 50% of cases it gradually disappears.[11]

Residual contracture following fasciectomy may be substantial in the treatment of PIPJ contractures of over 60 degrees, and intraoperative gentle manipulation after completion of fasciectomy has been found to have the same outcome as surgical division of the flexor sheath, check reign, and collateral ligaments.[15] Temporary K-wiring after full release offers no benefits, most likely because of the central slip attenuation that often develops in severe PIPJ contractures. On another note, a residual PIPJ contracture is often compensated by hyperextension at the MCPJ and therefore it is not such a functional problem. Finally, it is good to realize that full extension of all joints of the fingers is not necessary for good hand function. Saffar has advocated the total anterior tenoarthrolysis for the treatment of severe PIP (and DIP) contractures. It consists in releasing the entire flexor apparatus and a subperiosteal dissection. The volar plates of PIP and DIP are released as a whole with the flexor apparatus. The extended finger and flexor apparatus are thereafter allowed to heal in a new relationship. Straightening of the finger is always possible. The range of motion is maintained or increased. This technique can also be used in stiff PIP joints and in certain serious forms of Dupuytren's contracture. In his paper in 1983, Saffar reviewed 56 cases with 78% providing good or fair results.[16] We have no experience with this technique and no comparative studies are available to reveal the true value of this technique.

Stiffness defined as impaired flexion of the operated ray or worse of the operated hand as part of or without other signs of complex regional pain syndrome (CRPS) is a tragedy, especially if it proves hand therapy resistant, and may leave the patient more incapacitated than preoperatively. Its incidence is low, but yet it is one of the more serious complications, which has made LF unpopular among those who suffer from it and it was one of the reasons why the authors for primary cases moved to less invasive treatments such as segmental fasciectomy (SF), PNF, and collagenase injections.

Recurrent contracture is not really a complication of LF, but part of the normal chronic disease course and something the patient should be warned for. It is one of the unpredictable sides of the treatment of DD and especially cumbersome if it occurs shortly after treatment. Some surgeons reoperate early in a vain effort to try and correct these early recurrences, but often find themselves confronted with even more severe recurrences. We believe that it is best to try and treat such unfortunate cases with maximal conservative care, including static night splinting in combination with intensive hand therapy and exercises during the day. Trials testing the benefits of additional local or systemic treatments are needed to disclose their efficacy.

Notwithstanding all these adverse events of LF, patients in general should be informed that the chance of a recurrence following treatment for DD is inversely related to the aggressiveness of the treatment. So, if a patient chooses for LF, the statistical chance of a recurrence is much lower than after PNF.[17]

20.2.2 Specific Complications of Segmental Fasciectomy (SF)

In SF, strategically chosen segments of the Dupuytren cords are removed. This minimally invasive surgical technique was popularized by Moermans, by using semicircular incisions.[18] Through this approach, short Dupuytren cord segments of about 10 mm are excised to regain finger extension, but the pathology in between the areas of SF is left untouched. In nodular forms with clearly hindering nodules, these prominent tumors are preferably removed with the underlying cord in this segmental technique, leaving only nondiseased strands that may even disappear spontaneously after surgery, once the traction on the cords is resolved. The SF can be looked upon as an augmented fasciotomy: the segment removal creates a firebreak within the Dupuytren cords. These firebreaks may at their turn be augmented by the interposition of an inert implant such as cellulose to prevent fibrotic bridging of the segmental gap and to isolate the overlying skin from the scarring process. This has been found to improve outcome in the short term with improved motion gain.[18]

Other surgical approaches are also possible for SF: multiple transverse incisions are an alternative, which avoid longitudinal scar contracture. To lengthen the skin up to 75%, Z-plasty skin closure may be used in SF after longitudinal incision.

The overall complication rate in SF is very limited, with cumulative complication risk reports of 0 to 5.6%. Mostly mentioned are hematomas, skin necrosis, nerve lesions, and CRPS.[19]

The advantages of SF are in line with those of other minimally invasive surgeries and are mainly a more swift recovery with less pain. However, no surgical procedure is without risk. In this form of minimally invasive surgery, the exposure of the diseased tissue and the neurovascular bundles is more limited than during LF. As explained earlier, these neurovascular structures are often displaced from their normal anatomical position. Therefore, the surgeon needs to take care that the risk of damaging them does not outweigh the benefit of a more limited approach with the more limited visualization, and be prepared to extend any incision if needed. However, some feel that limited exposure of the neurovascular structures may be better than no exposure at all as in percutaneous techniques, and therefore, nerve lesions are rare (less than 1%). Nerve injuries will become visible during SF, and are just as in LF best treated with immediate microsurgical repair. Neuropraxia is not mentioned in the literature, but obviously, transient sensory loss may occur in some cases.

Wound healing is usually faster than after more extensive surgery, and mobilization is easier, fast, and immediate. The risks of secondary reactive pain syndromes (associated with DD, common after surgical treatment) are lower, since CRPS is associated with more extensive trauma. In the literature, this complication following SF hardly exists at all (less than 1%). Hematoma, limited skin necrosis, and transient superficial wound infection are mentioned in less than 3% and local treatment usually resolves the problem in 2 to 4 weeks.[19]

6

Whether or not this incomplete cord resection is prone to higher recurrence of contracture remains controversial, and comparative studies have not been performed.

20.2.3 Specific Complications of Dermofasciectomy (DF)

In dermofasciectomy (DF) as developed by Hueston, overlying skin is removed together with the underlying Dupuytren cords and nodules.[18,20] In some cases, the skin is not replaced and left open for secondary healing. McCash introduced the latter technique. Usually, in DF the amount of resected skin is more substantial and replaced by a full-thickness skin graft, taken from the ulnovolar side of the proximal forearm or upper arm. In our practices, we mostly apply the technique in recurrent cases and remove the skin of the proximal phalanx from one midlateral line to the other with a small rim of distal palm and midphalanx skin. Obviously, DF is a rather invasive extensive surgical procedure. The advantage is that skin shortage, certainly if the skin is completely adherent and involved in the Dupuytren pathology, is resolved, and affected or scarred skin is replaced by a skin graft from the forearm, where DD does not occur. Moreover, removing the affected skin and replacing it with healthy skin with different properties than that of the palm of the hand adds to the completeness of the removal of all affected Dupuytren tissue. This reflects in lower reported recurrence rates underneath the skin grafts in the long term.[21] Unfortunately, comparative studies are lacking at present to substantiate its value, so it is very much an expert opinion that leads to its application in selected cases.

The procedure is more invasive than the other surgical interventions and therefore requires a longer and more intense rehabilitation. The risk for complications is accepted to be higher than in lesser invasive procedures, and the severity of these unwelcome events is greater. However, pooled complication incidences rated them somewhat lower: 11.6% versus 78% in collagenase treatment and 19% in PNF, 17.4 in LF.[22] This bizarre difference in incidence is, however, very inconsistent and unreliable, due to the high variability in reporting, follow-up, and definitions.

In short-term prospective follow-up, temporary hypesthesia is present in about half of the patients, although most fingers have complete sensory recovery within 3 months.[23] CRPS is present in 5%. Regional anesthesia possibly lowers the incidence of CRPS compared to general anesthesia. Hand therapy is usually successful in these cases but some residual stiffness is often unavoidable. In the donor site of the skin graft at the arm, the morbidity is usually limited to a rare wound dehiscence, which may be prevented by protecting the wound using suture strips, or a hematoma risk (less than 1%), which we try to prevent using a compressive bandage after surgery. If primary skin closure at the forearm is very tight, we remove the subcutaneous tissues while preserving the medial antebrachial cutaneous nerve.

An unsightly scar may remain in rare cases, but usually it is not cumbersome. In the hand, wound dehiscence (10%) or infection (18%) is more likely, requiring antibiotics and regular dressing changes. The period in which dressing is needed is also longer. Total graft failure is rarely reported, but partial graft loss is not that uncommon in our practices. We have slightly different approaches to prevent graft failure, but agree that any effort should be taken to remove blood from under the graft at the end of the surgery and keep it away by applying pressure and immobilization. If a wound-healing disturbance does occur, local dressing changed every 2 to 3 days will allow for healing by secondary intention.

Although the surgery is obviously more extensive in DF, motion gain in the long term does not appear to differ significantly from that following SF or LF. However, most reports focus on the gain of extension. A possible flexion loss is hardly ever even mentioned, but it is not farfetched following elaborate surgery such as DF. As said before, any flexion loss in the fingers may impact significantly on functional outcome. Therefore, careful monitoring is advised, and early hand therapy may be helpful and splinting needs to be indicated with proper caution.

20.3 General Complications of Fasciotomy

There are two ways to perform fasciotomy: openly and percutaneously. In general, the frequency and severity of complications following fasciotomy is lower than that following fasciectomy. It is conceivable that the chance of complications using a blade (such as during open fasciotomy [OF]) is greater than following needle fasciotomy and that the chance of complications in needle fasciotomy is directly dependent on the thickness of the needle used.

20.3.1 Specific Complications of Percutaneous Needle Fasciotomy (PNF)

PNF is a minimally invasive treatment modality that in the 1970s of last century was introduced in the literature by rheumatologists. The epicenter for these trainings has been Paris. Many hand surgeons who have published extensively on this technique where trained by Drs. Lermusiaux, Thyssedou, and Badois in l'Hôpital Lariboisière around the turn of the century. PNF entails the percutaneous division of cords responsible for contractures in DD using intradermal anesthesia only. Because of its minimal invasiveness, it can be performed as an office or treatment room procedure. Its efficacy in contractures of up to 90 degrees is just as good as that of LF, and most practitioners only apply it for MCPJ contractures, since they are afraid to damage the NV-bundles in the fingers.[24] This fear is understandable, but not supported by the literature.

Skin tears are relatively common and may occur in up to 50% of cases in recurrent cases where the skin may be affected.[9,10] Our personal skin tear rate is much lower, at least to some extent, thanks to the adaption of Denkler's technique: he advised to perform—what he calls—"subscision" a procedure in which the skin is freed from the underlying cords using a 19-gauge needle. If skin tears do appear, they usually can be left to heal secondarily. In extreme cases, a local skin flap can be employed to close a defect.

Most feared but infrequent are tendon and digital nerve injuries. For obvious reasons, their incidence is related to the thickness of the needle that is used. Using intradermal anesthesia only, and working from distal to proximal, allows the patient to warn the surgeon when the needle gets close to or in contact with a nerve. We always warn the patient for postoperative temporary anesthesia, which is caused by the spreading of the local anesthesia around the nerves, and specifically ask the patients to call us if sensibility remains disturbed the day after PNF. Only once in the 20 years that PW has been performing PNF, a complete nerve injury was feared since there was total numbness distal of the side of PNF and a positive Tinel's sign. At exploration, the nerve was nonetheless anatomically intact. In the literature, the reported incidence of nerve injury is 1 to 4% and as said and done: every persistent hypesthesia on the day after treatment should be explored. Neuropraxia does happen in 1% of cases but is by its nature temporary.

Flexor tendon injury is more common following PNF than after LF, since the flexor tendons are not directly visualized. Rates of tendon injury during PNF have been reported as occurring in 0.05% of cases. To prevent this, the patient should be asked to move the finger while the needle is placed at estimated maximal thickness of the cord. If it moves during that procedure, it is inside the tendon and should be withdrawn. At the end of the procedure, the patient should always be asked to make a full fist and a small fist to exclude tendon injury. If in doubt, exploration should follow and in worse case, repair. Until now we did not have to do this. A subclinical, partial injury to the tendons warrants the prohibition of heavy labor in the first 2 weeks following PNF.

Infection following PNF is rare. The reported percentage in the literature is 0.7%. Personally, we have seen one case of infection that needed surgical debridement. In that case, in hindsight, infection may have been related to inadvertent transection of a skin pit by the needle, causing it to become buried under the skin. The infection was only resolved after removal of this buried piece of skin.

Recurrence following PNF is much more frequent than after more invasive procedures, but this should not be seen as a complication, but rather a direct result of division of the cord only. The treatment can usually be repeated a number of times and thereby a more invasive procedure delayed. For many patients, this is an advantage big enough for them to accept the disadvantages of a lesser durability.[17]

20.3.2 Specific Complications of Open Fasciotomy (OF)

OF was first proposed by Henri Cline of London in 1787 for DD, although there is no record that he ever performed it. It was demonstrated during a lecture for medical students at l'Hopital Dieu in Paris on the 5th of December 1831 by Dupuytren himself. It was performed without anesthesia while standing behind the patient whose hand was elevated with the shoulder in 90 degrees abduction and the elbow in 90 degrees of flexion. It is not known how much collateral damage occurred during this procedure, nor in the years that followed and during which the technique was frequented, but it was stressed by Dupuytren that this disease did not affect the flexor tendons and that these therefore should be preserved.

In the last century, some surgeons revisited and refined the technique of Dupuytren and performed it openly using small skin incisions. It is conceivable that this technique is at least as effective as PNF, but has a slightly more elevated risk of injury to the neurovascular bundles.[25] It was reported to be especially effective for MCPJ contractures, with a durability after 5 years of 55%. Personally, we do not employ it, since the advantages over PNF on one hand and SF on the other seem limited.

20.4 Complications of Treatment with Collagenase (CCH)

The collagenase treatment is a minimally invasive (nonsurgical) enzymatic fasciotomy to treat Dupuytren contractures. This innovative treatment option was clinically introduced in the first decade of this century after a long duration of translational research by Hurst and Badalamente from Sunny Brook New York.[26] The cords in DD are rich in collagen, and this particular drug, produced by *Clostridium histolyticum*, is used to resolve them at strategically chosen injection sites to recover finger extension. The injectable drug consists of collagenases of class I and II, acting in concert to degrade collagen. Both types are present not only in the cords of DD, but also in the (flexor) tendons, but not in the neurovascular bundles which contain mostly collagen type IV in their basement membrane structure and therefore the blood vessels and nerves are spared.

The reported complication rate in collagenase treatment is higher than in any other treatment modality: up to 78%. However, most of these are debatable as complications: edema (62%) and hematoma (25%) are mentioned most frequently but are obviously also present following any other treatments. The reason for these reported numbers is the thorough prospective clinical research and follow-up of this innovative treatment option, which is hardly ever the case in more classic treatment options. Moreover, swelling and hematoma are obviously present in almost every operative case in the first days or weeks after surgery, but never mentioned. Skin tears may occur after the injection (in 24%), most often as the result of the manipulation of the fingers 1 to 7 days after the injection. This stretching is standard to regain full range of motion. The skin is affected by an inflammatory reaction at that moment and is often connected to the underlying Dupuytren cords. Firm manipulation and stretching regularly results in skin tears that can be quite large. However, dry dressings, changed every 2 or 3 days, usually allow for healing without further treatment within 5 to 10 days even in quite large tears. In 9% the inflammation, which can be considered a reaction to the collagenase, will cause a temporary axillary lymphadenopathy, which requires no treatment. The mostly feared and serious complication is a tendon lesion. Flexor tendon ruptures are reported in 4% of the patients, mostly in injections for PIP joint contractures of the fifth digit. Careful patient selection and avoiding injections into the tendons can minimize the risk for this serious adverse event. If it occurs, it depends on the wish of the patient if further treatment is chosen. Most patients prefer to accept the handicap of limited active flexion over secondary flexor tendon repair and long rehabilitation. In our practice, it occurred once in a severe case of hooked deformity in the fifth digit where the patient chose the collagenase treatment over surgery, although he was warned about this risk. The patient was satisfied that at least he could open his finger again and accepted the active flexion lack, and refused tendon repair.

A number of well-designed randomized controlled trial have shown that the recurrence rates of Dupuytren contractures after collagenase in the long term are not different than those of PNF, but higher than after surgery.[27] However, the patient satisfaction is very high and the clinical results are good to excellent, without limitations in repeat injection if needed in severe cases. Unfortunately, as of 2020 this elegant treatment option is not available anymore in Europe, sadly for the numerous patients that were very satisfied and even dependent on disease control with this enzyme. Another pharmaceutical company (Fidia Ltd, Milan) is currently performing a phase 1 trial to test an alternative collagenase for injection.

20.5 Complications after Treatment with Radiotherapy (RTX)

Radiotherapy as treatment for DD is still controversial. There are reports with debatable evidence that low-dose irradiation (30 Gy in five consecutive daily 3-Gy sessions, repeated after 6 weeks) prevents disease progression in early disease. This means that only patients with palmar nodules and emerging contractures may benefit from radiotherapy.[18] To date, prospective or randomizing trials with long-term follow-up of these patients are lacking.

Although high levels of satisfaction are reported in patients treated with hand radiation therapy in general, (mild) complications are common. A known early side-effect is acute erythema which is present in 40%. A late complication is skin atrophy in 10% of the patients. In general, a 0.02% malignancy risk increase is estimated. Due to the well-known universal radiotherapy side-effect of late-onset progressive fibrosis, a possible long-term increase in DD, which is a fibrotic process, is not unthinkable. As a side note, it needs to be highlighted that this therapy is only suggested in cases with nodules only, and very limited contractures. We have previously shown that prevalence of nodular disease in people over 50 is over 20%.[1] Recently, 7 years after the first investigation, we have reviewed this prevalence and found that only 20% of the cases with the nodular stage have progressed to the next Iselin state[28]. So, treating everybody with nodules would mean an absolute overkill. Therefore, we feel that the issue of overtreatment should be sufficiently weighed in view of possible benefits versus society health care costs and unknown long-term complication risks. Randomized controlled trials are currently under way coordinated by a group of radiation oncologists in New Castle, Australia to determine the exact place of RTX in the spectrum of treatments for DD.[29]

20.6 Complications of Local Treatment

Local nonsurgical treatment of Dupuytren contracture can be either mechanical (splinting) or chemical (ointments and infiltrations other than collagenase).[18] With external splinting, the contracture may be (partially) corrected or stabilized. Splints can be either static or dynamic (with springs), with tension or compression on the Dupuytren nodules/cords. It is controversial to use splints after (surgical) treatment to preserve or improve the clinical result of finger extension. One of the reasons for this is that postoperative splinting does not necessarily ameliorate the extension of the fingers, but carries the risk of causing stiffness and flexion loss. Evidence suggests that hand therapy consisting of active exercises and stretching is possibly just as effective for an optimal result. Next to the risk of stiffness, pain can be an issue of splinting. Since CRPS is associated with Dupuytren and surgery and CRPS is associated with (plaster) immobilization, splinting may also add to the risk of CRPS after treatment for DD. If splinting is used to try and correct finger contractures, pain, pressure sores, and consequently noncompliance (in up to 35%) are also not uncommon. However, these issues are less likely to occur when applying compressive (palmar) splinting, which is better tolerated by most patients.

Local infiltrations with steroids have been attempted in case series of Dupuytren's and Ledderhose's disease and in a randomized controlled trial in Dupuytren patients in Taiwan.[30] Softening and partial regression of the nodules was reported. This was explained by apoptosis and inhibition of collagen production. Side-effects were not mentioned.

Topical treatment is even less well studied. Only anecdotal or case series are available. Since anti-inflammatory drugs such as steroids may decrease myofibroblast activity, its local use has been advocated, but long-term follow-up is missing. Skin atrophy is a most known risk and thus long-term use is not recommended. Other anti-inflammatory topicals such as, for instance, diclofenac have never been properly studied in DD. Although complications are unlikely, local allergic reactions are possible but very rare. Systemic side-effects such as gastrointestinal ulceration, kidney insufficiency, hepatic toxicity, and anemia are listed in the pharmacologic compendium.

Next to anti-inflammatory topicals, the benefits of high vitamin E ointments are sometimes suggested (as used in cosmetics). In a small study performed by one of the authors, about 50% of the cases treated by vitamin E ointment mentioned that their Dupuytren nodules softened while using these products twice daily, but no prospective data is available.

20.7 Complications of Systemic Treatment

Systemic drug treatment is not yet common practice in DD. However, the fibrosis process is an inflammatory-like histological event. The (de-)activation of myofibroblasts and their collagen production may well be modified by certain drugs, as has been demonstrated in several in vitro studies. Also, a limited number of clinical trials in DD have been published.[18] Systemic steroid administration for short periods was attempted in the 1950s, but the benefit on outcome was controversial, while systemic use of corticosteroids and other immunomodulation drugs may have significant side-effects, certainly in long-term use. Osteoporosis, skin atrophy, bruising, cataracts, muscle weakness, and oral candidiasis or other infections are some of the numerous side-effects that are the reason that this therapy is not applied today.

Due to the histopathological similarities of DD with desmoids tumors, highly dosed tamoxifen was tested as neoadjuvant pharmacotherapy in a double-blinded randomized controlled trial versus placebo until 3 months after surgery in patients with severe fibrosis diathesis. Although there was evidence that this improved outcome significantly, long-term use was not considered due to the risk of serious systemic side-effects (such as thromboembolism and liver toxicity) and unfortunately the beneficial effect was lost after 2 years.[18] Nonetheless, this trial again holds strong argument to continue the surge to additional pharmacotherapy in severely progressive forms of DD. Many options have been suggested, limited trials are ongoing, but in any future systemic treatment, possible benefits will need to be strongly outweighed against its risks.

20.8 Take-Home Message

Treatment options for patients with DD are numerous, but none of them can guarantee a definite result and treatment side-effects and significant complications are not uncommon.

Disease controlling or stopping therapies with topical or systemic drugs have not yet reached adulthood. Collagenase injection therapy is probably as effective and durable as minimally invasive surgery.

Surgical treatment is unfortunately hampered by complications inversely related to its invasiveness: More invasive surgical treatment options (LF and DF) have more major complications than less or minimally invasive surgery (SF, OF, PNF). Shared decision-making and informed consent prior to embarking on treatment is paramount, as is prevention of complications. The latter is easier said than done and sometimes impossible, especially in secondary surgery. The operating microscope may increase efficiency and safety in challenging cases. If complications (mostly neurovascular damage) occur, action should be taken to treat them and details need to be reported to the patients as well as documented in the surgical notes for future surgeries.

A multidisciplinary DD treatment algorithm, including all options, is mandatory, fitting the needs of the population. Complex cases (higher recurrences, patients with diathesis) should be referred to Dupuytren specialists to offer the most appropriate treatment, preferred and consented by the patient.

The future will hopefully bring local treatments that will stop disease progression. Until that day, anatomical knowledge, surgical expertise, diligence, and humbleness are paramount.

References

[1] Lanting R, van den Heuvel ER, Westerink B, Werker PMN. Prevalence of Dupuytren disease in The Netherlands. Plast Reconstr Surg. 2013; 132(2):394–403

[2] Ng M, Thakkar D, Southam L, et al. A genome-wide association study of Dupuytren disease reveals 17 additional variants implicated in fibrosis. Am J Hum Genet. 2017; 101(3):417–427

[3] Mathieu S, Naughton G, Descatha A, Soubrier M, Dutheil F. Dupuytren's disease and exposure to vibration: systematic review and meta-analysis. Joint Bone Spine. 2020; 87(3):203–207

[4] Broekstra DC, Groen H, Molenkamp S, Werker PMN, van den Heuvel ER. A systematic review and meta-analysis on the strength and consistency of the associations between Dupuytren disease and diabetes mellitus, liver disease and epilepsy. Plast Reconstr Surg. 2018; 141 (3):367e–379e

[5] Lanting R, van den Heuvel ER, Werker PM. Clusters in short-term disease course in participants with primary Dupuytren disease. J Hand Surg Am. 2016; 41(3):354–361, quiz 361

[6] Haase SC, Chung KC. Dupuytren disease. Hand Clin. 2018; 34(3):1

[7] Zhou C, Ceyisakar IE, Hovius SER, et al. Surgeon volume and the outcomes of Dupuytren's surgery: results from a Dutch Multicenter Study. Plast Reconstr Surg. 2018; 142(1):125–134

[8] Denkler K. Surgical complications associated with fasciectomy for Dupuytren's disease: a 20-year review of the English literature. Eplasty. 2010; 10:e15

[9] Eberlin KR, Mudgal CS. Complications of treatment for Dupuytren disease. Hand Clin. 2018; 34(3):387–394

[10] Therkelsen LH, Skov ST, Laursen M, Lange J. Percutaneous needle fasciotomy in Dupuytren contracture: a register-based, observational cohort study on complications in 3,331 treated fingers in 2,257 patients. Acta Orthop. 2020; 91(3):326–330

[11] McKirdy SW, Jacobs N, Nassab R, Starley IF. A retrospective review of cold intolerance following corrective surgery for Dupuytren's disease. Hand Ther. 2007; 12:55–59

[12] van der Avoort DJ, Hovius SE, Selles RW, van Neck JW, Coert JH. The incidence of symptomatic neuroma in amputation and neurorrhaphy patients. J Plast Reconstr Aesthet Surg. 2013; 66(10):1330–1334

[13] Malsagova AT, Zwanenburg RL, Werker PMN. New insights into the anatomy at the palmodigital junction in Dupuytren's disease: the palmodigital spiralling sheet. J Hand Surg Eur Vol. 2019; 44(9):972–978

[14] Hettiaratchy S, Tonkin MA, Edmunds IA. Spiralling of the neurovascular bundle in Dupuytren's disease. J Hand Surg Eur Vol. 2010; 35(2):103–108

[15] Breed CM, Smith PJ. A comparison of methods of treatment of pip joint contractures in Dupuytren's disease. J Hand Surg [Br]. 1996; 21(2):246–251

[16] Saffar P. Total anterior teno-arthrolysis. Report of 72 cases. Ann Chir Main. 1983; 2(4):345–350

[17] van Rijssen AL, Ter Linden H, Werker PMN. Five-year results of a randomized clinical trial on treatment in Dupuytren's disease: percutaneous needle fasciotomy versus limited fasciectomy. Plast Reconstr Surg. 2012; 129(2):469–477

[18] Moermans JP. Segmental aponeurectomy in Dupuytren's disease. J Hand Surg [Br]. 1991; 16(3):243–254

[19] Werker PMN, Degreef I. Alternative and adjunctive treatments for Dupuytren disease. Hand Clin. 2018; 34(3):367–375

[20] Hueston JT. Dermofasciectomy for Dupuytren's disease. Bull Hosp Jt Dis Orthop Inst. 1984;44(2):224–232

[21] Armstrong JR, Hurren JS, Logan AM. Dermofasciectomy in the management of Dupuytren's disease. J Bone Joint Surg Br. 2000; 82(1):90–94

[22] Krefter C, Marks M, Hensler S, Herren DB, Calcagni M. Complications after treating Dupuytren's disease. A systematic literature review. Hand Surg Rehabil. 2017; 36(5):322–329

[23] Ullah AS, Dias JJ, Bhowal B. Does a "firebreak" full-thickness skin graft prevent recurrence after surgery for Dupuytren's contracture? A prospective, randomised trial. J Bone Joint Surg Br. 2009; 91(3):374–378

[24] van Rijssen AL, Gerbrandy FS, Ter Linden H, Klip H, Werker PM. A comparison of the direct outcomes of percutaneous needle fasciotomy and limited fasciectomy for Dupuytren's disease: a 6-week follow-up study. J Hand Surg Am. 2006; 31(5):717–725

[25] Stewart C, Davidson D, Hooper G. Re-operation after open fasciotomy for Dupuytren's disease in a series of 1077 consecutive operations. J Hand Surg Eur Vol. 2014; 39(5):553–554

[26] Hurst LC, Badalamente MA, Hentz VR, et al. CORD I Study Group. Injectable collagenase clostridium histolyticum for Dupuytren's contracture. N Engl J Med. 2009; 361(10):968–979

[27] Scherman P, Jenmalm P, Dahlin LB. Three-year recurrence of Dupuytren's contracture after needle fasciotomy and collagenase injection: a two-centre randomized controlled trial. J Hand Surg Eur Vol. 2018; 43(8):836–840

[28] van den Berge BA, Werker PMN, Broekstra DC. Limited progression of subclinical Dupuytren's disease. Bone Joint J. 2021;103-B(4):704–771

[29] https://www.genesiscare.com/au/depart-clinical-trial/?gclid=CjwK-CAjw1uiEBhBzEiwAO9B_HZy8L4PW1ZsWufEvEP7ZEzfu6rRiyvjhI-QeXDSePmtGdVnKiIa3m9hoCgpgQAvD_BwE

[30] Yin CY, Yu HM, Wang JP, Huang YC, Huang TF, Chang MC. Long-term follow-up of Dupuytren disease after injection of triamcinolone acetonide in Chinese patients in Taiwan. J Hand Surg Eur Vol. 2017; 42(7):678–682

6

21 Management of Complications in the Treatment of Fingertip Injuries

Florian S. Frueh and Maurizio Calcagni

Abstract

The fingertip is the most frequently injured part of the hand. Accordingly, complications after fingertip injuries are very common and knowledge about their treatment is important for hand surgeons. Nail deformities, such as nail ridges, split nails, or hook nails can be challenging to correct. While nail ridges are relatively easy to address, split nails and hook nails are difficult problems and may also be solved with nail eradication and skin grafting. Painful neuromata are another common and potentially debilitating complication of fingertip injuries. Traditionally, the surgical treatment includes resection of the neuroma with nerve shortening and relocation. However, a multitude of treatment strategies has been described without a single technique providing superior results. Finally, tendon or bone infection, cold intolerance, and hypotrophic digital pulps may occur after fingertip injuries. While exarticulation and finger shortening can always be performed, specific and more sophisticated surgical procedures should be part of the armamentarium of hand surgeons to maintain digital length and function.

Keywords: cold intolerance, fingertip injuries, hypotrophic fingertip, infection, nail deformity, neuroma

21.1 Introduction

The fingertip is defined as the part of a finger distal to the insertion of the extensor and flexor tendons on the terminal phalanx.[1] With a unique anatomy, it is essential for highly specialized functions such as sensation, protection, or fine manipulation. Due to its high mechanical exposure during hand use, it is the most commonly injured part of the hand.[2] Hence, managing fingertip injuries and their complications is among the most frequent problems encountered by hand surgeons. Injuries to the fingertip can be classified according to their etiology (i.e., Guillotine vs. crush vs. crush avulsion injury[3]) or according to the extent of tissue loss. For that purpose, the fingertip has been divided into different zones (▶ Fig. 21.1).[4,5] While very distal fingertip injuries commonly undergo uneventful healing by secondary intention, more proximal injuries with significant bone and nail bed loss (i.e., >Hirase IIA and Allen II type amputations) exhibit a higher risk for complications. In order to prevent potentially severe sequelae, each anatomical component of an injured fingertip should be addressed meticulously during the primary treatment. In the present chapter, we discuss the most important complications after fingertip injuries and their surgical management.

21.2 Nail Deformities

Except for very distal injuries involving only the pulp, the nail bed is always affected in fingertip injuries. Nail bed lacerations can be open and obvious (i.e., lacerations or amputations) or closed and more challenging to recognize, for example, when associated with crush injuries and fractures of the terminal phalanx. Nail deformities after fingertip injuries are very common and highly disturbing for patients due to a frequently eye-catching aesthetic abnormality. Moreover, fragile nail plates with sharp edges may result in significant functional impairment. From a morphological point of view, three different types of nail deformities can be found: nail ridges, split nails and hook nails.[6] Nail ridges occur after missed or uneven repairs of the nail bed or following dorsally displaced fractures of the subungual bone. Split nails, in contrast, are found after scarring of the germinative matrix. Finally, hook nails occur following insufficient volar bony support, for instance, in oblique fingertip amputations. If the nail bed is not trimmed back meticulously, the lack of bone support results in a volarly curved nail growth with aesthetical and functional impairment.

21.3 Painful Neuroma

The formation of a painful terminal neuroma is a common complication of fingertip injuries. Many cases can be managed conservatively by means of desensitization

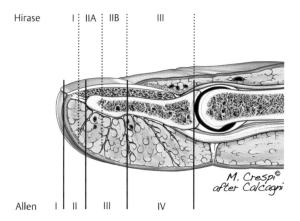

Fig. 21.1 Classification of fingertip amputations according to Hirase and Allen. Hirase classification: I = distal to digital artery termination, IIA = distal to terminal division of central artery, IIB = distal to nail fold, type III = distal to DIP joint. Allen classification: I = distal to nail bed, II = distal to terminal phalanx, III distal to lunula, IV = distal to DIP joint.

exercises and the temporary use of protection devices instructed by a trained hand therapist. However, if severe neuropathic pain develops, surgical treatment may be indicated. The clinical presentation of painful terminal neuromas of the digital nerves is predominantly characterized by pressure pain and hypersensitivity.[7] The diagnostic algorithm includes a digital block with a local anesthetic, after which the patient should be pain-free or experience significant pain relief. In case of persistent pain after nerve block and when abnormal local trophism is present, the surgeon should think of a complex regional pain syndrome type II as differential diagnosis.

Frequently, the surgical treatment of painful digital neuromas is delayed, and the function of the affected digit and hand is markedly limited with often significant socioeconomic consequences, in particular for blue-collar patients. Time is an important factor when treating patients with highly symptomatic neuromas. Hence, we recommend early and aggressive surgical treatment of debilitating digital neuromas. A multitude of methods for the surgical management of digital neuromas has been described, including shortening and nerve relocation in bone or muscle, end-to-side neurorrhaphies, nerve capping, local flaps or—more recently—the use of regenerative peripheral nerve interfaces (RPNI).[6,7,8,9] However, none of these techniques is accepted as gold standard and outcomes of revision surgery are difficult to predict. In our experience, patients with debilitating and chronic neuropathic pain are at highest risk for permanent symptoms even with revision surgery. Hence, this point should be clarified when the consent for surgery is obtained from the patient because unrealistic expectations may jeopardize the compliance during the early and critical phase of recovery, where hand therapy should be attended with maximal discipline.

21.4 Infection

Severe infections after fingertip injuries are rare. However, destructive osteomyelitis of the terminal phalanx or pyogenic flexor tendon synovitis can occur with potentially fatal consequences for the function of a hand. Osteomyelitis after contaminated open injury is often polymicrobial and requires a combined treatment including surgery and antibiotic therapy.[10,11] The diagnostic algorithm includes X-ray images of the affected finger and bone biopsies with detection of characteristic pathology and positive cultures.

21.5 Cold Intolerance and Fingertip Hypotrophy

Cold intolerance and significant hypotrophy of the digital pulp are common complications of fingertip injuries. In the pertinent literature, rates from 30 to 100% have been reported for cold intolerance.[12,13] According to our experience, these problems are more often found after the conservative treatment of proximal fingertip amputations using occlusive dressings. Hypotrophic fingertips are a particularly disturbing problem because patients suffer from limited mechanical robustness of a single finger in an otherwise normal hand. Cold intolerance is difficult to treat and commonly ameliorates over time and with support of a hand therapist. In contrast, hypotrophic fingertips commonly profit from soft tissue augmentation with local flaps or—usually less effective—injection of autologous microfat.

21.6 Authors' Own Experience and Preferred Technique

21.6.1 Nail Deformities

Nail ridges can be managed straightforward with nail plate removal and resection/reconstruction of uneven nail bed areas. Larger nail bed defects can be reconstructed using acellular dermal matrices or nail bed transplants harvested from the toes. In contrast, the surgical management of split nails is more challenging. Depending on the size of the destructed matrix area, the scar can be resected with direct repair in small defects. If the matrix defect is extensive, reconstruction is difficult and ablative procedures such as nail eradication with subsequent full-thickness skin grafting may be more suitable. Finally, hook nails can be corrected in selected cases, but the patients should be informed about considerable surgical investment with the risk of recurrent nail deformity. Hook nails can be corrected with restoration of bone support, such as bone transplantation in combination with local flaps. However, many patients prefer a faster solution with nail ablation. Taken together, nail deformities should be avoided by a thorough primary assessment and treatment with anatomical reconstruction of the damaged nail structures.

21.6.2 Painful Neuroma

Prevention is key: To minimize the risk of symptomatic terminal neuroma formation after fingertip injuries, we recommend aggressive shortening of lacerated digital nerves with sufficient soft tissue coverage during the primary treatment. Furthermore, the nerve stump can be infiltrated with a local anesthetic and sealed with bipolar cautery. Our standard surgical approach to painful digital neuromata of the fingertip includes neuroma resection with nerve shortening and proximal relocation. Notably, we have made convincing first experiences with RPNI for the treatment of larger nerve neuromas, but this novel technique will have to be tested in randomized clinical studies before a broader application can be suggested.

21.6.3 Infection

Pyogenic flexor tendon synovitis is commonly treated with aggressive surgical debridement, including rinsing of the flexor tendon sheath and intravenous antibiotics. Selected cases such as early stage infection without sonographic evidence of peritendinous pyogenic collections can be managed conservatively with intravenous antibiotics alone.[14] However, these cases should be monitored closely by a hand surgeon to verify clinical improvement within reasonable time (i.e., within 24–48 h).

Osteomyelitis of the terminal phalanx can be managed with exarticulation of the distal interphalangeal joint. If digital reconstruction is feasible, aggressive debridement of the affected bone with subsequent bone transplantation and adequate soft tissue reconstruction should be performed. For this purpose, the distal radius or the iliac crest are suitable donor sites. Key to a good result is a solid soft tissue coverage after bone transplantation. In our hands, local neurovascular island flaps, such as Venkataswami or dorsal finger perforator flaps,[15] are reliable work horses for the reconstruction of insufficiently covered fingertips.

21.6.4 Fingertip Hypotrophy

Insufficient soft tissue of the digital pulp following conservative treatment of fingertip injuries may lead to pain while pinching and is particularly disturbing for patients who are dependent on precision work, such as musicians. Commonly, the terminal phalanx is only covered with a thin layer of scarred dermis and epidermis without a subcutaneous layer, which is critical for shock absorption during pinching (▶ Fig. 21.2a–d). The reconstruction of hypotrophic fingertips can be achieved with local neurovascular island flaps, such as VY advancement (▶ Fig. 21.2e–h) or Venkataswami flaps with reliable results. In addition, a frequently present and aesthetically disturbing short nail can be improved using an eponychial flap[16] (▶ Fig. 21.2i, j). From a technical point of view, this flap is simple and only results in ~10 min of additional operating time. Full loading of the reconstructed pulp is allowed after ~4 weeks (▶ Fig. 21.2k, l).

In the thumb, extensive traumatic loss of the pulp is a rare but challenging problem and commonly requires microsurgical tissue transfer. For this purpose, we have used neurovascular hemipulp flaps harvested from the great toe.[17] The glabrous skin of this flap exhibits the unique advantage of *like with like* reconstruction of the thumb pulp which is crucial for pinching and fine manipulation (▶ Fig. 21.3).

21.7 Take-Home Message

Nail deformities, painful neuromas, infections, cold intolerance, and hypotrophic digital pulps are common complications of fingertip injuries. Importantly, the majority of these problems can be avoided by a meticulous primary surgery with anatomical reconstruction of nail bed defects and adequate soft tissue coverage of exposed structures.

6

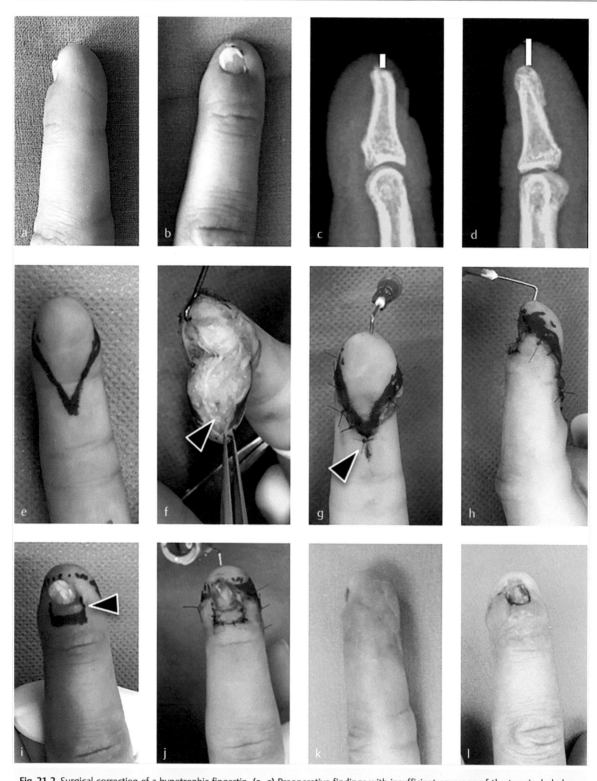

Fig. 21.2 Surgical correction of a hypotrophic fingertip. **(a–c)** Preoperative findings with insufficient coverage of the terminal phalanx. **(d)** Normal fingertip. Scale bars: **c** = 1 mm; **d** = 3 mm. **(e–h)** Design and dissection of an extended neurovascular VY flap (**f**, *arrowhead*) with appropriate advancement (**g**, *arrowhead*). **(i,j)** Eponychial flap with optical elongation of the nail plate for ~1.5 mm (**i**, *arrowhead*). **(k,l)** Result 4 weeks after surgery.

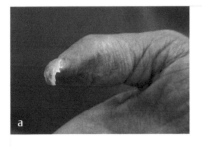
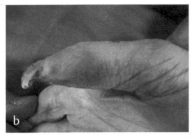
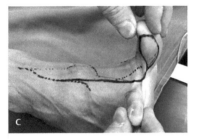
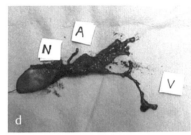
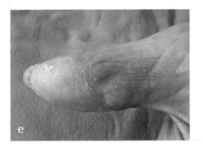
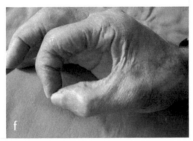

Fig. 21.3 Microvascular great toe hemipulp for thumb reconstruction. **(a,b)** Hypotrophic and painful thumb pulp after extensive volar amputation. **(c,d)** Design and harvest of a neurovascular lateral hemipulp from the great toe providing ideal soft tissue reconstruction. **(e,f)** Clinical result with uneventful healing of the reconstructed pulp allowing physiological pinching.

6

References

[1] Lemmon JA, Janis JE, Rohrich RJ. Soft-tissue injuries of the fingertip: methods of evaluation and treatment: an algorithmic approach. Plast Reconstr Surg. 2008; 122(3):105e–117e

[2] Panattoni JB, De Ona IR, Ahmed MM. Reconstruction of fingertip injuries: surgical tips and avoiding complications. J Hand Surg Am. 2015; 40(5):1016–1024

[3] Yamano Y. Replantation of the amputated distal part of the fingers. J Hand Surg Am. 1985; 10(2):211–218

[4] Hirase Y. Salvage of fingertip amputated at nail level: new surgical principles and treatments. Ann Plast Surg. 1997; 38(2):151–157

[5] Allen MJ. Conservative management of finger tip injuries in adults. Hand. 1980; 12(3):257–265

[6] Lee DH, Mignemi ME, Crosby SN. Fingertip injuries: an update on management. J Am Acad Orthop Surg. 2013; 21(12):756–766

[7] Elliot D, Sierakowski A. The surgical management of painful nerves of the upper limb: a unit perspective. J Hand Surg Eur Vol. 2011; 36 (9):760–770

[8] Kakinoki R, Ikeguchi R, Atiyya AN, Nakamura T. Treatment of post-traumatic painful neuromas at the digit tip using neurovascular island flaps. J Hand Surg Am. 2008; 33(3):348–352

[9] Hooper RC, Cederna PS, Brown DL, et al. Regenerative peripheral nerve interfaces for the management of symptomatic hand and digital neuromas. Plast Reconstr Surg Glob Open. 2020; 8(6):e2792

[10] Honda H, McDonald JR. Current recommendations in the management of osteomyelitis of the hand and wrist. J Hand Surg Am. 2009; 34(6):1135–1136

[11] Pinder R, Barlow G. Osteomyelitis of the hand. J Hand Surg Eur Vol. 2016; 41(4):431–440

[12] Buntic RF, Brooks D. Standardized protocol for artery-only fingertip replantation. J Hand Surg Am. 2010; 35(9):1491–1496

[13] van den Berg WB, Vergeer RA, van der Sluis CK, Ten Duis HJ, Werker PM. Comparison of three types of treatment modalities on the outcome of fingertip injuries. J Trauma Acute Care Surg. 2012; 72 (6):1681–1687

[14] Frenkel Rutenberg T, Velkes S, Sidon E, et al. Conservative treatment for pyogenic flexor tenosynovitis: a single institution experience. J Plast Surg Hand Surg. 2020; 54(1):14–18

[15] Besmens IS, Guidi M, Frueh FS, et al. Finger reconstruction with dorsal metacarpal artery perforator flaps and dorsal finger perforator flaps based on the dorsal branches of the palmar digital arteries: 40 consecutive cases. J Plast Surg Hand Surg. 2020; 54(4):248–254

[16] Fakin RM, Biraima A, Klein H, Giovanoli P, Calcagni M. Primary functional and aesthetic restoration of the fingernail in distal fingertip amputations with the eponychial flap. J Hand Surg Eur Vol. 2014; 39 (5):499–504

[17] Guelmi K, Barbato B, Maladry D, Mitz V, Lemerle JP. [Reconstruction of digital pulp by pulp tissue transfer of the toe. Apropos of 15 cases]. Rev Chir Orthop Repar Appar Mot. 1996; 82(5):446–452

Section 7

Rehabilitation: How to Prevent and Manage Complications by Hand Therapy

22 Flexor Tendon Repair in Zone 2: Prevention and Management of Complications by Hand Therapy

Gwendolyn van Strien

Abstract

Therapists, like surgeons, make choices regarding the details of each patient's rehabilitation program to get the best possible outcome. For a rehabilitation program after flexor tendon repair, the choices made by the therapist are based initially on information from the hand surgeon, including mechanism of injury, zone of repair, type of suture material and suture technique used, and pulley status, and then other issues are factored in, related to the work of flexion (WOF), pain, and patient adherence. The aim of this chapter is to propose that early active motion approaches that are patient-centered or individualized rather than protocolled may lead to better flexor tendon repair outcomes.

Keywords: flexor tendon repair, early active motion, rehabilitation, work of flexion (WOF), outcomes, patient-centered approach, patient motivation, splint

22.1 Wound Healing—A Paradigm Shift

Wong et al[1] have given us a renewed perspective on healing of a repaired flexor tendon and its surrounding tissue (ST). These researchers observed that collagen production starts in the ST about day 3, with the tendon following about a week later, catching up with the ST around day 21. This early healing of the ST and sheath before the tendon translates to ST adhesions which limits repaired tendon glide within the first 3 weeks of injury. These observations coupled with the use of stronger suture materials and repair techniques (4+strand repairs) suggest that the tendon needs to start moving actively within the first 3 to 5 days.

22.2 Complications

22.2.1 Adhesions versus Ruptures

Adhesions and ruptures are both failed results since both will need secondary surgery. Tenolysis is a more common complication than rupture after flexor tendon repair, with re-repair having better outcomes than tenolysis.[2] The rate of tendon rupture is not much different whether early passive motion (4%) or early active motion (EAM) (5%) is used. Yet the difference in tendon glide/excursion achieved with EAM (9%) is significantly greater than that achieved with early passive motion (6%), suggesting when possible, EAM should be the chosen program.[3]

22.2.2 Bowstringing

Stronger repair techniques are more bulky, consequently pulley venting is being done so not to interfere with proximal and distal tendon glide/excursion. Pulleys were once thought to be a biomechanical necessity, we know now that this is not entirely true as observations with sonography showed only minimal bowstringing 1 year after pulley venting.[4] Surgeon communication of details including the number of repair strands, pulley(s) status vented or repaired, and how well the repair was actively or passively gliding intraoperatively are essential for the hand therapist to develop an individualized postoperative plan.

22.3 Prevention of Complications

22.3.1 Early Active Motion

Work of Flexion and Tendon Glide

An early active motion (EAM) program initiates active tendon excursion within the first 7 days after repair. The objective of safe EAM is to use the least amount of force to achieve enough tendon glide to minimize adhesions. Under normal conditions as fingers actively flex, resistance or work of flexion (WOF) is encountered.[5] The WOF is influenced by edema, stiffness, and position of the wrist and fingers, tight pulleys, all important considerations to avoid repair rupture.

Edema and WOF

Edema management is key as EAM starts within the first postoperative week, and edema increases WOF. Wu and Tang[6] estimated that the tissues on the volar aspect of the finger plus edema contribute 20 to 25% of total WOF.
- Compression wraps are often used to control edema; however, a single study found that the WOF increased with the application of these wraps.[7] Consider compression wrap removal during exercise to possibly lower the WOF.

Stiff Joints and WOF

After repair, stiff finger joints and friction from tendon swelling and repair bulkiness (internal WOF) account for about 25 to 30% of total WOF.[6] This resistance is reduced when passive range of motion of the interphalangeal joints is done prior to active motion exercises.[6]
- Passive range of motion *always* before active motion.
- Active motion *beyond* what has been achieved passively puts the repair at risk.

Wrist Position and WOF

WOF for an intact tendon increases significantly (flexor digitorum superficialis [FDS] more than flexor digitorum profundus [FDP]) with the wrist positioned in flexion when the fingers are flexed (Kleinert splint position). However, WOF during finger flexion can be lowered for both tendons if the wrist is positioned in neutral or slight extension.[8] The Manchester short splint, which allows the wrist to move freely, was used with EAM and four-strand FDP repairs with no increase in tendon ruptures and fewer proximal interphalangeal (PIP) joint contractures.[9]

- To minimize risk of repair rupture in the postoperative cast *and* the dorsal protective splint, position the wrist in slight extension, never flexion.
- To lessen repair risk, fabricate the *Manchester short splint* to restrict wrist extension at 45 degrees and advise patients not to simultaneously flex wrist and fingers.[9]

Finger Position and WOF

During active finger flexion, the passive tension imposed by the dorsal extrinsic extensor tendons accounts for about 15% of total WOF.[6] As discussed, positioning the wrist in extension affects passive tension from the long extensors. Equally as important is that WOF by FDP and FDS can lower further, depending on the position of the metacarpophalangeal (MCP) joints. Flexor tendon WOF was lowest at 15-degree MCP joint position; however, when MCP joint angles were greater than 45 degrees, WOF substantially increased in both tendons.[8]

- Since this chapter advocates individualized treatment, the author recommends that one can choose the 15-degree position when the surgeon is confident about the repair and the therapist is experienced in using an EAM approach. A position between 30 and 45 degrees is best practice for less experienced therapists or when the surgeon feels the repair needs a more protected approach.
- Some patients can benefit from more MCP joint flexion (30–45 degrees) to make PIP and distal interphalangeal (DIP) extension easier and prevent flexion contractures. Keep in mind that full extension is rarely achieved in the first 7 to 10 days postoperatively but, when safe, strive for full IP extension as early as possible.
- Later during the initial 4 postoperative weeks, the angle of MCP joint flexion can always be adjusted to further reduce WOF and achieve optimal tendon glide.

Pulleys and WOF

After tendon repair, pulleys contribute about 30% of total WOF with active finger flexion.[6] WOF can be reduced by venting of the pulleys and/or resecting one slip of the FDS tendon.

Another important consideration is that by allowing too much active composite finger flexion early on, the rate of tendon ruptures has been shown to increase.[6] There were less tendon ruptures when active composite finger flexion was limited to one-third compared to two-thirds, and full flexion. In the same study, after pulley resection, the increased rate of rupture seen with two-thirds to full active composite finger flexion was reduced.

- To avoid potentially harmful WOF, the surgeon is advised to communicate key details of the surgery to the hand therapist, such as repair bulk, pulley status, vented or not, quality of intraoperative tendon glide through the pulleys.
- Do not encourage active full finger flexion until 3 to 4 weeks after repair. A one-third to a one-half fist active composite finger flexion requires less WOF and permits enough tendon glide to discourage adhesions.

22.4 Effective Exercising—Tips and Tricks to Improve Outcomes

22.4.1 Move from the DIP and Not from the PIP

Strickland[10] reported that after repair, FDP excursion was decreased by 65%, while FDS excursion was decreased by only 10%. Clinically, this loss of FDP glide results in less DIP joint flexion as tendon excursion is redistributed to hyperflex the MCP joint, especially in the ulnar digits. To identify how well a zone 1 or 2 FDP repair is gliding, it is important to calculate total active motion by excluding the MCP joint measurement altogether, using only measurements of PIP and DIP joint motion (▶ Fig. 22.1). The cause of limited FDP glide can be attributed to tightness

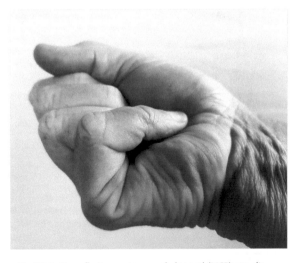

Fig. 22.1 Hyperflexion metacarpophalangeal (MCP) can disguise a loss of distal interphalangeal (DIP) flexion when the formula to calculate total active motion (TAM) includes all three finger joints.

of the A5 pulley usually due to repair bulk, or the repair getting caught as the two FDS slips at the decussation narrow during PIP flexion.[11]

- Best practice is for the surgeon to communicate when the location of the FDP repair is near the FDS decussation (when slip of FDS is not resected) so that the therapist knows to avoid FDP trapping exercises, such as a straight fist/PIP joint flexion, and will instead advise "DIP flexion first" exercises.
- Surgeon communication regarding intraoperative observation of FDP glide at the A5 pulley is helpful so that the therapist can prescribe the exercise that is most effective for FDP tendon glide.

22.4.2 Make Sure the "Right" Tendon Is Moving

There are two ways to make a fist: (1) the intrinsic dominant way which initiates movement from the MCP joint and is observed in about 30% of normal subjects, and (2) the extrinsic dominant way which initiates movement from the IP joints, and observed in about 70% of normals.[12] After tendon repair, digits are swollen and sometimes painful, so when patients are asked to flex their fingers they will do their best to move, but will avoid pain. As a result, flexion from the MCP joint using an intrinsic dominant pattern will more than likely be observed over flexing from the IP joints. If this intrinsic pattern continues, it will convert into a normal motor cortex pattern of movement within 48 to 72 hours.[13] Once established as a normal pattern, it is difficult to change, especially during the early weeks after tendon repair when extrinsic flexor tendon gliding not intrinsic activity is critical.

- The surgeon, therapist, and patient should observe and correct any tendency to use the "wrong" finger flexion pattern to make sure the right tendon(s) is gliding.
- To discourage MCP joint flexion and encourage an extrinsic flexion pattern and DIP joint first motion, position the splint's palmar bar or strap a bit more distal.

22.4.3 Postoperative Exercise—Keep It Simple, Functional, and Relatable

Issuing protocolled handouts is not better; in fact, exercises that resemble our daily motion provide the opportunity for more repetition and better outcomes.[14,15] The first step is the understanding that one exercise protocol does not work for all patients because each patient reacts to injury differently and is motivated differently. The second step is to carefully watch how the patient is—or is not—moving so that a best-fit exercise program can be designed. During the initial 4 weeks, the exercises will need to be on pace with repair healing, so changes will be required in exercise prescription based on therapist observations and appreciation of WOF variability.

- To improve patient motivation, use a few effective exercises versus too much information.
- Provide visual reminders like a video of the patient doing the exercise correctly so the patient can imitate this again at home.
- To motivate, use the patient's cell phone to take photos while doing the therapy exercises correctly to serve as a "handout" for home and work.
- Purposeful activities, integrating familiar objects, should be used to make exercises functionally friendly to the cortex. "Half a fist" can be done as the patient's hand is intuitively placed around a bottle or a mug (▶ Fig. 22.2).
- The bonus of using every day activities and objects for exercises is the mental jog it gives the patient, e.g., to do the exercise when sitting down for a drink with a mug of coffee or bottle of water is much more effective than a piece of paper stuck to the refrigerator at home!
- A functional exercise to use in the later phases of healing to achieve final DIP joint flexion is a "hook fist" around the width of a smartphone. Millennials are known to check their phone 150 times daily, so asking for three to five repetitions of "hook fist" every time they look at their phone will give a lot of repetitions! (▶ Fig. 22.3).
- To block the intrinsic pattern of finger flexion (especially with an adhered repair), try using a relative motion extension splint (RMES). The RMES limits 15 to

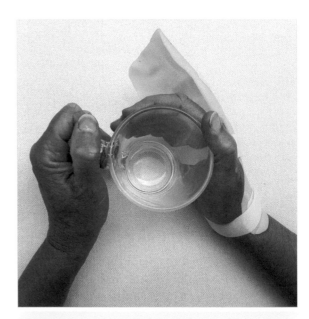

Fig. 22.2 *Placing* the digit(s) around a glass/mug/bottle, which equals one-third or one-half fist feels "natural," less effort is often needed. Using the command, "*touch* the mug with your fingertips" automatically recruits distal interphalangeal (DIP) joint flexion. Because the exercise is linked to an activity that is repeated many times a day (having a drink), it will be done naturally and often during the day.

20 degrees of MCP joint motion to engage more excursion of the FDS/FDP (▶ Fig. 22.4). The bonus of the RMES is that the patient exercises and uses the hand normally without impeding motion. For an adhered repair, daytime wearing an RMES may help avoid a tenolysis later.

22.4.4 Patient-Centered versus Protocol-Driven Care

A protocol limits the therapist's option to individualize the exercise prescription based on what is observed and in line with how the repair is healing. Dosage is one element of exercise prescription that can change; for example, early on if the repaired tendon is showing exceptional gliding, there is no need to exercise 10 times every hour

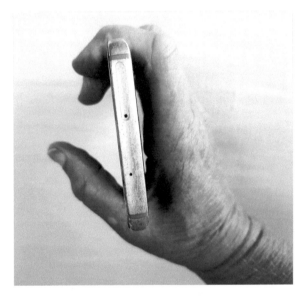

Fig. 22.3 Distal interphalangeal (DIP) joint flexion is encouraged when done around the edge of a smartphone.

as the tendon is healing with minimal adhesions and too many repetitions may attenuate/rupture the repair. Another example of a protocolled exercise that may not be appropriate is "place and hold" especially when done by the *overly motivated patient* who passively places the finger in *more* flexion than the repaired tendon is able to "hold"/glide, putting the integrity of the repair at risk as the motivated patient flexes the finger with *more* force to achieve the "hold." On the other hand, the *easily discouraged patient*, who places the finger *beyond* what the repaired tendon can "hold" will get demotivated and give up as he/she realizes they cannot "hold" flexed position.

This author prefers to start EAM by instructing the patient on how to move (from the DIP joint first—focus on FDP glide), considering the WOF variables and adjusting or adding "tricks" when the tendon glide is not coming along as expected. It has been this author's experience that once the patient feels and sees the repaired tendon "actually work," even if only a few degrees of DIP joint flexion, it motivates most patients. The therapist's responsibility is to find what exercise safely moves the repair and motivates the patient, because ultimately patient participation leads to better outcomes.

22.5 Take-Home Message

If the aim is to get better outcomes, one needs to cater to each patient individually. Patient-centered care relies on the ability to communicate with each other, including the patient, as well as a working knowledge of flexor tendon anatomy, tendon healing, and WOF all of which impact clinical decision-making.

Acknowledgment

I would like to express my very great appreciation to Julianne W. Howell for her valuable and constructive help while writing this chapter.

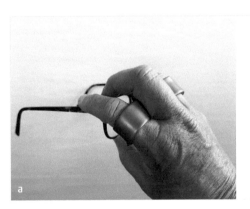
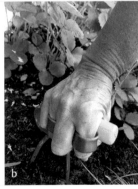

Fig. 22.4 (a, b) The relative motion extension splint (RMES) in this picture limits long finger metacarpophalangeal (MCP) joint flexion to permit more flexor digitorum superficialis (FDS)/flexor digitorum profundus (FDP) excursion to be disbursed to interphalangeal (IP) joint flexion. RMES can be worn all day and normal activity exercises can be done as motion is not impeded.

References

[1] Wong JKF, Lui YH, Kapacee Z, Kadler KE, Ferguson MWJ, McGrouther DA. The cellular biology of flexor tendon adhesion formation: an old problem in a new paradigm. Am J Pathol. 2009; 175(5):1938–1951

[2] Dy CJ, Hernandez-Soria A, Ma Y, Roberts TR, Daluiski A. Complications after flexor tendon repair: a systematic review and meta-analysis. J Hand Surg Am. 2012; 37(3):543–551.e1

[3] Starr HM, Snoddy M, Hammond KE, Seiler JG, III. Flexor tendon repair rehabilitation protocols: a systematic review. J Hand Surg Am. 2013; 38(9):1712–7.e1, 14

[4] Reissner L, Zechmann-Mueller N, Klein HJ, Calcagni M, Giesen T. Sonographic study of repair, gapping and tendon bowstringing after primary flexor digitorum profundus repair in zone 2. J Hand Surg Eur Vol. 2018; 43(5):480–486

[5] Amadio PC. Friction of the gliding surface. Implications for tendon surgery and rehabilitation. J Hand Ther. 2005; 18(2):112–119

[6] Wu YF, Tang JB. Tendon healing, edema, and resistance to flexor tendon gliding: clinical implications. Hand Clin. 2013; 29(2):167–178

[7] Buonocore S, Sawh-Martinez R, Emerson JW, Mohan P, Dymarczyk M, Thomson JG. The effects of edema and self-adherent wrap on the work of flexion in a cadaveric hand. J Hand Surg Am. 2012; 37(7):1349–1355

[8] Kursa K, Lattanza L, Diao E, Rempel D. In vivo flexor tendon forces increase with finger and wrist flexion during active finger flexion and extension. J Orthop Res. 2006; 24(4):763–769

[9] Peck FH, Roe AE, Ng CY, Duff C, McGrouther DA, Lees VC. The Manchester short splint: a change to splinting practice in the rehabilitation of zone II flexor tendon repairs. Hand Ther. 2014; 19:47–53

[10] Strickland JW. Development of flexor tendon surgery: twenty-five years of progress. J Hand Surg Am. 2000; 25(2):214–235

[11] Walbeehm ET, McGrouther DA. The "Chinese Finger"; is the FDS Decussation a Trap? J Hand Surg Am. 1994; 19(1) suppl:38

[12] Al-Sukaini A, Singh HP, Dias JJ. Extrinsic versus intrinsic hand muscle dominance in finger flexion. J Hand Surg Eur Vol. 2016; 41(4):392–399

[13] Weibull A, Flondell M, Rosén B, Björkman A. Cerebral and clinical effects of short-term hand immobilisation. Eur J Neurosci. 2011; 33(4):699–704

[14] Guzelkucuk U, Duman I, Taskaynatan MA, Dincer K. Comparison of therapeutic activities with therapeutic exercises in the rehabilitation of young adult patients with hand injuries. J Hand Surg Am. 2007; 32(9):1429–1435

[15] Thomas JJ. Materials-based, imagery-based, and rote exercise occupational forms: effect on repetitions, heart rate, duration of performance, and self-perceived rest period in well elderly women. Am J Occup Ther. 1996; 50(10):783–789

7

23 Peripheral Nerve Surgery: Prevention and Management of Complications by Hand Therapy

Ton A. R. Schreuders

Abstract

Meticulous surgical repair is only the first step after nerve injury after which a long process of rehabilitation will be required to regain a good hand function. After an initial period of protection of the nerve, many hours of training will have to follow to provide sufficient motor and sensory function and prevent complications. This chapter discusses the complications that can be avoided or treated by appropriate hand therapy.

Keywords: complications nerve surgery, hand therapy, nerve injuries, sensory re-education, relearning, hand rehabilitation

23.1 Introduction

The value of hand therapy has been shown in patients with peripheral nerve injuries; those who are treated by a hand therapist have a 3.5 times higher chance to return to work within a year than those who have not received this specialized form of therapy.[1]

Although it is common practice to protect the sutured peripheral nerve in the first 3 to 4 weeks by immobilization with a plaster cast, studies show contradicting results. The primary goal is to minimize tension on the repaired nerve(s) which has been proven to be harmful in experiments in dog trials.[2] Some advocate even longer periods of immobilization, i.e., 6 weeks for wrist-level nerve injuries.[3] In contrast, other studies have shown no beneficial effect of immobilization on the recovery of digital nerves.[4] Further research is warranted to evaluate if, and how, repaired nerves can be mobilized earlier.

After this initial protection phase, the splint is weaned of while tension on the nerve is gradually increased. Controlled movements to regain mobility must be exercised in combination with nerve gliding exercises to prevent short scars around the nerve.

23.2 Complications

23.2.1 Edema

Nerve injuries, like many other hand injuries, suffer from excessive swelling of the hand. Besides the nerve, often other structures like tendons and blood vessels are also damaged, causing poor circulation and subsequent swelling.

Treatment

For the management of edema, the usual care of elevation, compression gloves, movement, and massages are done, keeping in mind that patients should move their injured arm slowly and take account of what they feel when moving their arms, since the regular instruction of elevating the arm can cause tension on the sutured nerve. For example, a sutured median nerve will be stretched when the elbow is extended for elevation. In general, any pain and/or tingling sensation must be avoided in this early phase. Tight splint straps or bandages should also be avoided, especially at the suture sight of the nerve.

23.2.2 Pain

This is crucial and needs to be addressed in a multidisciplinary fashion and commences when the patient is undergoing nerve surgery. In order to prevent upregulation of the pain directly postoperatively, adequate pain regimes, preferably regional techniques, are imperative.

After a few days, the therapy protocol also needs to focus on minimizing pain when optimizing functional return, with the emphasis on active range of motion. In later stages, sensory and motor-relearning activities should be used to treat the pain.

After a peripheral nerve lesion, a non-noxious stimulus is sometimes perceived as being noxious, which is called allodynia.

Treatment

Electrical stimulation, e.g., transcutaneous electrical nerve stimulation (TENS), as used in chronic back pain, can be beneficial in patients with hyperesthesia. In desensitization strategies, different surfaces or textures are used to lower the pain caused by touching of the hand. The concept is similar to sensory re-education such that different types of stimulation, like vibration, and textures are used to re-educate and desensitize the area of hyperesthesia.

In contrast of desensitization strategies, somatosensory rehabilitation (SSR) of pain avoids stimulating the hypersensitive, painful area.[5] In the SSR method, the skin area of the allodynia is mapped by allodynography and its severity by the rainbow pain scale which categorizes the severity with a series of monofilaments. Thereafter, a comfortable tactile or vibratory "counterstimulation" is given at a distant proximal zone and in time the painful area will become smaller.

Mirror therapy has also been shown to be effective in the treatment of complex regional pain syndrome (CRPS) type 2 caused by neuromas.

23.2.3 Muscle Strength Loss

Data supports the view that training protocols specifically addressing the relearning process substantially increase the possibilities for improved functional outcome after nerve repair.[6] Trends in hand rehabilitation focus on modulation of central nervous processes rather than on peripheral nerve factors. Language learning is a thought-provoking metaphor to use when explaining this process of recovery to the patient, explaining the necessity of many hours of practice.[7] Principles are being evolved to maintain the cortical hand representation by using the brain capacity for visuotactile and audiotactile interaction during the initial phase following nerve injury and repair.[8]

Full muscle power recovery is still rarely seen. Expectation management is important to prepare the patient for this. Fortunately, many patients learn to compensate for the loss of strength, although this automatic compensation can be counterproductive for the recovery.

The so-called disuse phenomenon is a very strong mechanism which can be observed in all patients. Patients learn quickly all kinds of trick movements and use compensatory movements to get the job done. Some of these movements help the patient to perform their activities of daily living but some can be counterproductive as the muscle power is not needed anymore.

Treatment

Like language learning, it takes hours of training and if possible can be used in a meaningful and purposeful way. In the first phase, muscle exercises are not the traditional fitness type of training but concentrated, short sessions of getting control of the right stimuli to the right muscle. Imagery and mirror therapy can also be helpful in this phase.

Therapists need to be aware of the disuse phenomenon mechanism and might consider treatment strategies like the constraint-induced movement therapy (CIMT) in which the noninjured arm is obstructed, e.g., with a splint or glove, which has been shown to be effective, e.g., in children with brachial plexus lesions.[9]

Electrical stimulation (ES) is common practice in some countries. The literature does not present strong clinical evidence to support the use of ES to maintain the muscle viability for reinnervation following a long duration of denervation. The mechanisms by which ES and/or exer-cise enhance nerve regeneration remain poorly understood; however, they do show accelerating nerve regeneration.[10]

A form of ES can be helpful in a phase when the nerve has reached the muscle but the patients cannot actively contract the muscle. In this situation, ES is used as a relearning option "finding" the right muscle.

23.2.4 Contractures and Shortening (E.g., Muscle Tightness)

In ulnar nerve lesions, especially in the supple hypermobile hands, there is a danger for progressive proximal interphalangeal (PIP) joint contractures due to inability to extend the PIP joints. The overaction of the extensor digitorum communis (EDC) creates hyperextension in the metacarpal phalangeal (MCP) joints of the fourth and fifth finger. Similarly, flexor tightness occurs which by itself increases the risk for PIP flexion contractures and vice versa. In longstanding intrinsic minus hands, even boutonniere deformities and extensor tendon luxation at the MCP joint level can occur.

In median nerve lesions, there is a danger of thumb web adduction contractures in the very early phase. In high median nerve palsy (Pointing Finger, ▶ Fig. 23.1), an extension contracture of the IP joints of the index finger and IP joint of the thumb often takes place.

In radial nerve palsy, wrist flexion contractures and flexor tightness are the complications to be prevented.

Treatment

Range of motion exercises need to be performed regularly to prevent these joint stiffness and muscle tightness. Splinting is used in many cases like an intrinsic plus night splint (▶ Fig. 23.2), a knuckle bender, and a thumb web

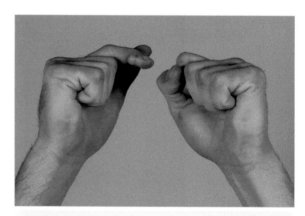

Fig. 23.1 A patient with a high median nerve palsy and typical Pointing Finger.

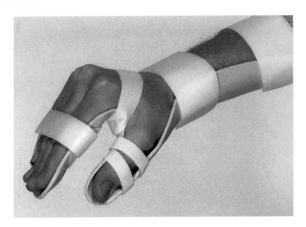

Fig. 23.2 Intrinsic plus night splint used to prevent proximal interphalangeal (PIP) flexion contractures and thumb web adduction contractures.

splint. A simple cock-up splint for patients with a radial nerve lesion helps in their daily activities and also to prevent wrist joint pain and stiffness.

23.2.5 Sensory Loss

Loss of protective sensation can cause wounds by sharp and hot objects. Patients need to be educated how to avoid these wounds and burns.

Treatment

Sensory re-education programs are routinely applied to facilitate sensory recovery. It is a cognitive behavioral therapy technique that helps the patient with a nerve injury to meaningfully interpret the altered profile or neural impulses reaching their conscious level after the altered sensation area has been stimulated.[11] Quiet surroundings and concentration are important.

Regaining sensation is similar to the motor function: a matter of concentrated exercises done at regular bases.

23.2.6 Autonomic Nerve Function Loss

Loss of sweating and loss of circulation control can cause pain and/or cold intolerance.

Treatment

Gloves are often useful besides instructions to avoid change in temperature especially from warm room to cold atmosphere temperature. Some patients find cold-warm baths to be useful.

23.2.7 Psychological Stress

Patients with peripheral nerve injuries suffer a great deal of psychological stress.[12] An intake by the psychologist should be standard within the rehabilitation program rather than just hand therapy.[13]

23.3 Future

The rehabilitation following nerve transfer requires strategies to augment cortical remapping and regain muscle balance. Because in a nerve transfer the reinnervated muscle is motored from a new proximal nerve source, the patient must establish and relearn new motor patterns. Studies that have evaluated the motor cortex and remapping have shown alteration in cortex following nerve transfer and thus the importance of sensorimotor relearning.[14]

23.4 Take-Home Message

To optimize recovery of hand function and sensibility, patients with peripheral nerve injury need to be guided by an experienced hand therapist. Expectation management is very important. In addition, determinants of success of therapy are:

- Pain: During the whole revalidation period a multidisciplinary treatment to minimize pain is important. Upregulation of pain should be avoided by TENS, desensitization, or SSR.
- Edema: Especially in the acute phase, treatment of edema is important while avoiding high pressure or traction on the repaired nerve.
- Function: After the acute phase, mobilization and re-education strategies combined with splints to avoid formation of contractures become important.
- Sensation: Re-education programs should be used. Like for function, training at regular bases and with full concentration is important to get results as good as possible.

References

[1] Bruyns CN, Jaquet JB, Schreuders TAR, Kalmijn S, Kuypers PD, Hovius SER. Predictors for return to work in patients with median and ulnar nerve injuries. J Hand Surg Am. 2003; 28(1):28–34

[2] Lee WP, Constantinescu MA, Butler PE. Effect of early mobilization on healing of nerve repair: histologic observations in a canine model. Plast Reconstr Surg. 1999; 104(6):1718–1725

[3] Dahlin LB, Wiberg M. Nerve injuries of the upper extremity and hand. EFORT Open Rev. 2017; 2(5):158–170

[4] Clare TD, de Haviland Mee S, Belcher HJ. Rehabilitation of digital nerve repair: is splinting necessary? J Hand Surg [Br]. 2004; 29(6):552–556

[5] Packham TL, Spicher CJ, MacDermid JC, Quintal I, Buckley N. Evaluating a sensitive issue: reliability of a clinical evaluation for allodynia severity. Somatosens Mot Res. 2020; 37(1):22–27

[6] Rosén B, Björkman A, Lundborg G. Improved sensory relearning after nerve repair induced by selective temporary anaesthesia: a new concept in hand rehabilitation. J Hand Surg [Br]. 2006; 31(2):126–132

[7] Lundborg G, Rosén B, Dahlin LB, Holmberg J, Karlson B. Functional sensibility of the hand after nerve repair. Lancet. 1993; 342(8882):1300

[8] Rosén B, Vikström P, Turner S, et al. Enhanced early sensory outcome after nerve repair as a result of immediate post-operative re-learning: a randomized controlled trial. J Hand Surg Eur Vol. 2015; 40(6):598–606

[9] Zielinski IM, van Delft R, Voorman JM, Geurts ACH, Steenbergen B, Aarts PBM. The effects of modified constraint-induced movement

therapy combined with intensive bimanual training in children with brachial plexus birth injury: a retrospective data base study. Disabil Rehabil. 2019; •••:1–10

[10] Gordon T, Sulaiman O, Boyd JG. Experimental strategies to promote functional recovery after peripheral nerve injuries. J Peripher Nerv Syst. 2003; 8(4):236–250

[11] Taylor KS, Anastakis DJ, Davis KD. Cutting your nerve changes your brain. Brain. 2009; 132(Pt 11):3122–3133

[12] Ashwood M, Jerosch-Herold C, Shepstone L. Learning to live with a hand nerve disorder: a constructed grounded theory. J Hand Ther. 2019; 32(3):334–344.e1

[13] Jaquet JB, Kalmijn S, Kuypers PD, Hofman A, Passchier J, Hovius SER. Early psychological stress after forearm nerve injuries: a predictor for long-term functional outcome and return to productivity. Ann Plast Surg. 2002; 49(1):82–90

[14] van Zyl N, Hill B, Cooper C, Hahn J, Galea MP. Expanding traditional tendon-based techniques with nerve transfers for the restoration of upper limb function in tetraplegia: a prospective case series. Lancet. 2019; 394(10198):565–575

7

24 Bone and Joint Surgery: Prevention and Management of Complications by Hand Therapy

24.1 Part A: Hand Therapy: Prevention and Management of Complications in Bone and Joint Fractures

Gertjan Kroon and Elske Bonhof-Jansen

Abstract

Common nondisplaced hand fractures without soft tissue injuries can be treated with cast immobilization or a protective or buddy splint. Complications such as joint stiffness, tendon adhesion, and nonunion or malunion are rarely seen. However, stiffness as complication can occur due to inadequate or prolonged immobilization. Complex fractures often require surgical treatment. In open or crush injuries, surgery can be considered to be a "secondary trauma" and potentially these injuries are prone to scar formation and motion deficits. To prevent and manage these complications, timely referral and close collaboration between hand surgeon and hand therapist is essential. Hand therapy focuses on safe, progressive motion with control of pain within the timeline of the healing process. This is done with the aim to provide the patient with functional use of the hand and to resume daily activities as quickly as the injury allows. This chapter provides insights into the tools available to the hand therapist to prevent and manage common complications after hand fractures.

Keywords: hand therapy, fracture, timing, communication, early motion, stiffness, splinting

24.1.1 General Principles

Timing of Treatment

When preventing or minimizing complications, the goals are to maintain joint and soft tissue mobility while protecting fracture stability. The risk of stiffness depends on the location and stability of the fracture and increases with concomitant soft tissue injury or surgery. It is known that the extent of soft tissue damage is directly correlated with functional outcome.[1,2,3,4] Also, patient factors such as higher age, comorbidities, smoking, and psychosocial context (e.g., pain, anxiety, or catastrophizing) can influence outcome negatively.[5,6] In case these negative predictive values are present, early and timely referral to hand therapy is essential to prevent stiffness. Unfortunately, rehabilitation after fracture stabilization is sparsely described in scientific literature. Hand therapy consists of supportive or protective splinting and exercises, allowing safe, progressive motion with control of pain, based on the stages of fracture and soft tissue healing. By embedding purposeful movements in exercises, functional use of the hand will be improved in order to resume daily activities, work, sports, and hobbies.[7] Hand therapy is most effective when started in the first week after surgical fracture stabilization, since it is easier to prevent stiffness and edema in the initial phase of fracture and soft tissue healing. The greatest recovery of active range of motion is seen within the first 6 weeks.[8] Common nondisplaced fractures without soft tissue injury are commonly treated nonsurgically with or without cast immobilization. Stiffness as complication can occur due to inadequate or prolonged immobilization. Hand therapy is not routinely indicated, as it may be expected that full range of motion will be restored within 2 weeks after cast removal. Informing the patients about goals, expected recovery time, and outcomes will improve self-management. However, when pain persists, or gain of motion or functional recovery is delayed, easy access to a surgeon or hand therapist is recommended.

Communication

Besides the technical aspects, communication is an important key to successful rehabilitation.[9] Close collaboration between surgeon, hand therapist, and patient is essential for effective treatment. The hand therapist will need information on fracture stability in order to initiate an appropriate rehabilitation program within the most effective but safe limits of fracture management.[7] Specifically, in cases where the surgical result is not optimal; for example, insufficient fracture stability, soft tissue weakness, perioperative or expected limited motion, and required splint support. In addition, patient information provided by surgeon and hand therapist can manage expectations and support the patients' self-management. Topics are pain and edema management, specific exercises, allowed functional use, expected recovery time, and outcome.

24.1.2 Complications

In open or crush injuries, surgery can be seen as a "secondary trauma," increasing the risk of scar formation and motion deficits. These risks, with associated costs, have to be considered in fractures where surgical management is not proven beneficial compared to conservative fracture management.[10] This chapter will describe complications that can be prevented or managed by hand therapeutic interventions.

Infection

In percutaneous fracture fixation with Kirschner wires or external fixation methods, pin-track infection may occur in 6 to 7% of cases.[11,12] In the majority of these cases, infections were superficial and resolved by oral antibiotics or removal of the infected pins. There is insufficient evidence that warrants a specific pin-site care strategy to minimize infection rates.[13] Risk factors that predispose an individual to a pin-site infection has not been determined yet.[12] Due to a lack of evidence, general strategies to reduce the infection risk are advised.[13] The hand therapist can inform the patient of infection prevention and give instructions for wound inspection to monitor for signs of inflammation.

Nonunion/Malunion

Local forces surrounding a fracture will influence bone generation.[14] Excessive strain will result in nonunion or malunion, taking into account the tendency of the fracture to deviate in a potentially instable fracture.[7] Fracture stability allowing active motion is assessed by the surgeon. When additional support is required during the first month, a three-point splint can be used in metacarpal fractures, a dorsal intrinsic plus splint in proximal phalanx fractures (▶ Fig. 24.1) and a dorsal finger splint in midphalanx fractures (▶ Fig. 24.2).

In case of intra-articular fractures, protected early motion will prevent joint stiffness and optimize remodeling of the articular surface. Insufficient stabilization or using too much force in the early stages of fracture healing may lead to nonunion or malunion. In stable hand fractures, buddy splints may be used to prevent forces from causing deviation during the early phase of fracture healing.

Tips and Tricks

- Absence of pain and tenderness at the fracture site on palpation is a clinical sign of fracture healing.[15]
- Early motion supports fracture healing and reduces edema.
- Scissoring of the fingers can be a sign of malrotation or a muscle imbalance; assess the intrinsic muscle function (intrinsic tightness or loss of coordination) to differentiate.
- Use additional splint support in case of insufficient stabilization to allow early motion with X-ray check-up to assess fracture alignment.
- Provide practical patient information on do's and don'ts in functional use in order to prevent overuse.

Stiffness

General

The cause of stiffness is often multifactorial. Initially, stiffness is due to edema. When edema is not controlled, the hand positions itself in metacarpophalangeal (MCP) joint hyperextension and proximal interphalangeal phalanx (PIP) joint flexion. This will lead to shrinkage of capsule and ligaments. Stiffness may also be due to arthrogenic limitations, resulting from either the trauma itself or from

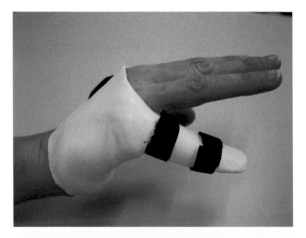

Fig. 24.1 Intrinsic plus immobilizing/exercise splint.

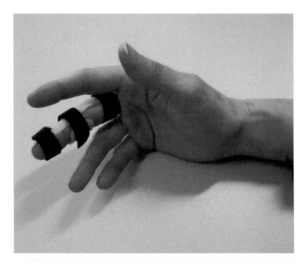

Fig. 24.2 Finger immobilizing/exercise splint.

prolonged immobilization with capsule and ligament shrinkage. Adhesions may prevent tendon gliding or restrict motion. Shortening of bone may lead to a misbalance of the muscle/tendon complex. Finally, psychosocial factors should not be underestimated,[6] since pain and fear to move or to use the hand during daily activities may also be a cause of stiffness, and overuse may cause swelling.

Joint Stiffness

Joint stiffness is characterized by MCP extension and IP flexion with limited range of motion in opposite direction. Often there is no obvious difference in active and passive joint motion. The opposite position, also known as "intrinsic plus position" or "the position of safe immobilization," can prevent stiffness by positioning the joint ligaments in elongated position. Here, the MP joints are positioned in 60 to 70 degrees of flexion and IP joints in 0 degrees of extension. Prevention of contractures starts with positioning the joints in this position.

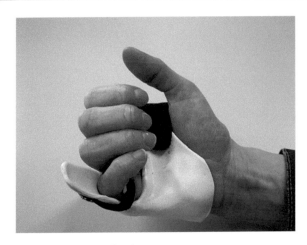

Fig. 24.3 Exercise with splint support.

A combination of early controlled motion and intrinsic plus splinting during rest is indicated for all stable fractures that show a tendency of stiffness.

A dorsal intrinsic plus splint is able to support insufficient fracture stability, allowing early active motion (▶ Fig. 24.3). For postoperative PIP flexion due to hydrops, step-wise redressing to intrinsic position combined with active range of motion exercises is recommended. In case of intra-articular fractures, it is recommended to keep the immobilization period as short as possible. Recent literature shows that treatment with a dorsal intrinsic plus splint (restricting MCP extension when allowing full range of motion of the PIP joints) is safe in proximal phalanx fractures and prevents range of motion limitations.[16]

When joint stiffness occurs, static progressive splints and sometimes dynamic mobilizing splints can be used around 6 weeks in fractures with enough structural strength; after which this may be alternated with a blocking splint to stimulate movement during activities in the limited direction. Relative motion splints are a user-friendly and effective supplement to support and improve active range of motion. If PIP flexion contractures occur, serial casting is indicated when other treatments have failed to regain extension; be sure that there is no flexion deficit prior to casting.

Tips and Tricks

- Control edema with pressure therapy (elastic-bandage wrapping or a pressure glove), elevation and massage.
- When immobilization is indicated, use intrinsic plus position.
- Use an intrinsic plus splint combined with early active motion in case of stable fractures.
- Use a mobilizing splint around 6 weeks in case of joint stiffness, if consolidation is confirmed, and alternate with active motion.

Tendon Adhesion

Hand fractures combined with soft tissue injury or surgery increase the risk of tendon adhesions. This is especially known for proximal phalangeal fractures because of the close relation of bone and tendons. When active motion is more impaired than passive motion, restrictive tendon adhesion is present. Prevention of restrictive adhesions is based on achieving stable (near) anatomic fracture position and early motion focused on tendon gliding, ideally started within 5 days after surgical fracture fixation.[7] All tendon-gliding restricting factors such as edema, pain, and fear to move must be attended.

In case of proximal phalangeal fractures, dorsal intrinsic plus splinting can contribute to prevention of tendon adhesions since the splint has several advantages. The extensor hood moves distally with MP joint flexion, providing circumferential compression to the proximal phalanx, hyperextension at the MP joint with proximal extensor tendon glide is prevented, and extensor tendon tension focuses at the PIP joint.[7] The splint can be combined with several types of joint motion: active, assisted-active, or passive motion. In the remodeling phase, blocking splints or relative motion splints can be applied to exert more stretch on the restrictive scar tissue during exercise and daily activities. When an extensor tendon adhesion occurs, with severe impaired flexion, a mono- or polyarticular mobilizing splint may be used. In case of muscular weakness, strengthening exercises are used to increase the influence of these forces on the adhesions. The greatest effect can be achieved by improving the flexor force for flexor and reducing extensor tendon adhesions. Depending on fracture healing and local tissue response, the force is increased in terms of duration and intensity.

Tips and Tricks

- Start early motion/tendon gliding exercises within 5 days after surgery.
- Intrinsic plus splinting supported with exercises is useful to prevent a PIP extensor lag.
- When placing Kirschner wires, tendon-gliding exercises should remain possible.
- In case of long-standing and noncorrectible deformities, hand therapy can improve functional outcome.

24.1.3 Conclusions

"Hand fractures can be complicated by deformity from no treatment, stiffness from over treatment and both deformity and stiffness from poor treatment."[17] Fracture management can be compared with a balance exercise between fracture stability and joint/soft tissue mobility for all involved disciplines. Conservative management must be considered in fractures where surgical management is not proven beneficial to decrease the risk of stiffness.

Surgeons have to consider if safe early motion is allowed after fracture stabilization. Hand therapists can support patients in performing an effective rehabilitation regimen adapted to fracture and patient-specific characteristics. Close collaboration between the disciplines involved in fracture management enables effective and efficient fracture management in pursuing individual patient goals.

24.1.4 Take-Home Message

Early controlled motion is one of the key aspects to prevent complications, such as stiffness. Together with a well-timed referral to hand therapy and a close collaboration between the patient and the disciplines involved, this can ensure optimal patient-specific functional outcomes.

24.2 Part B: Rehabilitation after Joint Arthroplasties in the Hand

Paul De Buck

Abstract

In practice, Swan neck or Boutonniere deformity and functional problems with joint arthroplasties in the hand, e.g., loss of range of motion, are often seen but not all are consistently mentioned in research. When a rehabilitation program is described, it is not detailed and lacks simple clinical reasoning and solutions. This section will present some general considerations and easy-to-use solutions for the treatment of functional complications seen with joint replacements in fingers used by our team. It is not the aim to address all existing rehabilitation programs used after a joint arthroplasty. The most frequently seen arthroplasties in our center are the pyrocarbon arthroplasties for proximal interphalangeal (PIP) joint and CMC-1 joint. These are the main subjects of this section. Each postoperative treatment should be adjusted based on symptoms and clinical reasoning. The use of different types of orthoses can be advocated to optimize the healing process and minimize the complications in combination with proper education of the patient. Because, in the end the patient needs to learn to accept the "new" joint with his possible limitations.

Keywords: hand therapy, joint arthroplasty, pyrocarbon, PIP joint, CMC-1 joint, relative motion splint, clinical reasoning

24.2.1 General principles

There are many types of joint arthroplasties, all with their own advantages and disadvantages. A lot of research is published about the biomechanics, the surgical protocols,

and the outcome, but few are written about rehabilitation programs after these arthroplasties. Research and clinical experience of the surgeons mentioned few complications after arthroplasties. The most frequent surgical complications described are failure or displacement of the prostheses. Nevertheless, in clinical practice patients complain often about the loss of function.

Patient Education

Patients are treated frequently by surgery.[18] The first choice of treatment should be conservative with the use of protective orthoses, exercises, occupational guidelines, and supportive devices.[19] These programs could postpone or even prevent surgery because patients have less pain with preservation of function.

A first and very important step in the conservative treatment and the rehabilitation of joint arthroplasties is patient education. As health care professional, it is important to create realistic expectations leading indirectly to better outcome satisfaction.[20] Patients need to be taught that the main purpose of an arthroplasty is pain reduction instead of full restoration of mobility. They need to realize that recovery will take a long time and pain will be felt up to 3 to 6 months postoperative. In order to give a patient a more realistic idea of the effect of the operation and evolution through the rehabilitation process, a preoperative baseline assessment of joint range of motion, grip force, and functionality level is crucial.

Choice of Postoperative Treatment

Depending on the joint that is being replaced and the pathology causing the need for replacement, different approaches, surgically and therapeutically, are needed. Some additional stability (stiffness) in the CMC-1 arthroplasty is favorable, and therefore an immediate active program is not necessary. In contrast, in metacarpophalangeal (MCP) and proximal interphalangeal (PIP) joint arthroplasties, there is a need for early movement. Techniques that allow early active mobilizations (for example, do not cut the central slip transversally) are favorable. Frequent therapy sessions are not mandatory in many cases. Hand therapists need to adjust therapy frequency considering the patient's sociodemographic characteristics, compliance, how many and which finger(s) operated, surgical method, and underlying pathology. For example, patients with osteoarthrosis need less intensive rehabilitation programs and protection compared to patients with rheumatoid arthritis.[20]

A rehabilitation program based on healing of the "damaged" surrounding, stabilizing, moving soft tissue is crucial because these new articulations are rather shallow. Incorrect loading can rapidly cause strain and eccentric loading, which will be harmful for the already operatively "damaged" soft tissue.[21] For example, a dorsal approach of the PIP joint with a longitudinal division of the extensor tendon needs a tendon-like protocol with appropriate protection and tendon gliding.

24.2.2 Complications

In general, therapists need to protect the "damaged" soft tissue and on the other hand they need to avoid loss of mobility, which is one of the most reported complaints. Therefore, regardless of an early active program or a period of complete immobilization, edema reduction and scar tissue treatment should be started in the early stages of the rehabilitation and should be monitored more closely. Non-involved joints should be kept mobile, especially the fingers. Stiffening of one finger will reduce the ability of all neighboring fingers leading to an additional loss of function based on impairment of the quadriga phenomenon.

In the following section, I will give an overview of frequently seen complications accompanied with useful rehabilitation advices.

Complications in PIP Arthroplasty

Loss of Range of Motion

Due to surgical changes of the extensor apparatus and the healing process, an altered movement pattern can occur resulting in two possible functional complications: a Swan neck deformity with loss of flexion and an extension lag with a flexion contracture over time, (pseudo) boutonniere deformity. Literature states that Swan neck deformities more often occur with PIP-joint surface replacing arthroplasties (pyrocarbon), especially with the dorsal approach.[22] This could be caused by shortening of the extensor tendon due to scar tissue shrinkage or adhesion in the postoperative wound-healing process, or a dorsal shift of the lateral bands, implicating that too much extension in the early postoperative phase could be a risk factor as well. These complications need to be avoided and a good balance between protection and movement is necessary, making it crucial to monitor the rehabilitation and adjust when needed.

This implicates that the rehabilitation protocol should focus on avoiding adhesions, shortening or lengthening the extensor hood, and overuse of the dorsal and palmar Interosseous muscles. All can be avoided by using a well-controlled, early, active protocol such as the Short Arc Motion protocol.[23,24] The protocol combines protective immobilization and tendon gliding within a protective range. Progression is based on the healing process of the soft tissue and the clinical representation.

Loss of Flexion

If a Swan neck deformity does occur, a PIP-joint hyperextension blocking orthosis could be used (▶ Fig. 24.4). When the deformity exists alongside a reduced PIP-joint flexion, this orthosis can be combined with a relative motion extension splint (▶ Fig. 24.4) as in the rehabilitation protocol for extensor tendons, zone 4 injuries.[25,26] Because the MCP joint is in a relative extended position compared to the adjunct nonoperated fingers, the focus of finger flexion will move to the PIP joint. In addition, the interosseous muscles of the finger is lengthened and the extensor tendon is protected.[27]

Loss of Extension

It is obvious when extension is lost, the onwards progression toward active PIP-joint flexion is postponed and more protection is given by using a static resting extension splint. To avoid complete stiffening of the finger or a pseudo boutonniere deformity, it is essential to keep the DIP joint mobile. Therefore, it should not only be left free within the protective PIP-resting splint, but the patient should also be trained how to keep the DIP joint mobile. Although the movement of the DIP joint is very important as it creates gliding of the flexor and extensor tendon, and lengthening of the Landsmeer ligament and lateral slips, it is often forgotten in rehabilitation exercises.

When the DIP joint has a good mobility, there is another possibility to restore the extension loss in a more dynamic and still safe way by using the relative motion flexion splint. The idea is simple and based on the use of

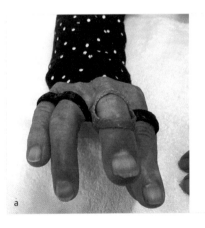
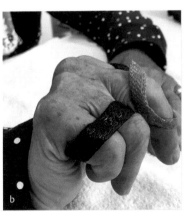

Fig. 24.4 (a, b) Relative motion extension splint (*black*) protecting the extensor tendon zone 4 and lengthening the interosseous muscles of the finger. Combined with a proximal interphalangeal (PIP) joint hyperextension blocking orthosis (*blue*).

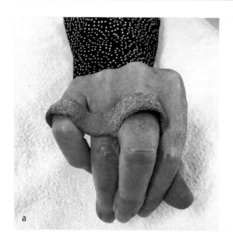 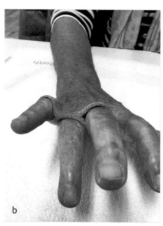

Fig. 24.5 (a, b) Relative motion flexion splint used to restore extension loss in an active way.

the extensor tenodesis. By blocking the MCP joint of the operated finger in a slightly flexed position, the focus during extension in this finger will be on the PIP joint. Hereby active extension can be trained (▶ Fig. 24.5).

Deviating Finger

In case of radial or ulnar deviation in the PIP joint, we propose to use a buddy-strap connecting the second phalanges of the neighboring finger. Personally, I prefer to make them out of thermoplastic material because this material does not lose stiffness and the space between neighboring fingers can be maintained.

Tips and Tricks

- Early active treatment is necessary with edema reduction, scar tissue treatment, and tendon gliding as key elements.
- Avoid adhesions, shortening or lengthening of the extensor hood, and overuse of the interosseous muscles of the finger.
- Maintain DIP-joint mobility.
- Find a balance in flexion gain and extension loss.
- Consider the use of the relative motion splint to maintain the balance. Adapt treatment when necessary.

Complications in CMC-1 Surgery

Overuse-Related Complaints: Quervain Syndrome

Thumb CMC-1 joint arthroplasties (pyrocarbon and Apreprotheses) have in general good results. A frequent functional complication is an aggravation of pain between 3 and 6 months postoperatively, especially in the first extensor compartment. A possible explanation is the increase in activities during this period, leading to over-use and the tendency of making compensatory wrist movements by which the muscles of the first extensor compartment are being stressed even more.

In order to prevent overuse, patients should be informed in advance and get a proper training. They should be treated with coordinative and proprioceptive exercises to master a correct muscular cocontraction of the thumb and wrist musculature. The treatment should address the whole kinetic chain of thumb and wrist. This should be projected on activities of daily living, teaching the patient how to prevent overload. The use of corrective braces or reminder tapes could support this. Depending on the compensations made, different tapes can be applied.

Trigger Thumb

Although trigger thumb is not often seen in our clinic as a complication after a CMC-1 joint replacement, it is sometimes found. In a case of flexor tendon tenosynovitis, a conservative treatment should be offered.[28] A splint will be advised for 4 weeks, immobilizing the IP joint of the thumb. Nevertheless, sometimes the trigger is provoked by flexion of the MCP joint, directing our treatment toward an immobilization of the MCP joint. The patient will be instructed to use the thumb correctly in order to prevent and to treat the trigger thumb. If this is not effective, a steroid injection into the tendon sheath is a possible option.

Tips and Tricks

- More stability is favorable, less need for early active treatment.
- Avoid overuse especially toward the third month of rehabilitation.
- Monitor compensatory movements during activities with increasing loading.
- Train thumb and wrist as a kinetic chain.

24.2.3 Conclusions

In general, patients need to learn to use the "new" joint and need to accept that the new joint will not be the same as the original joint but it will be better than the destructed one. Acceptance of some loss of function and some reduction in loading capacity, knowing that pain will decrease, is essential for a good recovery.

24.2.4 Take-Home Message

When conservative treatment does not give expectable pain relief, surgical treatment could be the next option. Patients need to be educated to have realistic outcome expectations. Pain is the main reason for surgical treatment, with regaining of function being secondary. Each postoperative treatment should be adjusted based on symptoms and clinical reasoning, with the focus on optimizing the healing process, especially of the extensor apparatus, and minimizing functional complications. It is very important to monitor the change in balance in the extensor apparatus of the finger. The use of the relative motion splint can be a part of the postoperative treatment either for regaining PIP joint extension or flexion. With CMC-1 joint arthroplasties, additional care should be taken to prevent the overload of the first extensor compartment. In the end, the patient needs to learn to accept the "new" joint with his possible limitations.

References

[1] Chow SP, Pun WK, So YC, et al. A prospective study of 245 open digital fractures of the hand. J Hand Surg [Br]. 1991; 16(2):137–140
[2] Duncan RW, Freeland AE, Jabaley ME, Meydrech EF. Open hand fractures: an analysis of the recovery of active motion and of complications. J Hand Surg Am. 1993; 18(3):387–394
[3] Shimizu T, Omokawa S, Akahane M, et al. Predictors of the postoperative range of finger motion for comminuted periarticular metacarpal and phalangeal fractures treated with a titanium plate. Injury. 2012; 43(6):940–945
[4] Swanson TV, Szabo RM, Anderson DD. Open hand fractures: prognosis and classification. J Hand Surg Am. 1991; 16(1):101–107
[5] Day CS, Stern PJ. Fractures of the metacarpals and phalanges. In: Wolfe SW, Hotchkiss RN, Pederson WC, Kozin SH, eds. Green's operative hand surgery. 6th ed. Part number: 9-9960-4987-6 (Vol. 1). Philadelphia: Churchill Livingstone Elsevier; 2011:239–290
[6] Keogh E, Book K, Thomas J, Giddins G, Eccleston C. Predicting pain and disability in patients with hand fractures: comparing pain anxiety, anxiety sensitivity and pain catastrophizing. Eur J Pain. 2010; 14(4):446–451
[7] Feehan LM. Early controlled mobilization of potentially unstable extra-articular hand fractures. J Hand Ther. 2003; 16(2):161–170
[8] Miller L, Ada L, Crosbie J, Wajon A. Pattern of recovery after open reduction and internal fixation of proximal phalangeal fractures in the finger: a prospective longitudinal study. J Hand Surg Eur Vol. 2017; 42(2):137–143
[9] Hays PL, Rozental TD. Rehabilitative strategies following hand fractures. Hand Clin. 2013; 29(4):585–600
[10] Giddins GEB. The non-operative management of hand fractures. J Hand Surg Eur Vol. 2015; 40(1):33–41
[11] van Leeuwen WF, van Hoorn BTJA, Chen N, Ring D. Kirschner wire pin site infection in hand and wrist fractures: incidence rate and risk factors. J Hand Surg Eur Vol. 2016; 41(9):990–994
[12] Hsu LP, Schwartz EG, Kalainov DM, Chen F, Makowiec RL. Complications of K-wire fixation in procedures involving the hand and wrist. J Hand Surg Am. 2011; 36(4):610–616
[13] Lethaby A, Temple J, Santy-Tomlinson J. Pin site care for preventing infections associated with external bone fixators and pins. Cochrane Database Syst Rev. 2013(12):CD004551
[14] Sathyendra V, Darowish M. Basic science of bone healing. Hand Clin. 2013; 29(4):473–481
[15] Cunningham BP, Brazina S, Morshed S, Miclau T, III. Fracture healing: a review of clinical, imaging and laboratory diagnostic options. Injury. 2017; 48 Suppl 1:S69–S75
[16] Byrne B, Jacques A, Gurfinkel R. Non-surgical management of isolated proximal phalangeal fractures with immediate mobilization. J Hand Surg Eur Vol. 2020; 45(2):126–130
[17] Swanson AB. Fractures involving the digits of the hand. Orthop Clin North Am. 1970; 1(2):261–274
[18] Gravås EMH, Tveter AT, Nossum R, et al. Non-pharmacological treatment gap preceding surgical consultation in thumb carpometacarpal osteoarthritis: a cross-sectional study. BMC Musculoskelet Disord. 2019; 20(1):180
[19] Wouters RM, Tsehaie J, Slijper HP, Hovius SER, Feitz R, Selles RW, Hand-Wrist Study Group. Exercise therapy in addition to an orthosis reduces pain more than an orthosis alone in patients with thumb base osteoarthritis: a propensity score matching study. Arch Phys Med Rehabil. 2019; 100(6):1050–1060
[20] Pratt AL, Burr N. Post-operative rehabilitation after PIP joint arthroplasty with early active motion: a retrospective review of outcomes. Br J Hand Ther. 2007; 12(1):22–27
[21] Wagner ER, Weston JT, Houdek MT, Luo TD, Moran SL, Rizzo M. Medium-term outcomes with pyrocarbon proximal interphalangeal arthroplasty: a study of 170 consecutive arthroplasties. J Hand Surg Am. 2018; 43(9):797–805
[22] Forster N, Schindele S, Audigé L, Marks M. Complications, reoperations and revisions after proximal interphalangeal joint arthroplasty: a systematic review and meta-analysis. J Hand Surg Eur Vol. 2018; 43 (10):1066–1075
[23] Evans RB. Early active short arc motion for the repaired central slip. J Hand Surg Am. 1994; 19(6):991–997
[24] McAuliffe JA. Early active short arc motion following central slip repair. J Hand Surg Am. 2011; 36(1):143–146
[25] Hirth MJ, Howell JW, O'Brien L. Relative motion orthoses in the management of various hand conditions: a scoping review. J Hand Ther. 2016; 29(4):405–432
[26] Howell JW, Peck F. Rehabilitation of flexor and extensor tendon injuries in the hand: current updates. Injury. 2013; 44(3):397–402
[27] Merritt WH, Wong AL, Lalonde DH. Recent developments are changing extensor tendon management. Plast Reconstr Surg. 2020; 145 (3):617e–628e
[28] Pencle FJ, Harberger S, Molnar JA. Trigger thumb. StatPearls Publishing; 2020: https://www.ncbi.nlm.nih.gov/books/NBK441854/

Section 8

CRPS

25 Debunking Complex Regional Pain Syndrome/Sudeck/Reflex Sympathetic Dystrophy

Francisco del Piñal

Abstract

The aim of this chapter is to demonstrate, that despite all our previous learning, we may have been misguided for many years as to the existence of the cryptic condition known as complex regional pain syndrome (CRPS), algodystrophy, Sudeck, or reflex sympathetic dystrophy. An in-depth study of each patient permits us to allocate each case in a named condition. The current arbitrary use of CRPS after surgery as "an unfortunate complication," or labeling conditions as CRPS because the surgeon ignores the actual diagnosis, is a clear disservice to the patient and to the progress of medicine.

Keywords: CRPS, chronic pain, RSD, Sudeck

25.1 Introduction

"Convictions are more dangerous enemies of truth than lies."

F. Nietzsche

CRPS—complex regional pain syndrome—(a.k.a. Sudeck atrophy, reflex sympathetic dystrophy [RSD], or algodystrohy) is an abnormal painful response after trauma or surgery, accompanied by vasomotor changes, and the lack of a plausible cause for its development. CRPS is an endpoint diagnosis, whose main treatment is medical in a Pain Clinic.[1,2,3,4,5,6]

The condition has evolved in its nearly 150 years of existence to include pathologies that were not initially part thereof, much depending on the moods of the age. What Silas Mitchell described as *causalgia* was the burning pain and vasomotor changes soldiers had in their limbs after sustaining major nerve trunk injuries. The condition had an evident inciting pathology, i.e., a nerve injury. This initial concept was somewhat distorted by Paul Sudeck in 1900, who extended the condition to cases with a similar clinical picture but caused by a minor or even a nontraumatic event (*minor causalgia*). Later, Leriche and Policard would attribute overactivation of the sympathetic nervous system as for the pathology resulting in the unusual clinical picture, hence the name Reflex Sympathetic Dystrophy. Recently, the taxonomy had to be revised in order to dodge the lack of sympathetic system involvement.[7,8] The new terms CRPS1 and CRPS2 emerged, parenthetically RSD for the former and causalgia for the latter.[9] In other words, RSD/CRPS1/Sudeck were additions to what Mitchell already had described in 1870. In his favor, Sudeck did not have tools such as CT scan, MRI, arthroscopy, and the like at his disposal to hone his diagnosis, and modifying the saying: all cats may have looked gray in the darkness of those times.

It may be wiser for me not to say that I firmly believe that CRPS1 is a convenient condition which shelters bad doctoring and our frustrations when we are at a loss.[10,11] Nevertheless, I am not alone in challenging the status quo. Several surgeons and neurologists[12,13,14,15,16,17,18] have written about the abuse and misdiagnosis of this condition. We may differ in the underlying pathology: some blame the nerves; others think there is a deep-rooted psychiatric problem, or a psychological issue. Yet, the message of all these authors is the same: CRPS is not a condition, in itself, but more so a constellation of signs and symptoms that needs proper identification and consequently effective treatment.

So, despite the place it has been afforded in the literature, its long existence, the multitude of papers in top journals and chapters in reference books, I am sticking to my guns and once again reiterate: *CRPS is a fabrication and as concocted should be radically excised from all medical practice.*

25.2 The Weakness of the CRPS Concept

Reading the literature, in my quest to understand CRPS, I have come across several weaknesses/inconsistencies/biases:

- It is astonishing that with today's medical advances,[2,3,19,20] the condition still has no clear-cut clinical picture, no specific diagnostic tests, an unknown pathophysiology, and lacks curative treatment. Thus, it is a condition underpinned on clinical lore not on scientific grounds.
- The criteria for diagnosing CRPS are exceedingly lax (Budapest criteria or Veldman's criteria).[1,21,22] Any painful condition with swelling and inflammation seems to fit under the umbrella. The most stringent criterion is the inability of the surgeon to provide an explanation for the patient's clinical picture. This item assumes that all doctors have the same ability to diagnose, which at this point of my career I can only grade as hilarious. Contrarily, as I have written, the only association I have been able to find was an exponential increase in CRPS cases in proportion to the ignorance of the surgeon who diagnosed the case.[11] This assertion seems to have irritated a fair number of people, when in fact all I did was to write a finding. Fortunately, I am again not alone here and others claim CRPS diagnosis to be a

consequence of "*lazy medicine*"[23] "by junior doctors who do not take into account the negative effect this diagnosis may entail."[24] Nevertheless, as I will discuss below this is fueled by an erroneously taught urgency to rush into the diagnosis in order not to miss a case.

- Some of the scientific backing of the condition comes from the assembly of an inexistent continuum from real conditions (causalgia) and imaginary ones (RSD-Psychogenic hand). It is surprising that most studies on the incidence and outcomes currently quoted were performed on distal radius fractures (DRF) on a time when suboptimal treatments for DRF were dispensed (simply cast, or at best supplemented with K-wires).[25,26,27] In a long-term study, it is claimed that the "reduction" was unrelated to the presence of CRPS, while in the same study osteoarthritis *was* ($p < 0.0001$).[26] This contradicts what we know today, i.e., that osteoarthritis is directly related to intra-articular malunion.

- Most current papers are review articles and are written by the same authors-institutions (Chicago-Cleveland-London-Mainz-Nijmegen-Vanderbilt) and in our field (Bristol-Poznan-London) as the most productive centers. The reviews are preceded by editorials: heaping hallelujahs on the review writing. In such reviews,[5,6,19] the dissident papers were systematically ignored, despite claiming in-depth reviews in PubMed. This is tantamount to pure denialism. Furthermore, the papers published in the higher impact journals are written by rehabilitation and pain doctors, when the only person who can decide if there is no explanation for a patient's pain in the realm of the hand is the hand surgeon.

- Authorities on CRPS[3,4,5,6,19,20,27,28,29] stress that early diagnosis is paramount to prevent the condition from evolving into the chronic stage. The review papers are full of claims such as: "better too much than too little," "better to overdiagnose than miss a case," "overdiagnosis is good," etc. This places enormous pressure on the clinician to lower the threshold to diagnose the condition to avoid missing a single case. Yet, *nobody has demonstrated that early diagnosis has any benefit on the outcome.*

Premature diagnosis swells the figures with cases that are not "CRPS" and, not surprisingly, studies on the natural history of the condition have shown spontaneous resolution in most cases.[25,30] In one of Zyluk's papers, none of the 15/120 patients who satisfied criteria for CRPS 6 weeks after the accident did so at 1 year; the final incidence was less that 1%! Thus, early diagnosis, linked to early treatment, may give the impression that early treatment is highly effective, when in fact *the patients may have been "cured" of a condition they had never had!* In keeping with the above, all available treatments are ineffective in the chronic stage.[4,5,6,19,29,31,32] This chronic group probably represents the only "true" CRPS cases—please note *true* is in inverted commas.

- Due to the lack of specificity of the criteria used to diagnose CRPS (Budapest's, Veldman's) some patients allocated in CRPS, in theory an end-point diagnosis, had surgical cure. There are many examples of this in the literature.[12,13,17,33,34,35,36,37] Unfortunately, most patients are not so lucky to find a surgeon who understands their claims, but are sent to the Pain Clinic, and there is no way back from there. This is not to say that the Pain Doctor is doing anything wrong. On the contrary, the mission of the Pain Doctor is to alleviate pain, not to know what the etiology of the pain is—this is the responsibility of the referral surgeon!

- This nonsensical sequence of events makes the number of CRPS cases soar to 50,000 a year in the United States alone.[38] Unfortunately, diagnosing CRPS lightly is not without its consequences. Psychiatrists, psychologists, and surgeons have warned that diagnosing CRPS has a deleterious effect on well-being and mental health, particularly of the most deprived population.[39] By being given this diagnosis, patients may find a reason for their complaints and actually become ill and unnecessarily medicalized.[18,23,24,40] It is thus crucial to narrow the diagnosis down to only those (if any) who develop this condition.

25.3 The Series

The weaknesses discussed and the blown-up figures were quite insufficient evidence to remove CRPS from our armamentarium. It is irrefutable that there were patients who had signs and symptoms making them eligible under Veldman's criteria, the Budapest Criteria, and who registered a high score on the CRPS severity score.[28] To unravel the conundrum, a prospective study was carried out. Beginning in January 2018 all patients attending the office for a second opinion having been diagnosed with and treated for CRPS were included. Our first purpose was to give them a fresh diagnosis and, if the patient accepted, to treat them surgically and assess the outcomes.

The study is still ongoing, so the breakdowns are under construction. Currently, there are 166 patients of whom 44 refused to be operated or failed to return to further follow-up. Some were disappointed or upset on being confronted with the fact they did not have CRPS. Some were sent to a psychiatric consultation, but never went. Sixteen good candidates for curative surgery, because they presented an irritative carpal tunnel syndrome, refused treatment counseled by their treating doctors (orthopaedic, rehabilitation, or pain doctors). I must admit that, albeit frustrating, there is nothing wrong with this choice, as papers and reference texts advise against surgery.[3,5,6,20,27,29,41,42] Some of those who refused surgery were overt cases of malpractice, and yet surprisingly still preferred to be treated by the original surgeon, perhaps dissuaded by the cost of private care. A further 28 did not need any surgery, they were cases of overdiagnosis, some

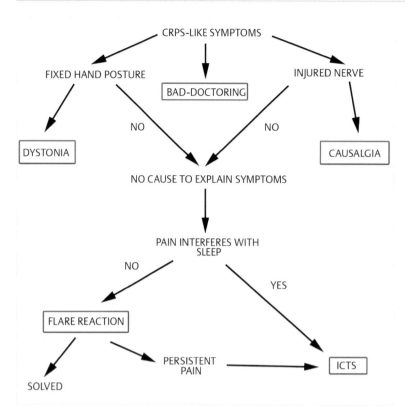

Fig. 25.1 Flowchart for allocating a patient with complex regional pain syndrome (CRPS)-like symptoms.

flare reactions, and at least four cases of misdiagnosis/ malpractice.

We had no drop-outs in the patients accepting to be operated or treated.

Considering only the treated patients (a population very similar to those who refused to be treated), the results demonstrate that there are only five categories in which to allocate patient with CRPS-like symptoms (▶ Fig. 25.1).

25.3.1 Flare Reaction

Some patients after trauma or surgery may have temporary pain, swelling, discoloration, and stiffness. They may have a great deal of difficulty in regaining motion. They tend to produce excessive fibrosis, but the process is somewhat self-limited but "may end in permanent stiffness."[43] The management consists of physical therapy, adding if needed low doses of pregabaline or gabapentin. Steroids can also be considered. There is no test to differentiate this group from a "true" CRPS, and my impression is that the vast majority of cases "cured" by the various CRPS regimens (bisphosphonates, DMSO, steroids, mannitol, ketamine, or even stellate ganglion blocks) are actually flare reaction cases, as no protocol has proved successful in chronic cases.[31,32,44] For me, what changes the whole picture and the indication for surgery is whether they have difficulty in sleeping. If despite the medication, the patient can't sleep, or the pain is not relieved, I would

be in favor of acting surgically (see Chapter 25.3.5). In this series, there were 26 patients wrongly diagnosed with CRPS who actually had or have had a flare reaction.

25.3.2 Causalgia

When trapped in scar, devascularized, kinked, or stretched, a nerve will elicit causalgic symptoms, namely: burning pain, allodynia, and dysesthesias. This is what was called CRPS type II, and corresponds to the original Mitchell description of wounded soldiers with unbearable pain. Several authors have shown that surgery, consisting in releasing the nerve from the scar and changing the devascularized nerve bed,[12,45,46,47] will ease the pain in about 80% of cases. This group also includes the so-called neurostenalgia described by Birch,[34] which can be a source of excruciating pain and responds to nerve release.[36,48]

25.3.3 Dystonic-Psychogenic Hand

Causalgic-CRPS[49] is thought, by neurologists, to result from some malfunction at the spinal cord. Good results have been reported in a case series with intrathecal baclofen.[50] The value of such an approach is disputed though,[51] and other neurologists consider the condition to be overtly psychologically mediated,[52,53,54] as do most surgeons.[55,56] Nevertheless, there is a gray line in dystonia-psychogenic hand-CRPS[15] in which patients may be allocated erroneously to one or the other,[54] and we have explored that "frontier." Five patients of 12 with dystonia-CRPS agreed to be operated: two of them were cured; another patient's pain disappeared and had some improvement in range of motion, and despite her satisfaction, to my mind, it was a poor result. Another had temporary improvement, while the final one's condition worsened. The difficulty in this group is that even in expert hands it is challenging to ascertain which patient will benefit from the operation. Currently, I consider locking postures a contraindication to proceed with surgery. Work-related injuries also seem to be a heads-up against operating. In any case, a psychological study[54] is needed as most of the dystonic-CRPS patients have depression and perhaps psychiatric consultation will be beneficial. Further studies are needed before we can advise on how to proceed in the dystonic-CRPS patient population. By the same token, what seems evident is that early identification of a true dystonic patient is paramount in order to eliminate the drain of medical resources and medicalization. These patients need psychiatric treatment, rather than being imprisoned in a Pain Clinic. In the current series, 12 dystonic patients were erroneously diagnosed as having CRPS.

25.3.4 Misdiagnosis–Bad Doctoring

Unfortunately, the symptoms and signs of CRPS are so unspecific and elusive that anything may be included. This could lead to lazy medicine and lax studying of patients with pain, or even worse, provide a shelter for bad practice. The patient is defenseless in such an outrage, as we, doctors, are supposed to be the experts. This series confirms the statement in Thimineur and Saberski's seminal paper: a clinical picture resembling CRPS should be the beginning of a proper study of any patient, not the sentencing of the patient to a Pain Clinic. Most patients in this category had been referred to the Pain Clinic or given the diagnosis of CRPS without ANY search into the root cause of their problem. This is a very unfortunate conclusion of this study, and very painful to put it in writing, but in our Hippocratic Oath we pledge to defend our patients not our colleagues. This review stresses that we need to study in depth the patient with unexplained pain.

In this series, 71 patients from one perspective or another fit in this heading. I include here four patients who probably had a flare reaction, and by the time of the visit had no pain and full range of motion. One patient denied having had any pain at any time, yet admitted to having felt some stiffness! This diagnosis had created anxiety and needed treatment with anxiolytics to control sleep deprivation in all four. Reassurance in the first visit with me relieved them from the heavy weight of an unnecessary label. One of them had his hardware removed without any incidence. Erring on the side of benevolence, at least 24 of the 166 were flagrant cases of malpractice (▶ Fig. 25.2).

25.3.5 Irritative Carpal Tunnel Syndrome (ICTS)

There was a remaining group of patients who had all the symptoms and signs of CRPS but that had nothing of the above. We have been working through the years on what I have termed "irritative carpal tunnel syndrome." The syndrome is a variant of the classic carpal tunnel syndrome (CTS) and responds well to carpal tunnel release (CTR). The chief complaints are pain and dysesthesias in the hand (not necessarily in the median nerve

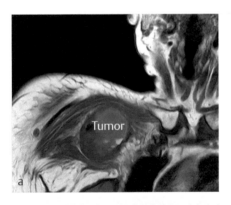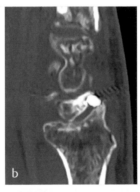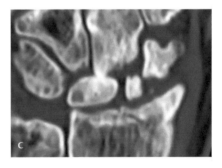

Fig. 25.2 Bad doctoring and malpractice labeled as complex regional pain syndrome (CRPS). (a) This lady had attended for 8 months the Pain Clinic diagnosed with CRPS. This was triggered by "overloading the right upper limb after a contralateral wrist fracture" (sic). The patient had a history of breast cancer operated 20 years before. Her surgeon failed to consider the possibility of the patient's pain coming from a local invasion of the brachial plexus as seen in the magnetic resonance imaging (MRI) of her first consultation with me. (b,c) Despite a computed tomography (CT) scan attesting to a prominent screw, destruction of the midcarpal joint, and persistent nonunion, the surgeon sent this patient to the Pain Clinic for "dystrophic changes and CRPS." The diagnosis was reinforced by a positive three-phase bone-scan.

distribution), worsening of the symptoms at night, and, frequently, inability to make a full fist. These features differed little from the ones presented by CRPS patients. I hypothesized that CRPS and irritative carpal tunnel syndrome (ICTS) were different intensities of the same condition as, in essence, the clinical picture was similar. The results of a subgroup of patients—those who could not make a full fist—have been presented in a recent publication.[57,58] Basically, if the surgeon is able to exclude other possible explanatory causes of pain, the outcome of CTR is outstanding. We have demonstrated that performing CTR procured lasting pain relief in 47/53 patients, who were categorized as CRPS and had been struggling with incapacitating pain for an average of 16 months. Disappointing results were obtained in borderline indications (dystonic-CRPS) and where there were ulterior motives, such as litigation or benefits. Needless to say, ill-advised CTR will make things worse.

25.4 Discussion

During the past few years that I have been on this crusade to wipe CRPS from our armamentarium, and eventually from the literature, I have received insults and bad press from patients and doctors alike. The patient understands that I refute they have a real pain or limitation, when the message is that we should be looking for their real problem in order to address it at its root, rather than treating the symptom, i.e., their pain. Included in the CRPS are true conditions, that respond to treatment, but also psychiatric conditions, malingerers, and patients who, one way or another, seek to benefit.[53,54,59] The resistance by some doctors may be due to the reluctance we all have to change, and out of respect for our teachers.

CRPS as an entity does not withstand a critical analysis. The evidence is weak even of its own existence, and in many cases the symptoms and signs may be the result of *simply disuse*.[60] In this study all patients were extracted from the CRPS bag, allocated into real conditions, and of those treated, most were weaned off neuropathic drugs. The classic principle of avoiding surgery in the CRPS scenario, or only operating exceptionally following the identification of a neurophysiologically proved nociceptive focus, which in turn has to have responded preoperatively to a sympatholytic block,[3,5,6,12,20,27,29,42,43,60,61,62] is unsubstantiated. On the contrary, our results prove that a significant number of patients benefit from properly formulated surgery.

25.5 Take-Home Message

In summary, the frivolity with which juniors and seniors alike give this diagnosis that has catastrophic consequences on the patient's well-being is appalling. This work points directly to us, surgeons, as the forerunners of this condition. Erasing the option of CRPS from our arma-

mentarium would oblige us to undertake an in-depth study of any patient with pain. Fortunately, an optimistic conclusion that can be drawn from this study: once the cases of misdiagnosis, dystonic-psychogenic hand, positive nerve damage, and occult nerve compressions are withdrawn from the "CRPS bag," there will be NO case left behind to be labeled as CRPS. CRPS is not needed in medicine.

References

[1] Veldman PH, Reynen HM, Arntz IE, Goris RJ. Signs and symptoms of reflex sympathetic dystrophy: prospective study of 829 patients. Lancet. 1993; 342(8878):1012–1016

[2] Marinus J, Moseley GL, Birklein F, et al. Clinical features and pathophysiology of complex regional pain syndrome. Lancet Neurol. 2011; 10(7):637–648

[3] Patterson RW, Li Z, Smith BP, Smith TL, Koman LA. Complex regional pain syndrome of the upper extremity. J Hand Surg Am. 2011; 36 (9):1553–1562

[4] Żyluk A, Puchalski P. Complex regional pain syndrome: observations on diagnosis, treatment and definition of a new subgroup. J Hand Surg Eur Vol. 2013; 38(6):599–606

[5] Bruehl S. Complex regional pain syndrome. BMJ. 2015; 351:h2730

[6] Birklein F, O'Neill D, Schlereth T. Complex regional pain syndrome: an optimistic perspective. Neurology. 2015; 84(1):89–96

[7] Schott GD. Interrupting the sympathetic outflow in causalgia and reflex sympathetic dystrophy. BMJ. 1998; 316(7134):792–793

[8] Straube S, Derry S, Moore RA, Cole P. Cervico-thoracic or lumbar sympathectomy for neuropathic pain and complex regional pain syndrome. Cochrane Database Syst Rev. 2013; 2013(9):CD002918

[9] Stanton-Hicks M, Jänig W, Hassenbusch S, Haddox JD, Boas R, Wilson P. Reflex sympathetic dystrophy: changing concepts and taxonomy. Pain. 1995; 63(1):127–133

[10] Del Piñal F. Editorial. I have a dream … reflex sympathetic dystrophy (RSD or Complex Regional Pain Syndrome—CRPS I) does not exist. J Hand Surg Eur Vol. 2013; 38(6):595–597

[11] del Piñal F. Reflex sympathetic dystrophy (RSD)/CRPS/Sudeck does not exist. IFSSH Ezine. 2019; 9(3):22–31

[12] Jupiter JB, Seiler JG, III, Zienowicz R. Sympathetic maintained pain (causalgia) associated with a demonstrable peripheral-nerve lesion: operative treatment. J Bone Joint Surg Am. 1994; 76(9):1376–1384

[13] Thimineur MA, Saberski L. Complex regional pain syndrome type I (RSD) or peripheral mononeuropathy? A discussion of three cases. Clin J Pain. 1996; 12(2):145–150

[14] Ochoa JL. Truths, errors, and lies around "reflex sympathetic dystrophy" and "complex regional pain syndrome". J Neurol. 1999; 246 (10):875–879

[15] Stutts JT, Kasdan ML, Hickey SE, Bruner A. Reflex sympathetic dystrophy: misdiagnosis in patients with dysfunctional postures of the upper extremity. J Hand Surg Am. 2000; 25(6):1152–1156

[16] Barth RJ, Haralson R. Differential diagnosis for complex regional pain syndrome. Am Med Assoc Guides Newsltt. September/October 2007; 12:1–4, 12–16

[17] Dellon AL, Andonian E, Rosson GD. CRPS of the upper or lower extremity: surgical treatment outcomes. J Brachial Plex Peripher Nerve Inj. 2009; 4:1

[18] Ring D, Barth R, Barsky A. Evidence-based medicine: disproportionate pain and disability. J Hand Surg Am. 2010; 35(8):1345–1347

[19] Birklein F, Dimova V. Complex regional pain syndrome-up-to-date. Pain Rep. 2017; 2(6):e624

[20] Goebel A, Barker CH, Turner-Stokes L, and the Membership of the Guideline Development Panel for 2018. Complex regional pain syndrome in adults: UK guidelines for diagnosis, referral and management in primary and secondary care. London: Royal College of Physicians; 2018

[21] Harden NR, Bruehl S, Perez RSGM, et al. Validation of proposed diagnostic criteria (the "Budapest Criteria") for complex regional pain syndrome. Pain. 2010; 150(2):268–274

[22] Harden N, Bruehl S. How to diagnose CRPS by utilizing the Budapest criteria. https://www.youtube.com/watch?time_continue=714&v=7-GI7cRL5lmw&feature=emb_title

[23] Basler MH, Rae CP, Stewart G. Diagnosis of complex regional pain syndrome needs to be tightened. BMJ. 2014; 348:g4029

[24] Bass C. Complex regional pain syndrome medicalises limb pain. BMJ. 2014; 348:g2631

[25] Bickerstaff DR, Kanis JA. Algodystrophy: an under-recognized complication of minor trauma. Br J Rheumatol. 1994; 33(3):240–248

[26] Field J, Warwick D, Bannister GC. Features of algodystrophy ten years after Colles' fracture. J Hand Surg [Br]. 1992; 17(3):318–320

[27] Merritt WH. Reflex sympathetic dystrophy/complex regional pain syndrome. In: Mathes SJ, Hentz RV, eds. Plastic surgery. Philadelphia: Saunders Pub Co.; 2006:823–874, Chap. 195

[28] Żyluk A, Mosiejczuk H. A comparison of the accuracy of two sets of diagnostic criteria in the early detection of complex regional pain syndrome following surgical treatment of distal radial fractures. J Hand Surg Eur Vol. 2013; 38(6):609–615

[29] Koman AL, Smith BP, Smith TL. A practical guide for complex regional pain syndrome in the acute stage and late stage. In: Wolfe SW, Hotchkiss RN, Pederson WC, et al., eds. Green's operative hand surgery. 7th ed. Philadelphia: Churchill Livingstone; 2017:1797–1827

[30] Zyluk A. The natural history of post-traumatic reflex sympathetic dystrophy. J Hand Surg [Br]. 1998; 23(1):20–23

[31] Schwartzman RJ, Erwin KL, Alexander GM. The natural history of complex regional pain syndrome. Clin J Pain. 2009; 25(4):273–280

[32] de Mos M, Huygen FJ, van der Hoeven-Borgman M, Dieleman JP, Ch Stricker BH, Sturkenboom MC. Outcome of the complex regional pain syndrome. Clin J Pain. 2009; 25(7):590–597

[33] Stein AH, Jr. The relation of median nerve compression to Sudeck's syndrome. Surg Gynecol Obstet. 1962; 115:713–720

[34] Birch R, St Clair Strange FG. A new type of peripheral nerve lesion. J Bone Joint Surg Br. 1990; 72(2):312–313

[35] Placzek JD, Boyer MI, Gelberman RH, Sopp B, Goldfarb CA. Nerve decompression for complex regional pain syndrome type II following upper extremity surgery. J Hand Surg Am. 2005; 30(1):69–74

[36] Camp SJ, Milani R, Sinisi M. Intractable neurostenalgia of the ulnar nerve abolished by neurolysis 18 years after injury. J Hand Surg Eur Vol. 2008; 33(1):45–46

[37] Dellon AL. Surgical treatment of upper extremity pain. Hand Clin. 2016; 32(1):71–80

[38] Bruehl S, Chung OY. How common is complex regional pain syndrome-Type I? Pain. 2007; 129(1–2):1–2

[39] Gupta A, Silman AJ, Ray D, et al. The role of psychosocial factors in predicting the onset of chronic widespread pain: results from a prospective population-based study. Rheumatology (Oxford). 2007; 46 (4):666–671

[40] Hayes PJ, Louis DS, Kasdan ML. Additional considerations in complex regional pain syndrome. J Hand Surg Am. 2012; 37(3):625–, author reply 625–626

[41] Noordenbos W, Wall PD. Implications of the failure of nerve resection and graft to cure chronic pain produced by nerve lesions. J Neurol Neurosurg Psychiatry. 1981; 44(12):1068–1073

[42] Jobe MT, Martinez SF. Peripheral nerve injuries. In: Azar FM, Beaty JH, Canale ST, eds. Campbell's operative orthopaedics. 13th ed. Philadelphia: Elsevier; 2017:3162–3224, Chap. 62

[43] Lankford LL. Reflex sympathetic dystrophy. In: Green DP, ed. Operative hand surgery. 2nd ed. New York: Churchill Livingstone; 1988:633–663

[44] O'Connell NE, Wand BM, McAuley J, Marston L, Moseley GL. Interventions for treating pain and disability in adults with complex regional pain syndrome. Cochrane Database Syst Rev. 2013; 4(4):CD009416

[45] Zhu SX, Lu SB, Yao JX, et al. Intrafascicular decompression in the treatment of causalgia with special reference to the mechanism. Ann Plast Surg. 1985; 15(6):460–464

[46] Jones NF, Ahn HC, Eo S. Revision surgery for persistent and recurrent carpal tunnel syndrome and for failed carpal tunnel release. Plast Reconstr Surg. 2012; 129(3):683–692

[47] Adani R, Tos P, Tarallo L, Corain M. Treatment of painful median nerve neuromas with radial and ulnar artery perforator adipofascial flaps. J Hand Surg Am. 2014; 39(4):721–727

[48] Simpson CK, Butt AM, Power D. Neurostenalgia as a cause of pain after tendon and nerve repair at the wrist. J Hand Surg Eur Vol. 2013; 38(6):687–688

[49] Bhatia KP, Bhatt MH, Marsden CD. The causalgia-dystonia syndrome. Brain. 1993; 116(Pt 4):843–851

[50] van Hilten BJ, van de Beek WJ, Hoff JI, Voormolen JH, Delhaas EM. Intrathecal baclofen for the treatment of dystonia in patients with reflex sympathetic dystrophy. N Engl J Med. 2000; 343(9):625–630

[51] Raja SN. Motor dysfunction in CRPS and its treatment. Pain. 2009; 143(1–2):3–4

[52] Verdugo RJ, Ochoa JL. Abnormal movements in complex regional pain syndrome: assessment of their nature. Muscle Nerve. 2000; 23 (2):198–205

[53] Hawley JS, Weiner WJ. Psychogenic dystonia and peripheral trauma. Neurology. 2011; 77(5):496–502

[54] Schrag A, Trimble M, Quinn N, Bhatia K. The syndrome of fixed dystonia: an evaluation of 103 patients. Brain. 2004; 127(Pt 10):2360–2372

[55] Louis DS. Recognizable dysfunction syndromes. Hand Clin. 1993; 9 (2):213–220

[56] Kasdan ML, Stutts JT. Factitious injuries of the upper extremity. J Hand Surg Am. 1995; 20(3 Pt 2):S57–S60

[57] del Piñal F. CRPS does not exist. Keynote lecture. 74th Annual Meeting of the American Society for Surgery of the Hand. Las Vegas. Sept 5–7, 2019

[58] del Piñal F. Irritative carpal tunnel: a new syndrome helping to solve the CRPS/reflex sympathetic dystrophy/Sudeck enigma. Plast Reconstr Surg. (Submitted)

[59] Ochoa JL, Verdugo R. Focal dystonia associated with pain. Brain. 2005; 128(Pt 4):E24

[60] Singh HP, Davis TR. The effect of short-term dependency and immobility on skin temperature and colour in the hand. J Hand Surg [Br]. 2006; 31(6):611–615

[61] Hobelmann CF, Jr, Dellon AL. Use of prolonged sympathetic blockade as an adjunct to surgery in the patient with sympathetic maintained pain. Microsurgery. 1989; 10(2):151–153

[62] Veldman PH, Goris RJ. Surgery on extremities with reflex sympathetic dystrophy. Unfallchirurg. 1995; 98(1):45–48

8

Section 9

Social Issues

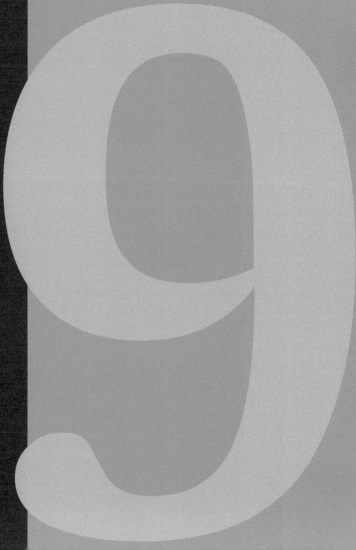

26 Managing Expectations/Factitious Disorders

Randy Bindra and Luke McCarron

Abstract

As a surgeon, it is not always easy to gauge if an operative procedure has been completely understood by the patient—this can lead to a gap in patient expectations. Patients are primarily concerned about getting better and often their considerations of the final aesthetic and functional outcome are not adequately voiced or discussed preoperatively. After surgery, this can lead to disappointment for the patient, even though the surgeon considers the surgery successful. Understanding the patients' needs and setting the expectations are critical to procedure selection and the consent process. Unmet or unrealistic expectations lead to dissent and can progress to litigation even after a seemingly minor complication. Involvement of a hand therapist in the process is advantageous.

The second part of the chapter deals with factitious disorders (FD) of the hand. These patients feign illness or willingly create a physical disorder for the sole purpose of assuming the sick role. These patients can be quite devious, can mimic classic physical signs, and will dispute laboratory and other tests and readily seek surgery. The patients are unnaturally difficult in the postoperative period as they seek to prolong their affliction. It is critical to identify these patients and avoid operating on them wherever possible. The management of these patients is multidisciplinary with larger role played by a clinical psychologist or psychiatrist in more severe cases with underlying psychiatric disorder.

Keywords: expectations, disappointment, outcome, factitious disorders, Munchausen, Secretan's disease, nonhealing ulcer

26.1 How to Set the Right Patient Expectations before Surgery

Over the past two decades "consumer experience" has emerged as a major contributor to patient perception on their care following surgery.[1] Clinicians have a dual responsibility of providing a high standard of clinical care, while also meeting the individual expectations of each patient.

Surgery to the hand is a team approach that involves the surgeon, the therapy team, and the patient. Greater post-surgery satisfaction is obtained when recovery expectations and roles of the care team are clearly defined, and then carried out to the preagreed standard.[2] Therefore, a detailed understanding of the patient's individual expectations for surgery can be more predictive of patient satisfaction than the surgeon's perceived level of success.

While not essential for every case, in complex hand deformities and in patients with comorbidities, close communication of the team including the surgeon, hand therapist, and physician and psychologist is often necessary. As part of the consent process, there should be ample opportunity to freely ask questions, identify any barriers to recovery, and identify solutions to mitigate these concerns. Strategies for managing daily activities while immobilized after surgery, such as driving, eating, and showering, must be in place prior to surgery, especially for the person living alone. ▶ Table 26.1 provides a list of potential presurgery discussion topics for the surgeon and patient. These include, though should not be limited to, conservative treatment options, timeframes for recovery following surgery, rehabilitation stages and expectations, financial costs and time burden to the patient, expected return to work or other gainful employment, and potential complications from surgery.

26.2 Importance of Patient Expectations with Relationship to Outcome and Unhappiness/Litigation

Patients present to a surgeon primarily for problems with pain, loss of function, or correction of deformity—patients are often reluctant to discuss the fact that they are also concerned by the appearance of the hand or finger and their ability to resume their hobbies. The primary problem, for example, pain, remains the focus of discussion and treatment, and issues like surgical scars, persistence of bony enlargement, and loss of motion are not adequately discussed. In a study of patients seeking litigation after maxillofacial surgery, medical errors were the least common cause of the discontent. The majority of complaints related to poor explanation of the proposed procedure or unrealistically high patient expectations.[3]

A lot of importance is paid to likely complications of surgery, but it is equally important that the preoperative discussion should include and must document: surgical scars, patient verbalization that they understand the procedure, pain management, and postoperative rehabilitation and recovery time. When treating patients with fractures and injuries, while keeping an optimistic attitude, the surgeon must be realistic about the scarring, number of operations that may be needed, expected motion, and if they would be able to return to their preoperative level of activity.

26.3 Role of the Therapist in Preoperative Counseling

Patient communication is the extent to which important information is delivered from health professional to

Table 26.1 Surgeon and patient presurgery discussion topics

- What are the conservative treatment options for the injury or condition in question?
- Do you live alone, or with another, who could assist you following surgery?
- Who are the members of your therapy team, and what roles do they play?
- How will you manage your transportation needs following surgery, including attending all medical and therapy appointments?
- Who will assist you with your activities of daily living, such as preparing meals, showering, and self-care activities?
- What are the financial costs of this procedure, including postsurgery therapy costs and time away from work?
- What is the likely timeframe for recovery, in weeks, months, or years?
- What does the phrase "complete recovery" mean to you?
- What are the rehabilitation requirements expected for the patient following surgery: how many therapy sessions over how many weeks?
- When is a return to work or other gainful employment likely to occur, in weeks, months, or years?
- What are the potential complications for surgery, and how can these be mitigated?

patient, and vice versa.[4,5] In addition, the time spent with the therapist will far exceed the time spent with the surgeon, enabling more opportunity to explore rehabilitation elements using depth and detail, with time for patients to think of and ask probing questions. The therapists' answers must be accurate, while also taking into consideration their individual role within the treatment team, and future interaction with the surgeon and other team members. The therapist is often asked to clarify surgical or rehabilitation information provided by the surgeon or other treatment team member by the patient. This is an opportunity for the therapist to demonstrate their injury, surgery, or anatomy knowledge, while reinforcing the treatment plan laid out by the surgeon. Pictorial, written, and verbal information should be utilized to ensure the patient better understands what was previously unclear. Rehabilitation goals should be discussed clearly using days or weeks as milestones for recovery.

As cost-effective patient care continues to integrate a multidisciplinary team approach, regular and meaningful surgeon-patient and therapist-patient communication interaction opportunities will increase.[6]

The surgeon-patient communication relationship is usually limited by time and occurs semiregularly, with increasing duration common between appointments. The surgeon possesses the injury knowledge and surgical information required to guide patient recovery and make patient-centered and injury-specific rehabilitation decisions. The information provided by the surgeon must be comprehended by the patient in a relatively short time, with some patients feeling unable to question or ask the surgeon for clarification during their scheduled review appointments. This can leave the patient feeling unsatisfied with their level of care, potentially causing conflict later in recovery. Answering patient questions is a core therapist skill, which can reassure and calm an anxious patient. Anecdotally, some patients have reported feeling more comfortable asking questions to their therapist, rather than the treating surgeon. The therapist-patient interaction occurs more regularly and is not usually limited by the same time restriction as the surgeon. The therapist can discuss the injury, rehabilitation plan, some general aspects of the surgery, using the time and detail required to ensure patient comprehension is achieved.

26.4 Factitious Disorders: Definition and Classification

Surgeons are accustomed to seeing patients for a defined problem and generally expect an "organic" disorder—where the condition has a known pathology, is supported by imaging and other investigations, and generally responds well to appropriate medical or surgical intervention. However, every surgeon will occasionally encounter a patient with a "nonorganic" disorder, with symptoms or signs that cannot be explained or supported by investigations, with emotional response of the patient varying from a lack of distress or extreme exaggeration.

Nonorganic disorders often relate to an underlying psychological disorder such as depression, personality disorder, or may have a psychiatric problem such as schizophrenia. The various types of nonorganic disorders include somatization disorder, where the patient focuses on a physical illness; conversion disorder, presenting as unexplainable paralysis or weakness; pain disorder simulating fibromyalgia or hypochondriasis, with phobia that a lump is cancerous.

Factitious disorders (FD) are a specific subset of nonorganic disorders where the patient feigns a physical illness or willingly creates a physical problem for the purpose of assuming the sick role and seeking medical attention. Unlike conversion disorder or hypochondriasis where the condition is not voluntarily produced, patients with FD knowingly feign symptoms, may actively create physical problems, such as wounds or swelling to deceive the medical team. Patients with FD are generally not seeking financial gain, merely seeking sympathy or attention from being unwell, and will often readily undergo a surgical procedure. They are not aware of any self-motivating factors and lack insight into their condition. This contrasts with a malingerer who will willingly exaggerate symptoms or signs following an injury to seek compensation for financial or nonfinancial gain such as access to drugs, delay return to work, or to avoid criminal prosecution.

9

Factitious disorders are included in the 2020 ICD-10-CM with diagnosis Code F68.10 as "Factitious disorder imposed on self, unspecified." The *Diagnostic and Statistical Manual of Mental Disorders*, Fifth Edition (DSM-5) classifies factitious disorders into factitious disorder imposed on self and factitious disorder imposed on another, in order to replace Munchausen's syndrome and Munchausen by proxy, respectively.[7]

The diagnosis of FD is by exclusion after every possible organic cause for the presenting symptoms is ruled out. For example, a patient with hand paresthesias with a nonanatomical pattern and inconsistent signs on clinical examination will need repeated clinical assessment, neurophysiological testing, magnetic resonance imaging (MRI), and possibly even a neurologist work-up. Cost of additional investigations, multiple specialist consultations, and hospital visits can amount to high costs in excess of 50,000 US dollars.[8] Although every patient is unique and requires individualized treatment, the following discussion includes the four types of FD presentations to the hand clinic.

26.4.1 Self-Mutilation

Self-mutilators create physical signs by covertly injuring themselves with blunt trauma or by injecting various substances under the skin, varying from air, liquids or physical objects such as needles. The term "Munchausen syndrome" applies to a patient with additional features of peregrination (wandering from hospital to hospital) and pseudologia fantastica (exaggerated irrelevant stories of self-importance).[9] Patients with Munchausen syndrome are twice as likely to be male and generally have more severe disease and worse prognosis. A variation of this disorder is Munchausen by proxy, where the illness is created in a dependent such as a child, with repeated hospital presentations requesting surgical intervention on the child for minimal symptoms.

A common type of presentation to the hand clinic is a nonhealing ulcer created by the patient (▶ Fig. 26.1). The patients typically have a lack of concern about the problem that often has been going on for several months and after treatment at multiple hospitals. Clinical examination, cultures, and biopsy are necessary to exclude a malignant ulcer before making the diagnosis. An X-ray may reveal inexplicable foreign bodies lodged in the deeper tissues inserted through the ulcer. These patients will typically manipulate the wound to prevent it from healing and will resist casting or other occlusive dressing that will preclude wound interference.

In contrast, "passive mutilators" seek out a surgeon who will create a wound for them. These patients are often highly intelligent and research medical conditions they can exploit. They are very manipulative and will begin their visit with the positivity that they have selected the surgeon due to local reputation and exper-

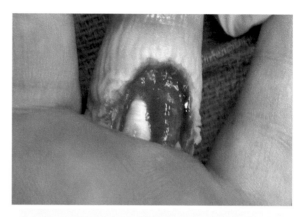
Fig. 26.1 Nonhealing base of finger ulcer created by the patient.

tise and convince the surgeon that they are good candidates for surgery. If the investigations do not corroborate their fabricated physical signs, they will dispute the results and insist on alternative testing centers or other less accurate options that might be supportive. After the procedure, these patients generally become very disruptive, noncompliant, and will prolong their hospitalization and delay recovery. They will occasionally turn against the treating team and blame the surgeon for doing an operation that has made them worse. After a breakdown in the doctor-patient relationship, they will generally move on to another surgeon in a different region and resist any attempts by the new team to secure previous medical records. This sad, hostile, anxious, frustrating, and tenacious behavior has been referred to by the acronym, SHAFT syndrome.[10]

26.4.2 Factitious Edema

Swelling in the soft tissues of the hand can be caused by constriction from tight dressings, splints, elastic bands, or tourniquets; injection of air or fluid under the skin; or by repetitive blunt trauma.[11] The level of constriction is usually concealed and the patient seems unaware of the causation; they simply seek care to resolve the swelling and will generally seek surgery (▶ Fig. 26.2). Clinical examination in most cases reveals a clear cut-off mark where the edema ends and the ligature is likely applied. Admission to hospital for observation results in temporary improvement of the swelling as the patient can no longer worsen the problem.

Hand edema from repetitive trauma creates a firmer, more localized area of swelling and was first described by Secretan[12] in 1901. In the original series, 11 patients with work compensation presented with persistent hard edema on the dorsum of the hand following a traumatic episode. He noted that the swelling did not resolve after the usual period of immobilization. Subsequent authors have pointed out that the condition is an FD and is caused

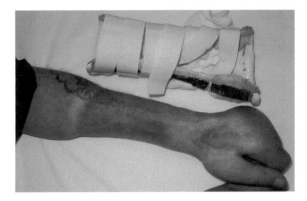

Fig. 26.2 Edema of the hand caused by constriction using the splint in picture.

by repeated self-inflicted contusions to the dorsum of the hand.

MR scans show evidence of diffuse fibrosis around the extensor tendons extending to the interosseous muscles. Surgery when undertaken inadvertently will reveal peritendinous fibrosis. Histological examination reveals evidence of acute changes of hemorrhage on a background of chronic fibrosis with hemosiderin deposition, a sign of repetitive trauma to the area.

26.4.3 Dystonic Posturing

Patients with FD will occasionally develop and maintain unusual hand or wrist posture after a seemingly trivial injury, infection, or another inciting episode (▶ Fig. 26.3). The posturing may be fixed or dystonic. In the latter condition, hand movements are slow, deliberate, and unnatural, and vary with different clinical visits. In the more severe static deformity or clenched fist syndrome, the ulnar two or three digits are held tightly clenched in the fist. The patient is apparently unable to straighten the fingers and passive extension is resisted with demonstrable contraction in the long flexors—the condition has been referred to as the psychoflexed hand or clenched fist syndrome.[13] In severe cases, the skin in the palm is macerated and the fingers may develop fixed contractures. The posturing and flexion is easily correctable under regional anesthesia but recurs immediately when the patient regains volitional control. The posturing can improve with splinting but recurs if the underlying psychological disorder is not addressed.

26.4.4 Diagnosis of FD

A patient with FD is not usually detected at the outset as they often present with a known clinical problem such as a wound, swelling, hand pain, or numbness. The diagnosis is sometimes made too late after the surgeon has been led down the path of surgery and the patient has developed postoperative complications and has turned hostile.

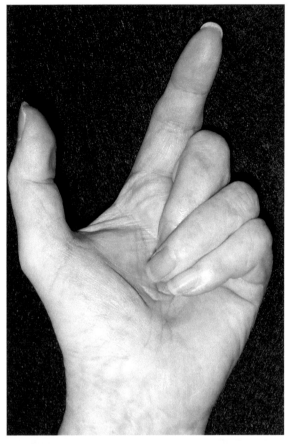

Fig. 26.3 Dystonic hand posture following incidental trauma.

The differential diagnosis varies with the different manifestations of FD and includes CRPS, malignant ulcer, Dupuytren's contracture, lymphedema, and subclavian vein thrombosis. In general, the following warning signs listed in ▶ Table 26.2 should alert a surgeon to the possibility of a patient with FD.

26.4.5 Management of FD

Once FD is suspected, the surgeon must avoid surgery as far as possible. Management is multidisciplinary and in collaboration with a psychologist or psychiatrist and hand therapist. The patient must be explained that the treating team is aware of the factitious nature of the problem in a nonconfrontational manner. Once the patient is accepting and prepared to commence psychologic counseling, any essential surgery such as debridement of nonhealing ulcers and removal of foreign bodies can be performed.

A close therapist-surgeon communication is vital when managing patient recovery, especially when the patient has been identified as "difficult." Valid patient outcome measures should be selected and implemented as appropriate to track patient progression. A written progress report from the therapist or joint appointment of the

Table 26.2 The warning signs of FD

- Dramatic and variable medical history
- Different clinical symptoms and signs on different visits
- Lack of concern over apparent loss of function
- Patient unusually aware of medical terminology and diagnostic signs and tests
- Presence of multiple surgical scars from different surgeons
- Patient disputes test results that do not support the diagnosis
- Change in posture of hand or ability to use the hand when patient is not aware they are being observed
- Seek surgical solution for seemingly minor problems
- Unusually willing to undergo invasive tests or surgery
- Resist access to test results, medical records, or surgical notes from previous treating institution
- Resist casting or other forms of immobilization that will preclude wound interference
- Angry or hostile behavior if surgery is denied
- Oppose psychological or psychiatric evaluation

Abbreviation: FD, factitious disorder.

patient with the therapist and surgeon will ensure that no miscommunication occurs, especially in patients with FD.

26.5 Take-Home Message

When seeing a patient with an inconsistent injury history, ambiguous physical signs, and unrealistic expectations, it is important to proceed with caution. Surgery should not be offered as a first option in most cases and should certainly be delayed for difficult patients, as it is important to identify potential factitious disorders. Repeat clinic visits to look for inconsistencies in signs and symptoms, review of medical records from previous treating practitioners, consultation with other members of the treatment team, and sometimes a second opinion from a senior colleague will help a surgeon avoid from falling victim to a manipulative patient.

References

[1] Johnson PJ. Understanding and improving patient satisfaction in orthopaedic surgical procedures: a review. Univ N M Orthop Res J. 2019; 8(1):19

[2] Swarup I, Henn CM, Gulotta LV, Henn RF, III. Patient expectations and satisfaction in orthopaedic surgery: a review of the literature. J Clin Orthop Trauma. 2019; 10(4):755–760

[3] Krause HR, Bremerich A, Rustemeyer J. Reasons for patients' discontent and litigation. J Craniomaxillofac Surg. 2001; 29(3):181–183

[4] Ha JF, Longnecker N. Doctor-patient communication: a review. Ochsner J. 2010; 10(1):38–43

[5] Stewart MA. Effective physician-patient communication and health outcomes: a review. CMAJ. 1995; 152(9):1423–1433

[6] Longstaffe R, Slade Shantz J, Leiter J, Peeler J. Surgeon–therapist communication: do all members see eye-to-eye? Phys Sportsmed. 2015; 43(4):381–387

[7] Edition F. Diagnostic and statistical manual of mental disorders. American Psychiatric Association; 2013

[8] Grunert BK, Sanger JR, Matloub HS, Yousif NJ. Classification system for factitious syndromes in the hand with implications for treatment. J Hand Surg Am. 1991; 16(6):1027–1030

[9] Folks DG, Freeman AM, III. Münchausen's syndrome and other factitious illness. Psychiatr Clin North Am. 1985; 8(2):263–278

[10] Wallace PF, Fitzmorris CS, Jr. The S-H-A-F-T syndrome in the upper extremity. J Hand Surg Am. 1978; 3(5):492–494

[11] Smith RJ. Factitious lymphedema of the hand. J Bone Joint Surg Am. 1975; 57(1):89–94

[12] Secretan H. Hard edema and traumatic hyperplasia of the dorsum of the metacarpus. Rev Med Suisse Romande. 1901; 21:409

[13] Frykman GK, Wood VE, Miller EB. The psycho-flexed hand. Clin Orthop Relat Res. 1983(174):153–157

9

27 Informed Consent/How to Prevent Medicolegal Issues

Ridzwan Namazie and Randipsingh Bindra

Abstract

Informed consent is a process by which a patient makes a voluntary decision on treatment based on the information provided by the treating physician. This should include details of the diagnosis, treatment options available, alternatives, risks, and benefits. In some situations, financial consent must be included.

Consent is a process that gives the patient time to digest the information, ask questions, make their independent inquiry, and come to a decision. Patient education sessions, written handouts, and links to resources are all vital tools but are not, in isolation, enough to constitute informed consent. A signed form merely indicates that a discussion has taken place but this may be insufficient to medicolegally qualify as fully informed consent. Detailed records of the discussion in the medical records are equally important.

Every country has their own health delivery system and cultural beliefs—consequently there are varying legal requirements and professional obligations with regard to treating a patient. However, while practitioners are universally familiar with their moral obligation to deliver the best care to the patient and to do no harm, it is their legal responsibility to ensure that the patient is made fully aware of the problem, the treatment offered, and be a part of the decision-making process.

Medicolegal issues arise when there is a breakdown of communication. Avoiding medicolegal issues begins with properly informed consent. Detailed documentation, developing a good rapport with the patient, and being transparent are all vital to ensure that the doctor-patient relationship is maintained.

Keywords: informed consent, medicolegal issues, medical malpractice, doctor-patient relationship, treatment options

27.1 Informed Consent

27.1.1 Background

Treating a competent patient without their permission is a violation of a basic tenet in medicine and transgresses their constitutional rights. Even in Hippocratic times, great emphasis was placed on listening to the patient, careful and comprehensive evaluation, discussing treatment options, and the open disclosure of prognosis.[1] Subsequently, medieval Europe changed to a more active-passive model where patients were seen as helpless and the elite doctors knew what was best.[2] The paternalistic model evolved with improved patient access to knowl-edge and information leading to increasing levels of participation by the patient to a more patient-centric model that is practiced today.

The European Union has treaties and agreements that cover all EU Citizens. Article 5 of The European Convention of Human Rights and Biomedicine (ECHRB) which was signed in 1997 specifies that a doctor can only carry out medical procedures with the consent of the patient and that consent may be withdrawn.[3] Further strengthening this is the Charter of Fundamental Rights of the European Union which states that patients have a right to be informed. Article 3 establishes that a doctor can only act with the consent of the patient.[4]

The standards of what constitutes properly informed consent have undergone constant evolution; however, the principles are largely unchanged. Each country has different laws that dictate the extent of what is acceptable consent. In addition, patient factors, cultural beliefs, religious beliefs, personal beliefs, and moral attitudes will also determine whether the consent obtained is adequate.

The phrase "informed consent" was first credited to an American lawyer PG Gebhard in 1957. He introduced the term in an amicus brief filed on behalf of the American College of Surgeons in a 1957 case of Salgo vs Leland Stanford Jr University. The final judgment of that case outlined principles that form the foundation of informed consent.[5]

27.1.2 Elements of Informed Consent

Medical consent does not apply to surgery alone; even the act of taking a history and examining the patient requires consent, although the patient visiting the physician imparts an implied consent. Further medical treatment, medications, or procedures are to be undertaken with the patient's expressed consent. There are three key elements that need to be met as part of a valid informed consent.[5]

Capacity to Consent

The patient needs to understand the information provided, weigh potential consequences, and make a decision on whether to undergo treatment or otherwise. Other elements that affect capacity include information retention and the ability to communicate. The default position should always be that a person can consent unless proven otherwise.

If a patient is temporarily incapacitated following a head injury or is under the influence of drugs or alcohol, consent and treatment may be delayed to a later time unless in an emergency, in which case local guidelines

9

and laws will dictate how to proceed in the best interest of the patient. In general, the principle of preservation of life and limb should prevail.

Where patients have a permanent impairment, there generally will be an appointed legal guardian with a power of attorney or an agency that has been given authority to consent. In some countries, the decision of acting in the best interests of an incapacitated patient rests with the doctor. Diminished mental capacity or a psychiatric condition does not automatically exclude a patient from the ability to consent. If patient comprehension is in doubt, written advice should be sought from their usual physician or psychiatrist. In any case, it is always in everyone's best interest to include the patient as much as possible in the decision-making process.

There are some objective tools such as the MacArthur Competence Assessment Tool For Treatment (MacCAT-T) that have been developed to assess mental competence in giving consent. These tools, however, are not easy to administer and can be time consuming, taking up to 30 minutes to perform.

Consent Must Be Voluntary

The patient must decide to proceed with treatment without any coercion either from the physician, relatives, or a third party. It is difficult and, in some cases, impossible for the surgeon to know if the patient is completely free of external influences.

Just being in the hospital environment itself can be daunting and unfamiliar for many patients and can make patients feel pressurized into agreeing to treatment. Pressure from family on a patient to undergo treatment can be quite subtle. In most cases, family members feel that they have the patient's best interests at heart; however, it is always important for the doctor to first and foremost respect the patient's wishes especially when treating the elderly.

Surgeons treating a patient need to be aware of how advice is provided. An open dialogue between the surgeon and the patient which allows the patient to participate in the process is essential. Providing information in such a way that creates unnecessary urgency or in an unduly alarming manner could be viewed as coercion. The patient needs to be reassured that their consent is entirely voluntary and can be revoked, should they change their mind later.

The Patient Must Be Informed

The surgeon needs to be as comprehensive as possible in providing all the necessary information to the patient pertaining to their condition and treatment proposed using terminology that the patient understands. The patient should be informed of their diagnosis, differential diagnoses, and proposed investigations to confirm the diagnosis. The benefits of any intervention should be explained together with the adverse effects and risks. Specific mention should be made if the intervention is controversial or experimental. In a teaching institution, the person undertaking or supervising the intervention should be identified. Other possible treatment options and the option of not having any treatment should also be discussed together with the risks and benefits of each.

A surgeon is expected to tell a patient about the most common risks but not expected to list every conceivable complication following a surgery. In general terms, a known risk should be disclosed when an adverse outcome is a common event even though the detriment is slight, for example, skin tears after collagenase injection, or an outcome is severe even though its occurrence is rare, such as complex regional pain syndrome (CRPS) after carpal tunnel release. The discussion must include any outcomes that a reasonable person in the patient's position would consider significant and the surgeon should be aware what complications may be of particular significance to that patient. A key aspect of the consent conversation is to find out what is important to the patient in their vocation and hobbies and to inquire about anything the patient may be particularly worried about. For example, loss of flexion at the distal interphalangeal joint would have differing significance for a guitar player versus a manual laborer. Patients need to be aware of the potential for complications in any procedure. When quoting complication rates, practitioners need to be clear on whether the data they are presenting relies on their own experience or whether they are referencing the literature,[6] for example, when discussing loss of wrist motion after partial arthrodesis procedures.

The postoperative and rehabilitation protocols should be discussed, including details such as medications, restrictions on function, assistance needed at home, days in the hospital, casting requirements, splintage, and attendance at therapy sessions. Most patients would require an estimate of time off work, and if suitable, a staged return to work plan could be suggested. Further planned surgical intervention (e.g., removal of implants), prognosis, and expected outcomes should be discussed as well.

The use of patient information handouts, diagrams, charts, and educational models in explaining the treatment to patients is helpful. Directing the patient to reputable online resources (e.g., www.handcare.org) can help patients research common conditions with diagrammatic pictures of what to expect. Other techniques for patient explanation include drawings and cutouts on a rubber glove to explain flaps, and temporary fixation methods such as taping or splinting to simulate postoperative splinting or arthrodesis.[7]

It is necessary to declare any conflict of interest, especially when the surgeon is involved in product development or clinical research that involves a particular implant or device. Most countries now have frameworks to proactively deal with these conflicts and it usually forms part of the ethics approvals process. Off-label use or use of a product that has not been approved by the local licensing authority for that particular indication must also be clearly disclosed and documented in the consent form.

27.1.3 Consent in Children

Each country has a different definition of a child when it comes to informed consent. Age is usually but not always the deciding factor. If a person is classified as a minor or a child, generally they need a parent or guardian to give consent on their behalf. In some extenuating circumstances, consent need not be sought from parents, but this dispensation varies between countries. The child's age, maturity, and treatment sought are generally considered. Most countries have a pathway for a child to apply to a court to grant consent where parents have refused.[8]

The legal age for consent varies from country to country. The lowest age for medical treatment consent is in South Africa where a 12-year-old child may give independent consent for medical procedures and with parent's assent for surgery. The minimum legal age for consent in Europe varies from 14 in Latvia, 15 in Denmark, to 16 in the United Kingdom and the Netherlands. On the other hand, in Austria, Belgium, the Czech Republic, Estonia, Germany, Luxembourg, and Sweden, there is no fixed minimum age requirement for medical consent; instead, each situation is treated individually depending on the maturity of the child (▶ Table 27.1). In the United States, India, and Australia the legal age for consent is 18 years of age and parental consent is required with the assumption that the parent is acting in the best interest of the child.

Local laws and regulations often supersede the minimum age based on prior legal precedents. For example, the Gillick case established that the parental right to determine whether or not their minor child below the age of 16 will have medical treatment terminates if and when the child achieves sufficient understanding and intelligence to understand fully what is proposed. "Gillick competence" in determining a child's ability to consent has been adopted in the United Kingdom, Australia, New Zealand, and Canada.[9] In the United States, in some cases children over 14 can be considered capable of giving consent if they are living independently and demonstrate comprehension of the treatment choices offered.

27.1.4 Financial Consent

In countries where public health care is fully funded, patient copayment or out-of-pocket expenses are not an issue. However, when patients seek out private treatment or have to pay for their treatment, it is important that patients are fully informed of the cost of treatment—

implant costs, surgeon and hospital charges, as well as postoperative care including therapy visits—before the procedure is undertaken.[10] The estimate of costs should also advise on the likely additional expenditure for unforeseen circumstances or complications. Surgeons should disclose if they have a financial interest in the treating facility.

27.1.5 Exceptions to Informed Consent

Informed consent need not be obtained in some exceptional circumstances. The details vary between countries. It is generally accepted during emergency situations where the patient's life or limb is threatened, a limited discussion may take place to expedite treatment. If the patient is unconscious, a doctor can decide on the patient's behalf as stated in Article 8 of the ECHRB. If appropriate, a discussion should take place with the patient's next of kin; however, it should not be at the expense of delaying emergency treatment. If there is a clear advance directive that is legally valid, the doctor needs to respect it and there is provision for this in Article 9 of the ECHRB.

Rarely, the doctor may believe that a patient may be harmed by the consent process. A patient disagreeing with the doctor's advice or having opinions not widely supported by modern medicine does not qualify for an exception. There must be evidence that the patient may become so unsettled that they might take a course of action that is detrimental to themselves or others. Cases of therapeutic privilege can be difficult to navigate and a second opinion from another doctor or legal advice should be sought.

An abbreviated discussion may take place if the patient has prior knowledge of the risks involved. One trap to avoid though is to assume that a doctor or medical expert presenting as a patient is fully informed. In all cases, it would be appropriate to gauge the patient's comprehension and decide what depth of discussion should take place.

27.1.6 Refusing Consent for Treatment

Patients have the right to refuse consent for treatment even if it means they might suffer an adverse outcome. This is on the proviso that they have met the criteria of having capacity to give consent, are making the decision on their own volition, and the doctor has fully informed them of all possible outcomes.

In these cases, it is helpful to get a second opinion from a colleague and give the patient time to digest the information. Refusing one particular treatment does not mean that the patient refuses all treatment. The patient may still require other medical interventions such as splinting, closed reduction of a fracture, or medication for pain relief, and it is the doctor's responsibility to determine what level of treatment the patient will accept. The patient should be advised that they are free to change their mind at any time.

9

Table 27.1 Ages at which children can seek or consent to medical treatment without informing their parents

Country	Age at which children can consent to medical treatments, including diagnosis and surgery, without parental consent	Age at which children can seek medical advice without parental consent and without information passed to parents
Austria	Depends on maturity	Depends on maturity
Belgium	Depends on maturity	Depends on maturity
Bulgaria	18	16
Cyprus	18	Depends on maturity
Czech Republic	Depends on maturity	Depends on maturity
Germany	Depends on maturity	Depends on maturity
Denmark	15	15
Estonia	Depends on maturity	Depends on maturity
Greece	18	18
Spain	16	16
Finland	18	Depends on maturity
France	18	Depends on maturity
Croatia	16	Not regulated
Hungary	18	18
Ireland	16	16
Italy	18	Depends on maturity
Lithuania	16	16
Luxembourg	Depends on maturity	Depends on maturity
Latvia	14	Depends on maturity
Malta	18	18
Netherlands	16	16
Poland	16	18
Portugal	16	Depends on maturity
Romania	18	16
Sweden	Depends on maturity	Depends on maturity
Slovenia	15	15
Slovakia	18	18
United Kingdom (except Scotland)	16	16

Source: https://fra.europa.eu/en/publication/2017/mapping-minimum-age-requirements/consent-medical-treatments. Accessed June 8, 2020.

27.1.7 Documentation

The doctor needs to make notes in a contemporaneous fashion. It should be detailed and include all the information that was discussed as part of the consent process. Use of a checklist or template to ensure a thorough process is useful.

It is common practice for a consent form to be signed by the patient and the doctor. Ideally, the details discussed should be noted in the form. An alternative would be documentation in the patient's chart. However, it should be noted that a signed form without the details backing up what was discussed is insufficient to show as evidence that informed consent was obtained. The patient should be given ample time to consider the information provided and the signed consent may be deferred for a subsequent appointment in nonurgent procedures.

Procedure-specific consent forms detail common and significant complications for individual procedures and form a useful checklist, but not a substitute for a clinical discussion.[11]

27.2 How to Prevent Medicolegal Issues

Society in general is becoming increasingly litigious. In a survey conducted by the American Medical Association, 57% of surgeons reported experiencing a medical malpractice claim during the career.[7] Being sued can be a very stressful event for the physician and can occupy their time and resources for several months until the case is resolved. This drains various resources and takes a doctor away from their patients and family. To prevent medicolegal complaints, it is important to understand the factors that make a patient choose this pathway.

A survey of patients pursuing legal action revealed four main reasons: (1) concern with standards of care, (2) lack of explanation, (3) compensation for losses—both financial and suffering, and (4) the belief that the doctor or the system should be held accountable for their actions. They reported that patients taking legal action wanted greater honesty, an appreciation of the severity of the trauma they had suffered, and assurances that lessons had been learnt from their experiences.[12]

27.2.1 Nature of Malpractice Claims

The most common claims relating to hand surgery appear to relate to commonly performed procedures of carpal tunnel decompression and treatment of wrist fractures. The main complaint after performing carpal tunnel decompression is iatrogenic median nerve laceration,[13] and with distal radius fracture, care relates to malunion and hardware complication of intra-articular or long screws. Other causes of litigation in hand surgery include missed injuries such as ring and little finger carpometacar-

pal fracture dislocations and scaphoid fractures. Operating on the wrong side remains a common cause of litigation among all extremity procedures and in the hand operating on the wrong digit is not uncommon. A paper by Norum et al from Norway which looked at malpractice claims after wrist surgery found the most common reasons were pain, stiffness, reduced function, and weakness. Other reasons were patient's perception that they were denied surgery or underwent the wrong procedure.[14]

27.2.2 Preventing Medicolegal Issues

The one issue underpinning all patient complaints and misunderstandings stems from lack of communication from the surgeon and the subsequent breakdown of the doctor-patient relationship leading to the patient seeking recourse elsewhere. The following principles are useful in mitigating medicolegal issues.[13]

Avoid Obvious Errors

Wrong side and site surgery is clearly avoidable and inexcusable when they occur. Systems should be developed and be in place to ensure that every patient gets the correct operation. Preoperative review of the clinic notes and consent form, marking of the limb, and planned surgical incision(s) with the patient awake would serve the dual purpose of confirming the correct operative site and giving the patient a better understanding of the procedure and scars that are expected.[7] A time-out check list that confirms the patient identity, procedure title, side, and site immediately prior to commencing the procedure is mandatory in most countries, but in the end, it is the diligence of the surgeon that is key.

Transparency

Patients are more likely to sue if they have an unexpected outcome that was not properly explained to them during the preoperative consultation. If a complication does occur, the doctor should openly disclose what happened at the earliest opportunity and what measures they will be taking to diminish the effect of the complication. The patient should not feel abandoned and should be provided with a plan to manage the complication and the patient afforded the opportunity to be treated by a different doctor when appropriate. The patient should be offered an appointment for a second opinion with a colleague to further indicate that the surgeon has nothing to hide.

Build a Good Doctor-Patient Relationship

Doctors that are liked by their patients are less likely to be sued. It may be impossible to develop a good rapport with all patients, but some strategies can be employed to assist. Adequate patient visiting time, feedback from imaging studies and pathology reports, and casual conversations about nonmedical topics and patient interests increase patient satisfaction.[15] If an adverse outcome should occur, the physician should allocate more time for the patient and family and work closely with other providers involved with the care, such as hand therapists and pain management specialists.

Detailed Discussion and Documentation

A detailed discussion of risks of a procedure has to be documented; otherwise, the automatic assumption is that it did not occur. It then comes down to the patient's word against the doctor's word and a jury of peers will likely favor the plaintiff who bears the consequences of the complication. All information provided to the patient including handouts, referral to websites must be recorded.[16]

Setting Correct Expectations

Most patients expect complete recovery after a procedure, especially after surgical repair of trauma. To a patient, nerve repair implies they will regain normal sensation, and tendon repair or fracture fixation indicates they will recover full mobility. It is critical that the patient indicates that they understand the sensation will likely never be the same after a nerve injury and the joint movement may not be the same after tendon repair or fracture in a finger. The patient needs to understand the functional loss is not a complication but an expected outcome and relates to the severity of the injury they present with and not the quality of care provided.

Other Factors

Patients usually express dissatisfaction and may put in a complaint before launching a lawsuit. It is in the doctor's best interests to proactively deal with any patient issues before it escalates to lawyers. Inadequately addressed pain is another cause for dissatisfaction after surgery. Being comfortable in the postoperative period with the use of comfortable splints, judicious blocks, and analgesia with easy access to the surgeons' office when required is important in keeping patients happy. The patient should always feel that they can seek help from their doctor should they have a problem and there should be some mechanism by which patients with problems can be reviewed early on before the issues escalate especially in a larger institution such as a teaching hospital.

If an error or complication has occurred during surgery, the institution risk management team should be informed of the occurrence as soon as possible. After discussion with the patient and the family, the practitioner should seek advice of legal counsel or from their malpractice provider even though legal proceedings may not have commenced. Early notification will provide recommendations that the surgeon can put into place to avoid escalation into a lawsuit.

References

[1] Miles SH. Hippocrates and informed consent. Lancet. 2009; 374 (9698):1322–1323

[2] Kaba R, Sooriakumaran P. The evolution of the doctor-patient relationship. Int J Surg. 2007; 5(1):57–65

[3] Council of Europe. Convention for the protection of human rights and dignity of the human being with regard to the application of biology and medicine. In: CETS 164. Oviedo; 1997

[4] Council and Commission. European Parliament. Charter of Fundamental Rights of the European Union. Off J Eur Union. 2016; 202:389

[5] Faden RR, Beauchamp TL, King NMP. A history and theory of informed consent. New York: Oxford University Press; 1986

[6] Haysom G, Narsai U. Informed consent and communicating information. Avant Mutual. https://www.avant.org.au/news/informed-consent-and-communicating-information/. Accessed 30 June, 2020

[7] DeGeorge BR, Jr, Archual AJ, Gehle BD, Morgan RF. Enhanced informed consent in hand surgery: techniques to improve the informed consent process. Ann Plast Surg. 2017; 79(6):521–524

[8] Casby C, Lyons B. Consent and children. Anaesth Intensive Care Med. 2019; 20(1):52–55

[9] Lennings NJ. Forward, Gillick: are competent children autonomous medical decision makers? New developments in Australia. J Law Biosci. 2015; 2(2):459–468

[10] Professional Development and Standards Board. RACS Position Paper: Informed Financial Consent. Royal Australasian College of Surgeons; 2019

[11] Queensland Health. https://www.health.qld.gov.au/consent/html/for_clinicians. Accessed 30 June, 2020

[12] Vincent C, Young M, Phillips A. Why do people sue doctors? A study of patients and relatives taking legal action. Lancet. 1994; 343 (8913):1609–1613

[13] Pappas ND, Moat D, Lee DH. Medical malpractice in hand surgery. Review. J Hand Surg Am. 2014; 39(1):168–170

[14] Norum J, Balteskard L, Thomsen MW, Kvernmo HD. Wrist malpractice claims in Northern Norway 2005–2014. Lessons to be learned. Int J Circumpolar Health. 2018; 77(1):1483690

[15] Gross DA, Zyzanski SJ, Borawski EA, Cebul RD, Stange KC. Patient satisfaction with time spent with their physician. J Fam Pract. 1998; 47 (2):133–137

[16] Bono M, Wermuth H, Hipskind J. Medical malpractice. StatPearls Publishing LLC; 2020

9

28 Complications: What They Do to the Surgeon

David Warwick

Abstract

The effect that a complication has on a patient is obvious: extra pain, extra suffering, extra anxiety, and extra treatment. But a complication can, indeed should, affect the surgeon. That effect can be positive—a humbling learning experience—but it may be very negative with so much anxiety and rumination that the surgeon becomes the "second victim." No surgeon can avoid *all* complications but all surgeons can avoid *some* complications. When a complication happens, the surgeon should *always* feel responsible and own the problem. The surgeon should manage not only the complication and the patient's emotions, but also their own emotions. This is not easy but can be summarized as *honest reflection in a supportive environment.*

Keywords: complications, error, negligence, resilience, surgeon, coping, resilience

28.1 Introduction

Every surgeon has complications. If a surgeon says he never has a complication then he must be **D**elinquent (never operating), **D**eceitful (lying to others), **D**eluded (lying to himself) or **D**aft (too stupid to realize).

Every surgeon carries within himself a small cemetery, where from time to time he goes to pray—a place of bitterness and regret, where he must look for an explanation for his failures.

René Leriche, La Philosophie de la Chirurgie, 1951

In this chapter, we will examine complications—how they can be avoided, how they can affect the surgeon, how litigation can be avoided; we will look at strategies to help the surgeon cope and avoid becoming the second victim.[1]

28.2 Complications and Errors

28.2.1 What Is a Complication?

Not all negative outcomes are complications. Dindo defined negative outcomes as complications, sequelae, and failure to cure.[2] A *complication* would be a deviation from the normal postoperative course whereas a *sequela* would be an expected consequence (stiffness after a metacarpophalangeal [MCP] fusion, weak pinch after a trapeziectomy) and *failure to cure* would be when the original purpose of the operation is not achieved (residual flexion contracture after fasciectomy, residual tumor after excision biopsy, persisting nonunion after bone graft).

28.2.2 The Chance of a Complication

Why Is the Risk Important?

If we know the chance of a complication, then we can do two important things:
- Warn the patient by fully informed consent.
- Take all measures to reduce that risk.

Do not Trust the Literature

The chance of a complication occurring is more of a *guess* than a *fact*. We have some idea from the journals and textbooks but these publications are subject to *ascertainment bias* (does a surgeon always admit to every complication, let alone publish their high rate?) and *publication bias* (do Journals want to publish bad results?). Also, even if the complication rate seems low, remember that in a small series a *confidence interval* will reveal a potentially much higher risk.

Audit Your Work

A surgeon should monitor the outcome of their work—this should include a system to collect the complications that occur. Various electronic systems are available. It takes some effort and some integrity to record each and every complication, but the data which are collected will inform the surgeon how to improve their practice and will inform the patient of the risk they are taking with their own choice of surgeon.

28.2.3 When Is a Complication a Non-negligent Error and When Is It Negligence?

It is important to distinguish between a *complication*, an *error*, and *negligence*. An error can cause a complication, but not all complications are caused by an error. And not all errors are negligent. The patient, the surgeon, and indeed the lawyer should understand the distinction.

Some complications just happen—an unavoidable deviation from the expected outcome caused by a natural event, such as infection, complex regional pain syndrome (CRPS), failure of a bone to heal, a tender carpal tunnel scar, and extensor pollicis longus (EPL) rupture after Colles fracture. Some complications reflect risks which occur in a proportion of patients however well the surgery is performed, such as an unstable Sauve-Kapandji, midcarpal arthritis after scaphotrapeziotrapezoid (STT) excision, and nonunion of scaphoid fixation.

Some complications occur as a result of understandable and forgivable (non-negligent) surgical error: dividing a

9

nerve in complex revision Dupuytren surgery, a screw not quite perfectly placed in a comminuted fracture, a wound closure after a fasciotomy which is too tight, a broken drill tip, a K-wire impinging the lateral band causing proximal interphalangeal (PIP) stiffness.

Some complications are negligent and reflect *poor decision making*: an unstable silastic implant in the index finger PIP, a failed wrist replacement in a young heavy worker.

Some complications are negligent and reflect *poor surgical technique*: a distal radius screw penetrating the joint, damage to the median nerve during carpal tunnel release, CRPS after careless damage to a cutaneous nerve, failure to use X-rays for procedures involving metal.

Some complications are negligent and poor practice: wrong-site surgery, thrombosis or infection when prophylaxis is not used according to guidelines, failure to check imaging prior to surgery, inadequate postoperative splinting.

Some complications are caused by the surgeon's team but beyond the surgeon's control: infection caused by someone else's poor aseptic discipline in theater or clinic, inadequate anesthesia causing the patient to move, incorrect physiotherapy.

Some complications are the patient's fault: scaphoid nonunion in a patient who still smokes, infection in a patient who removes their own dressing, malunion in a patient who removes their own plaster or wires too soon.

28.3 Avoiding Complications and Consequences

28.3.1 The Competence of a Surgeon

A competent surgeon is not just defined by the technical skill of the operation itself but by the skill of preoperative decision making and consent, as well as the skill with which postoperative complications are managed. The latter skill needs not only *technical expertise* for the physical treatment but especially *psychological expertise* for essential emotional treatment.

28.3.2 How Can a Surgeon Avoid Complications?

No surgeon can avoid *all* complications but all surgeons can avoid *some* complications. When a complication happens, the surgeon should *always* feel responsible and *usually* feels unhappy. Therefore, for a surgeon to cope with a complication, they must be comfortable that they have done everything possible to avoid that complication.

- Choose the most suitable procedure for each *individual* patient—a gymnast will hate a fused thumb carpometacarpal (CMC) whereas a road digger will hate an unstable trapeziectomy.

- Choose an operation for which you are trained and with which you are experienced—*surgeons do operations better when they do lots of them.*
- Avoid experimentation—it takes many procedures by many surgeons in many centers before the technique is considered reliable and before the potential flaws are known. *Patients are not laboratory rats.*
- Understand the potential complications for each procedure and do what you can to avoid them—put the volar plate proximal to the watershed line to avoid tendon rupture, minimal resection of the distal pole of the scaphoid for STT osteoarthritis (OA).
- Use operating loupes—avoid damaging nerves and vessels.
- Operate meticulously—place tendon sutures perfectly, close the wound impeccably, check each screw length twice.
- Plan postoperative care carefully—ensure the therapist will see the PIP replacement within just a few days to avoid stiffness, do not change dressings too early which invites infection, apply the correct splint at the correct time.
- Follow established guidelines—WHO Checklist, handwashing, "bare below the elbows."
- Use evidence-based medicine not your own opinion—thromboprophylaxis and antibiotic prophylaxis should not be used on all patients but only when recommended.
- Warn patients not to smoke (they usually ignore this).
- Ensure diabetes and anticoagulation are controlled.

28.3.3 Consent

Consent Is Essential to Manage Complications

If the patient experiences an unavoidable complication—an unfortunate but recognized natural event—then they will share the surgeon's despair and disappointment *but only if they realize that it was a risk that they had been prepared to take.* This is why thorough preoperative consent is so important. If a complication occurs after surgery, then a properly consented patient will think the surgeon is wise for having warned them and will work with the surgeon as their partner in sorting it out; a patient who was not consented properly may see the surgeon as incompetent.

Realistic Expectations

Never set unrealistic expectations before surgery—if you do then you increase your chance of an unhappy patient because if the patient has an average result, they will think you are not as good as you promised. Instead, it is wise to predict a below average outcome and an above average risk of complication: when the patient does better than predicted without a complication, then the patient thinks you are a great surgeon. The patient will be more likely to accept a worse outcome or complication.

The Patient's Rights

Every patient has a right to be told three key points before deciding to have surgery:
- Surgery is almost never essential; it is an option. It is usually wise to consider doing nothing, or trying something simple like an injection or splint.
- For most conditions there is more than one surgical option, each with its own advantages and risks, each with its own rate of recovery. The *patient* should choose which is best for them, *not the surgeon*.
- Any operation can make you worse if there is complication and some complications cannot be reversed (nerve damage, severe CRPS) and may be worse than the original condition.

28.4 What to Do If a Complication Happens

28.4.1 Admit to Yourself a Complication Has Happened

Own the Complication

While the surgeon has an absolute duty to disclose the complication to the patient, the first duty is to disclose it to themselves. It is tempting for a surgeon to deny a complication especially if he or she made an error. The emotional reaction to a complication, something discussed below in more detail, can suppress acceptance that something has not gone well. Decide to *own* the complication—do not deny it from yourself, do not make it unimportant to you. Promise yourself you will deal with it.

Analyze

Whatever the complication, the surgeon must accept that the error has happened, and then understand exactly and honestly why it has happened. Analyze what happened—was it an *unavoidable* natural event, an a*cceptable* error, or a *negligent* error?

Whose Fault Was the Complication?

- The surgeon.
- Nature.
- The odds—a proportion will go wrong however well performed.
- The system.
- The team.
- The patient.

28.4.2 Tell the Patient That a Complication Has Happened

Most sensible patients will understand the distinction between *avoidable* and *unavoidable* complications and then work with the surgeon to improve the situation. A kind, forgiving patient will understand that we are all human and we can all make errors. Some patients will assume that any complication is always a negligent error and will find a lawyer.

So as soon as *any* complication occurs, the surgeon must share it with the patient.
- Explain that something has happened.
- Empathize with the patient.
- Let the patient realize that you, in your human and professional way, are as concerned as they are.
- Make them confident that you will admit if it is an error.
- You will work with them to make the problem better if you can.
- You will be with them for the journey—they can ask questions whenever they wish.
- If you need help from another colleague then you will ask for it; offer the patient a second opinion.
- Patients often blame themselves when they should not—the surgeon should always take away the patient's guilt if either nature or the surgeon is at fault.

Never, ever:
- Deny the complication has happened.
- Give a false explanation.
- Make the complication seem trivial—even if the surgeon thinks it is trivial, the patient does not.
- Blame the patient unfairly.

28.4.3 How to Deal with a Natural Complication

The surgeon has to explain the complication, what happened and why. The surgeon must be completely honest and explain why they think that the complication is a natural and unavoidable event; this must be done in a sympathetic and educational manner but never in a patronizing, evasive manner. The patient will notice when the surgeon tries to blame nature rather than to take responsibility for an error. The surgeon's own view is of course biased at this guilty, stressful, and disappointing moment.

Refer Back to the Indications and Consent

This conversation is never easy, especially with an angry, suspicious, and anxious patient. The initial indications for surgery should be reviewed in a *supportive and nondefensive*

9

way. It is at this stage that the *quality* of *preoperative informed consent* is so important—if the surgeon can refer back to this process then a realistic patient will realize that they are an unfortunate victim of bad luck. They will continue to trust the surgeon.

Second Opinion

Ask if the patient would like a second opinion very early on if this conversation seems to be failing. Sometimes even the legal process may be used if the patient does not feel the surgeon has fully explained matters.

28.4.4 How to Deal with an Error

If the surgeon lacks the personal integrity and psychological skills to deal with an error, then the patient will not *respect* the surgeon. The patient will *resent* the surgeon and might, quite rightly, find another surgeon or even a lawyer. The patient's anxiety and stress and doubts must be respected.

Non-negligent or Negligent Error?

The surgeon's own view is of course biased at this guilty, stressful, and disappointing moment. A second opinion from another surgeon and sometimes even the legal process may be required to distinguish between non-negligent and negligent error if the patient does not feel the surgeon is being straight.

Every patient has made some well-intentioned mistakes in their lives. Even if the surgeon has made a non-negligent or negligent error, a kind patient may forgive this error if the surgeon is truly honest, humble, apologetic, and respectful. The patient can still trust the surgeon even if the surgeon has made a mistake, if the surgeon works with the patient and explains how the error can be corrected or mitigated. Many patients want to feel that they can help to avoid similar harm to someone else in future.

Negligent Error

Sometimes, the patient deserves compensation because the error was too stupid, too avoidable, such as a K-wire penetrating the median nerve because X-rays were not used and an osteotomy for minor symptoms which then failed to heal because of poor technique. If the patient has come to real irreversible harm from an unacceptable error, then the surgeon should help the compensation process and never confuse it. This will eventually be less expensive, less stressful, and less confrontational for everyone. This has been elegantly proven in the Michigan Error Disclosure program.[3]

28.5 Effects of Complications on the Surgeon

28.5.1 The Second Victim

Uneasy lies the head that wears a crown.
(Shakespeare Henry IV)

The drastic consequences of our mistakes, the repeated opportunities to make them, the uncertainty about our own culpability when results are poor, and the medical and societal denial that mistakes must happen all result in an intolerable paradox for the physician.[4]
(Hilfiker 1994)

Natural disasters can affect anyone, such as a thunderbolt striking a house or a viral pandemic. But a natural surgical disaster involves the innocent surgeon. Surgeons are probably no more or less prone to errors than any other human but like a pilot, yet unlike perhaps a lawyer or an accountant, the consequences can be far greater and cannot always be fixed by money alone. A study of 7900 surgeons found that during the 3 months after a surgical error there was a higher prevalence of depression and a lower quality of life.[5]

We must never forget that it is the patient who suffers the complication. The patient's emotions must take priority. However, we cannot underestimate or ignore the effect that complications have on surgeons. Surgeons will react in their own way because each surgeon has their own personality. While some might be too heavily affected, others might not be affected at all. Neither is ideal. If a surgeon is *too sensitive* then they may experience unmanageable anxiety, guilt, and loss of confidence, spoiling their ability to return to being an effective surgeon. If a surgeon is *too insensitive* then they may not have the empathy which the patient needs for support or the insight the surgeon needs to become a better surgeon.

The surgeon can indeed become the second victim.[1]

28.5.2 Emotional Toil

Surgeons who experience complications are almost all affected emotionally.[6,7,8,9]

The depression and burnout syndrome developing in the surgeon due to surgical complications not only affect the surgeon and his family but also adversely affect the surgeon's clinical performance and patient safety.[10]
(Shanafelt et al 2009)

Even if the complication is not the surgeon's fault such as a joint infection, the emotional effect on the surgeon can be profound.[11]

Common reactions include:
- Guilt.
- Anxiety.
- Shame/embarrassment.
- Sadness.
- Anger.
- Crisis of confidence.
- Worry about reputation.
- Worry for the patient.
- Fear of litigation.
- Interference with professional and leisure activities.
- Rumination.
- Insecurity.

28.5.3 Risk of Depression and Burnout

Surgeons want to discuss with others for personal and professional reassurance. They want to learn and understand from the event. However, the surgeon may be inhibited from discussion because of many factors such as an institution's culture of blame, professional jealousy of colleagues, the risk of litigation, and the expectations for surgeons to be tough and nonemotional. These factors make the surgeon internalize the negative reactions—a perfect precursor for depression and burnout.[6]

28.6 Coping Strategies

28.6.1 Emotional Strategies

There are many ways to help the surgeon cope:
- Discuss the complication with a trusted mentor.
- Rationalize the complication and realize that the complication was unavoidable, that the patient had been properly consented.
- Accept that error happens to the best of us; if we are to have the emotional rewards of being a surgeon then we have to accept the emotional stress of our failure.
- Talk openly to patients as a way of finding closure.
- Learn more about the procedure—read about it, attend a course, do the procedure again with a senior colleague.
- Teach—publish a case report, write an article, incorporate your complication in to a lecture. You are mitigating your guilt by making sure others learn.
- Develop protocols to prevent the complication happening again.
- Do not withdraw—a rider who falls from the horse should get back in the saddle straightaway.

Other coping strategies for a surgeon throughout their professional life but especially after a complication include:

- Mindfulness.
- Time with family and friends.
- Exercise.
- Artistic creation.
- Absorbing hobby.
- Medication, alcohol, and substance abuse—not to be recommended.

28.6.2 Risk Aversion

Surgeons often become more averse to risk after a complication. Indeed, an older and more experienced surgeon is less likely to operate and is more likely to do a simpler procedure than a young, ambitious but inexperienced surgeon. This change over the years is probably driven by an accumulation of negative outcomes. This is a positive aspect of complications—keeping patients safer.

However, risk aversion can be negative because it may deny potentially valuable treatment in a suitably consented patient. A previous bad experience should not unwisely affect future decision making.

For example, there are advantages to wrist replacement over fusion, such as better movement, better cosmesis, and better patient satisfaction. However, a proportion fail soon after surgery (and in fact all will fail eventually) and require a technically complex fusion. If a surgeon has an early failure and denies all his future patients the choice of a replacement then his patients are deprived of a valuable option and have not been given their right to choose the procedure for themselves based on their own assessment of the real benefits and risks.

28.6.3 Institutional Culture

Many institutions have, or may be perceived by the second victim as having, a culture of blame and zero-tolerance of error and failure. This is unacceptable. An institution should have a system of mentoring, emotional support, and learning.[6,12,13]

28.6.4 Recovery

The surgeon's emotional recovery from a complication seems to follow a predictable order[14]:
1. Chaos and accident response.
2. Intrusive reflections.
3. Restoring personal integrity.
4. Enduring the inquisition.
5. Obtaining emotional first aid.
6. Moving on.

The sixth stage, moving on, led to one of three outcomes: dropping out, surviving, or thriving. Regardless of the final recovery, an adverse event is a life-altering experience that leaves a permanent imprint on the individual.

9

28.6.5 Resilience

Fortunately, most surgeons are resilient enough to move on from a complication and accepting that such occurrences were inevitable at some point in their career.[11]

The complication should help the surgeon become a better surgeon—better decision making, better consent, more careful technique, more empathetic, more self-aware. This learning process will, to some extent, reduce the guilt and create a valuable experience from a bad experience.

28.6.6 Summary

The coping strategy can perhaps be summarized as *honest reflection in a supportive environment.*

Suggested Reading

I would recommend the following two books which are beautifully written, emotionally intelligent, and profoundly wise:

[1] Gawande A. Complications. London, UK: Profile Books; 2003
[2] Marsh H. Do No Harm. London, UK: Orion, 2014

References

[1] Wu AW. Medical error: the second victim. The doctor who makes the mistake needs help too. BMJ. 2000; 320(7237):726–727
[2] Dindo D, Demartines N, Clavien P-A. Classification of surgical complications: a new proposal with evaluation in a cohort of 6336 patients and results of a survey. Ann Surg. 2004; 240(2):205–213
[3] Kachalia A, Kaufman SR, Boothman R, et al. Liability claims and costs before and after implementation of a medical error disclosure program. Ann Intern Med. 2010; 153(4):213–221
[4] Hilfiker D. Facing our mistakes. N Engl J Med. 1984; 310(2):118–122
[5] Shanafelt TD, Balch CM, Bechamps G, et al. Burnout and medical errors among American surgeons. Ann Surg. 2010; 251(6):995–1000
[6] Ullström S, Andreen Sachs M, Hansson J, Øvretveit J, Brommels M. Suffering in silence: a qualitative study of second victims of adverse events. BMJ Qual Saf. 2014; 23(4):325–331
[7] Pinto A, Faiz O, Bicknell C, Vincent C. Surgical complications and their implications for surgeons' well-being. Br J Surg. 2013; 100(13):1748–1755
[8] Han K, Bohnen JD, Peponis T, et al. The surgeon as the second victim? Results of the Boston Intraoperative Adverse Events Surgeons' Attitude (BISA) study. J Am Coll Surg. 2017; 224(6):1048–1056
[9] Srinivasa S, Gurney J, Koea J. Potential consequences of patient complications for surgeon well-being: a systematic review. JAMA Surg. 2019; 154(5):451–457
[10] Shanafelt TD, Balch CM, Bechamps GJ, et al. Burnout and career satisfaction among American surgeons. Ann Surg. 2009; 250(3):463–471
[11] Mallon C, Gooberman-Hill R, Blom A, Whitehouse M, Moore A. Surgeons are deeply affected when patients are diagnosed with prosthetic joint infection. PLoS One. 2018; 13(11):e0207260
[12] Pratt S, Kenney L, Scott SD, Wu AW. How to develop a second victim support program: a toolkit for health care organizations. Jt Comm J Qual Patient Saf. 2012; 38(5):235–240, 193
[13] Turner K, Johnson C, Thomas K, Bolderston H, McDougall S. The impact of complications and errors on surgeons: Do surgeons need support—and, if so, what kind? RCS Bull. 2016; 98:404–407
[14] Scott SD, Hirschinger LE, Cox KR, McCoig M, Brandt J, Hall LW. The natural history of recovery for the healthcare provider "second victim" after adverse patient events. Qual Saf Health Care. 2009; 18(5):325–330

29 Complications: What They Do to the Patient

Terry L. Whipple

Abstract

What complications from hand surgery do to the patient is more extensive than mere surgical challenge. Informed consent to submit to hand surgery requires educating a patient's expectations for outcomes and instilling trust in the surgeon and his team. Surgery complications inconvenience a patient's plans for return to function and comfort. A patient is ultimately responsible for the added expense of the complication and also suffers the cost of disrupting relationships with family, co-workers, and friends. The emotional stress of complications and potential loss of hand functionality add to surgical risks. As per Hippocrates, these personal patient matters also are the responsibilities of a good hand surgeon.

Keywords: trust, inconvenience, expense, functionality, Hippocratic oath, Responsibility, outcomes

29.1 Introduction

Everyone entering a surgical experience has expectations. Ideally, the expectations are identical, or at least very similar, for all parties involved—surgeon, nurses, patient, family, employers, attorneys, insurance carriers. At times, however, for whatever reason, outcomes of surgery do not match the expectations. Surgical treatment outcomes may exceed or fall short of expectations; or ultimate outcomes may be delayed or even substantially altered by complications.

No one expects complications, but they can occur unexpectedly. Even unexpected complications can have the same expected outcomes ultimately, but the course to that eventuality may be prolonged, and can entail additional or divergent treatments, additional surgeries, other specialty consultations, and often additional rehabilitation. If the ultimate outcome of the initial surgery is altered significantly by a complication of any nature, the impact for the patient may be profound.

Avoidance of complications, minimizing their risk, is the responsibility of every good surgical team. Each member of the team should assume that responsibility from the same page of protocol and benevolence. Hand patients—like any other patients—are consumers, usually contractual consumers, giving informed consent to the surgical intervention which guides their expectations. Emphasis on *informed* consent means more than just cataloging possible inadvertent tissue injuries on a preoperative signature form; it means educating a patient about the pros and cons of alternative treatment options and the rationale of selecting a surgical approach. Surgical preparation entails risk management—medication adjustment, diet, pre-habil-itation conditioning, sanitation, arrangements for postoperative care, splinting, and many others.

Hand surgery outcomes that are delayed or significantly altered by complications can be considered in a variety of categories, from the patient's perspective. For this chapter, we will divide them broadly into the issues of trust, inconvenience, cost, and functionality.

29.2 Trust

A hand surgery patient's relationship with his surgeon may be brief and emergent, or it may be cultivated over a longer period of time. It may stem from the hand surgeon on call for an emergency department, or begin with an Internet search, referral from one's primary care physician, or from the recommendation of a friend. In any event, the relationship is based in patient trust and confidence in the surgeon and his team. Why else would one lie down under anesthesia and entrust the future of his hand—his instrument of function, of expression, of productivity, of exploration—to someone else to do something surgical, something to alter his natural anatomy, about which he the patient has no familiarity, certainly no expertise and probably little or no personal experience? He must have *trust*; confidence in the ability of the surgeon to whom he entrusts his well-being. We surgeons are not mere technicians. We must be physicians first, dedicating ourselves to the benefit of our patients.

Surgical complications—or more inclusively, any complications from a surgical experience—can easily result in a breach of that patient trust. Diligently building that relationship of confidence firmly during the preoperative period helps enormously in preserving a patient's trust in the event of complications. Herein lies the importance of that informed consent; and also the importance of instilling into the patient a sense of human value in the eyes of the surgeon. That builds a relationship. It may need to be built speedily in emergent cases, or slowly but surely over time preoperatively in the clinical setting. But it must be built.

Loss of a patient's trust following a hand surgery complication can ruin a surgeon's reputation that took years to earn in the community or among peers. Disgruntled patients can be vociferous and negatively effective. For patients with surgical complications, laying blame is reflexive. Where would they turn first? To the surgeon or the hospital team. For the patient, a sense of having experienced wrongdoing, imagined surgical error, discourtesy, inattentiveness, any sense of unimportance, all make for ripe and convincing table-talk in the community. A patient's perspective of his complication, handled poorly, overshadows the problem he initially sought help for preoperatively.

9

29.3 Inconvenience

Hand surgery complications can cause temporary or endless inconvenience for patients. Previous chapters have surveyed common complications of various types associated with hand surgery procedures. Their immediate care can sometimes mitigate the impact of the complication by stabilizing a fracture or vein-wrapping a nerve repair during the initial surgery, for example. But if the complication occurs or is discovered late, rehospitalization, return to surgery, prolonged PT or OT, or antibiotics may delay one's return to function, return to productivity, or return to comfort. More time is required for treatment and recovery than what had been anticipated preoperatively.

Imposition on one's time cannot be summarily described. The hand is a functional terminal unit of the extremity. Disabling the function of even part of the hand is an impairment. One's hand dominance, age, lifestyle, family role, financial provision, and comorbidities merge to affect the inconvenience of prolonged hand impairment due to surgical complications. These effects extend beyond the patient. They involve co-workers, work project schedules, dependency on family or friends for transportation, delay of domestic responsibilities, independent activities of daily living, and a host of other matters that require the substitution or assistance of others. The complication is more than a personal matter. It produces inconvenience for many others in the patient's orbit of life.

The need for additional appointments for clinical evaluation and for rehabilitation is impositions on a patient's time and schedule that had not been anticipated. Patients' time has value. Their additional sacrifice or investment of that time deserves high regard by the surgeon and each member of his sympathetic team. That ability helps define good hand surgeons.

29.4 Expense

The costs associated with surgical complications alone would justify their preventative measures. Immeasurable time and efforts have been invested to determine the estimated monetary value an insurance company will pay for any given procedure. Complicating that procedure inflates the professional time and medical resources necessary to reach the initially anticipated outcome as nearly as possible. It inflates the expense of the procedure for the insurance carrier(s) and for the patient. All complications cost money.

Whether medically or surgically, mitigating or correcting a complication may require additional surgery procedures with attendant anesthesia professionals. Surgical suites or intensive care units compound the cost more so than additional physical therapy and occupational ther-apy, but any such treatments have additional costs. Consultation with medical specialists necessitated by surgery complications may introduce infectious disease specialists, cardiologists, urologists, general surgeons, vascular surgeons, neurologists, physiatrists, and even psychiatrists if the complication has serious emotional impact. All comes with a financially burdensome expense that must be covered by someone. Ultimately, though, the patient is responsible for the costs.

But finance is not the only expense to the patient. Emotional stress comes with uncertain outcomes of the complication and its potentially lasting effects. Stress takes its own toll. It may affect domestic or marital relationships, friendships, employment relationships, either through dependence, imposition, uncertainty or emotional instability, and frustration on the patient's part. These intangible costs also may be temporary or permanent. A good hand surgeon appreciates these emotional tariffs and should offer or direct such patients to appropriate assistance or counseling.

The security of a patient's employment may be jeopardized by a complication from hand surgery. The ability to provide for his family or maintain his mortgage or other debt obligations are no small consideration for disability. Financial assistance programs should be maintained as every surgeon's convenient resource. The need for such unanticipated financial dependence poses an additional stress for the patient.

29.5 Functionality

As is well known, the hand is a functional terminal unit of the upper extremity. It performs feats of creation, maintenance, molding, communication, protection, and emotional expression. From infant care to housekeeping, from typing to painting, from making payments to making surgery to changing tires or waiving "hello," the hand is used throughout every day. Especially because of the opposable thumb and the dense population of sensory nerves, the hand is uniquely useful to people. Patients treasure their hands as much as do surgeons. Every hand surgery encounter is a threatening experience for a patient's hand, with uncertain outcome. It is well that we hand surgeons should keep this foremost in mind.

Previous chapters have demonstrated that surgery complications resulting in hand stiffness, loss of sensibility, loss of stability or strength can significantly compromise a patient's functionality. Surgery complications often result in hand impairments. The *AMA Guide to the Evaluation of Permanent Impairment*[1] accords particularly high impairment percentages for the "whole person" as the result of impairments to the hand. If these complications can be mitigated or resolved, permanent impairment can also be spared. If not, the lasting functional impairment may have permanent effects on a patient financially and emotionally, as well. A patient's functional dependence on the hand cannot be underestimated.

Improved hand function and comfort are the most common reasons for surgical treatments. To the extent that surgical complications may further impair hand functionality, at least, prevention of surgical complications should be a deliberate surgical concern. Reference here recalls one of the principle tenants of the Hippocratic Oath, as rewritten in 1964 by Dr. Louis Lasagna, Academic Dean of Tufts University School of Medicine in Boston: "I will remember that I do not treat a fever chart, a cancerous growth, but a sick human being, whose illness may affect the person's family and economic stability. My responsibility includes these related problems, if I am to care adequately for the sick."[2]

Thus, may we hand surgeons practice for the betterment of our patients, first as humanitarians, second as physicians, and then as surgeons, in preventing all potential complications of our hand surgery and mitigating their many deleterious effects, should they ever occur.

References

[1] Rondinelli RD, ed. Guides to the evaluation of permanent impairment. 6th ed. USA: American Medical Association; 2008

[2] Practo. https://doctors.practo.com/the-original-and-revised-version/. Published March 10, 2015

9

Index

Note: Page numbers set *italic* indicate figures.